Clinical Fluid Therapy in the Perioperative Setting

Edited by
Robert G. Hahn
Södertälje Hospital, Södertälje, Sweden
Faculty of Health Sciences, Linköping University, Linköping, Sweden
and
Karolinksa Institute, Stockholm, Sweden

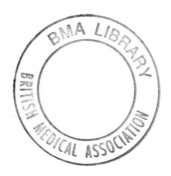

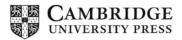

CAMBRIDGE
UNIVERSITY PRESS

CAMBRIDGE UNIVERSITY PRESS
Cambridge, New York, Melbourne, Madrid, Cape Town,
Singapore, São Paulo, Delhi, Tokyo, Mexico City

Cambridge University Press
The Edinburgh Building, Cambridge CB2 8RU, UK

Published in the United States of America by Cambridge University Press, New York

www.cambridge.org
Information on this title: www.cambridge.org/9781107000988

© Cambridge University Press 2011

First published 2011

Printed in the United Kingdom at the University Press, Cambridge

A catalogue record for this publication is available from the British Library

Library of Congress Cataloguing in Publication data
Clinical fluid therapy in the perioperative setting / [edited by] Robert G. Hahn.
p. ; cm.
Includes bibliographical references and index.
ISBN 978-1-107-00098-8 (pbk.)
1. Anesthesia–Complications.   2. Fluid therapy.   3. Therapeutics, Surgical.   I. Hahn, Robert G.
[DNLM: 1. Fluid Therapy.   2. Perioperative Care.   3. Rehydration
Solutions–therapeutic use. WD 220]
RD51.C55 2011
617.9′6–dc23   2011014909

ISBN 978-1-107-00098-8 Paperback

Clinical Fluid Therapy in the Perioperative Setting

Contents

List of contributors   *page* vi
Preface   ix

1 **Crystalloid fluids**   1
   Robert G. Hahn

2 **Colloid fluids**   11
   Robert G. Hahn

3 **Rules of thumb**   18
   Hengo Haljamäe

4 **Intra-abdominal surgery**   29
   Yifat Klein and Idit Matot

5 **Spinal anesthesia**   45
   Michael F.M. James and
   Robert A. Dyer

6 **Geriatric, obstetric and pulmonary
   surgery**   51
   Kathrine Holte

7 **Day surgery**   56
   Jan Jakobsson

8 **Pediatrics**   65
   Isabelle Murat

9 **Hypertonic fluids**   73
   Eileen M. Bulger

10 **Invasive hemodynamic
   monitoring**   82
   Philip E. Greilich and William E.
   Johnston

11 **Goal-directed fluid therapy**   91
   Timothy E. Miller and Tong J. Gan

12 **Non-invasive guidance of fluid
   therapy**   103
   Maxime Cannesson

13 **Hemodilution**   112
   Philippe van der Linden

14 **Microvascular fluid exchange**   120
   Per-Olof Grände and Johan Persson

15 **Body volumes and fluid
   kinetics**   127
   Robert G. Hahn

16 **Adverse reactions**   137
   Hengo Haljamäe

17 **Irrigating fluids**   148
   Robert G. Hahn

18 **Severe sepsis and septic shock**   157
   Palle Toft and Else Tønnesen

19 **Hypovolemic shock**   166
   Niels H. Secher and Johannes J. van
   Lieshout

20 **Uncontrolled hemorrhage**   177
   Richard P. Dutton

21 **Fluids or blood products?**   184
   Oliver Habler

Index   193

*Colour figures appear between pages 86
and 87.*

Contributors

Eileen M. Bulger
University of Washington, Seattle, WA, USA

Maxime Cannesson
Department of Anesthesiology and Perioperative Care, University of California, Irvine School of Medicine, Irvine, CA, USA

Richard P. Dutton
Department of Anesthesiology, University of Maryland School of Medicine, and R Adams Cowley Shock Trauma Center, University of Maryland Medical System, MD, USA

Robert A. Dyer
Department of Anaesthesia, University of Cape Town and Groote Schuur Hospital, Western Cape, South Africa

Tong J. Gan
Department of Anesthesiology, Duke University Medical Center, Durham, NC, USA

Per-Olof Grände
Department of Anaesthesia and Intensive Care, Lund University Hospital, Lund, Sweden

Philip E. Greilich
Division of Cardiothoracic Anesthesia, Department of Anesthesiology and Pain Management, University of Texas Southwestern Medical Center, TX, USA

Oliver Habler
Department of Anesthesiology, Surgical Intensive Care Medicine and Pain Therapy, Krankenhaus Nordwest GmbH, Frankfurt am Main, Germany

Robert G. Hahn
Södertälje Hospital, Södertälje, Sweden; Faculty of Health Sciences, Linköping University, Linköping, Sweden; and Karolinska Institute, Stockholm, Sweden

Hengo Haljamäe
Department of Anaesthesiology and Intensive Care, The Sahlgrenska Academy at Göteborg University, Sahlgrenska University Hospital, Gothenburg, Sweden

Kathrine Holte
Department of Surgical Gastroenterology, Hvidovre University Hospital, Hvidovre, Denmark

Jan Jakobsson
Institution for Physiology & Pharmacology, Department of Anaesthesia & Intensive Care, Karolinska Institute, Stockholm, Sweden

Michael F.M. James
Department of Anaesthesia, University of Cape Town and Groote Schuur Hospital, Western Cape, South Africa

William E. Johnston
Scott & White Healthcare, Temple, TX, USA

Yifat Klein
Department of Anesthesiology & Intensive Care, Tel-Aviv Sourasky Medical Center, Affiliated with Tel Aviv University, Israel

Idit Matot
Department of Anesthesiology & Intensive Care, Tel-Aviv Sourasky Medical Center, Affiliated with Tel Aviv University, Israel

Timothy E. Miller
Department of Anesthesiology, Duke University Medical Center, Durham, NC, USA

Isabelle Murat
MD, Department of Anesthesia, Hôpital d'Enfants Armand Trousseau, Paris Cedex, France

Johan Persson
Department of Anaesthesia and Intensive Care, Lund University Hospital, Lund, Sweden

Niels H. Secher
Department of Anaesthesia, Rigshospitalet, University of Copenhagen, Copenhagen, Denmark

Palle Toft
Department of Anaesthesiology and Intensive Care, Odense Universitetshospital, Odense, Denmark

Else Tønnesen
Department of Anaesthesiology and Intensive Care, Aarhus University Hospital, Kommunehospitalet, Aarhus, Denmark

Philippe van der Linden
Department of Anesthesiology, CHU Brugmann-HUDERF, Free University of Brussels, Brussels, Belgium

Johannes J. van Lieshout
Department of Internal Medicine and the Laboratory for Clinical Cardiovascular Physiology, AMC Centre for Heart Failure Research, University of Amsterdam, The Netherlands

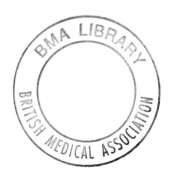

Preface

Intravenous fluid is a cornerstone in the treatment of the surgical patient. Perioperative management with intravenous fluids is a responsibility of the anesthetist but many others, including the surgeon, must be oriented in the principles that guide the therapy.

The clinical use of infusion fluids has long been overlooked as a science. There are several reasons for the neglect. One reason why fluids have not been considered to be drugs, is that many of the usual requirements for registration, such as the specification of a therapeutic window and detailed pharmacokinetics, have been overlooked. On the other hand, the experience of the clinical anesthetist is indeed that infusion fluids are drugs. Their appropriate use can be life-saving, while inappropriate use might jeopardize the clinical outcome and even be a threat to the patient´s life.

The scattered scientific basis for perioperative fluid therapy has necessitated the development of experience-based "rules of thumb," which still play an enormously important role in daily practice. They are usually based on a summation of perceived and measured losses and also include compensation for various factors, such as anesthesia-induced vasodilatation and protein losses due to inflammation.

Alongside the trial-and-error approach and theoretical calculations, scientific methods have been used to find evidence-based guidelines. In the 1980s, scientists tried to determine whether fluid therapy should be based primarily on crystalloid or colloid fluid. This was followed by a belief that invasive monitoring of pulmonary artery pressures could be the way to tailor optimal therapy.

The scenario has changed dramatically in the past decade. The amount of fluid infused has been shown to greatly affect the course of the postoperative follow-up, at least after some types of operations. Another important insight is that guiding fluid therapy by dynamic hemodynamic measures reduces the risk of postoperative complications. A changeover from relying on the pulmonary artery catheter to less invasive and even non-invasive tools for the monitoring of fluid administration is in full swing.

I am extremely proud to welcome the contributions from 23 colleagues around the world who are among the highest ranked researchers in the field of perioperative fluid therapy. They have written authoritative chapters about subjects in which every anesthetist should be updated when working with patients subjected to common types of surgery.

Each chapter should be read as an independent essay, which means that a topic discussed briefly by one author might be explored in more detail by another. The chapters are gathered in a sequence intended to give you an enjoyable journey into this fascinating field rather than grouping them into basic science, physiology and clinical applications.

This book does not have the ambition to provide full coverage of all special fields of surgery in which fluid therapy is being used. For more complete coverage the reader is recommended the more extensive presentation given in *Perioperative Fluid Therapy* by Hahn-Prough-Svensen (Informa Healthcare, 2007).

Chapter

1

Crystalloid fluids

Robert G. Hahn

The term *crystalloid fluid* refers to sterile water solutions that contain small molecules, such as salt and glucose, which are able to crystallize. These solutes easily pass through the capillary membrane, which is the thin fenestrated endothelium that divides the plasma volume from the interstitial fluid volume. This process of solute distribution brings along water. Hence, the volume of a crystalloid fluid is spread throughout the extracellular fluid (ECF) space.

Osmolality is the number of particles dissolved in the water solution. The osmolality of the body fluids is approximately 295 mosmol/kg and is a powerful driving force for water distribution. However, it is both the type of dissolved particles and the osmolality of the solution that determine the tonicity, i.e., to what degree the infusion fluid hydrates or dehydrates the intracellular fluid (ICF) space [1].

If the solutes in the infusion fluid remain outside the cells, as is the case for sodium and chloride, the osmolality and the tonicity agree. An iso-osmotic infusion fluid (295 mosmol/kg) is then isotonic. In contrast, osmolality and tonicity are not equivalent in the case where the solutes easily penetrate the cell membrane, which separates the ECF from the ICF. An example is ethanol, which markedly raises the body osmolality but without redistributing water. Therefore, ethanol is said to have low tonicity.

The cell membrane regulates the distribution of many other solutes across the cell membrane in a finely graded manner via energy-consuming pump mechanisms, which then also modify the water distribution. These pumping mechanisms operate slowly (minutes to hours) while changes in osmolality redistribute water within seconds.

The marketed crystalloid infusion fluids are usually isotonic or nearly isotonic. Hence, they expand the ECF volume but not the ICF volume.

Normal saline

A 0.9% solution of saline is isotonic and is therefore called physiological or "normal." The fluid still contains a marked surplus of chloride ions and no buffer (Table 1.1) and, hence, infusion of 2 l or more of the fluid causes hyperchloremic metabolic acidosis [2].

In adults, normal saline should be reserved for patients with hypochloremic metabolic alkalosis, as in disease states associated with vomiting. The fluid has a more accepted role for perioperative fluid therapy in children where the risk of subacute hyponatremia is a more serious concern than in adults (see Chapter 8 – Pediatrics).

Clinical Fluid Therapy in the Perioperative Setting, ed. Robert G. Hahn. Published by Cambridge University Press. © Cambridge University Press 2011.

Table 1.1. Composition of plasma and the most common crystalloid solutions.

	Osmolality (mosmol/kg)	pH	Na⁺ (mmol/l)	K⁺ (mmol/l)	HCO₃⁻ (mmol/l) equivalent	Cl⁻ (mmol/l)	Glucose (mmol/l)
Plasma	295	7.40	140	3.6–5.1	30	100	5
0.9% saline	308	5.0	154	0	0	154	0
7.5% saline	2400	3.5–7.0	1250	0	0	1250	0
Lactated Ringer's	274	6.5	130	4	30	110	0
Acetated Ringer's	270	6.0	130	4	30	110	0
Plasma-Lyte Aᵃ	294	7.4	140	5	27	98	0
Glucose (5%)	278	5.0	0	0	0	0	278
Glucose (2.5%) + electrolytes	280	6.0	70	0	25	45	139

ᵃ Plasma-Lyte A also contains 23 mmol/l of gluconate.
All infusion fluids may contain small amounts of electrolytes like magnesium and calcium.

When infused in healthy volunteers normal saline might cause abdominal pain, which is not the case for lactated Ringer's [3]. The fluid also has more undesired effects, including acidosis, when used during surgery [4].

Normal saline is excreted more slowly than both lactated and acetated Ringer's solution [5,6], increasing the volume effect ("efficiency") of the fluid to be about 10% greater compared with the Ringer's solutions [5].

Saline may also be marketed as hypertonic solutions at strengths of 3% and 7.5% solution. The first is mainly intended as a means of raising the serum sodium concentration in in-hospital patients, whereas the latter is used for plasma volume expansion in emergency care. In volunteers, 7.5% saline is four times more effective as a plasma volume expander than normal saline [5].

Ringer's solutions

Ringer's solution is a composition created by Sydney Ringer in the 1880s to be as similar as possible to the ECF. Alexis Hartmann later added a lactate buffer to the fluid and made it Hartmann's solution, or "lactated" Ringer's solution.

Lactate and acetate

Today Ringer's solution is used with the addition of buffer in the form of *lactate* or *acetate*, of which the former is most common. Both ions are metabolized to bicarbonate in the body, albeit with certain differences. Lactate is metabolized in the liver and the kidneys with the aid of oxygen and under production of bicarbonate and carbon dioxide. Acetate is metabolized faster and in most tissues, and it consumes only half as much oxygen per mole of produced bicarbonate compared with lactate. Hence, lactate slightly increases the oxygen consumption [7] and might also raise plasma glucose, particularly in diabetic patients [7,8]. Large amounts of lactated Ringer's confuse assays used to monitor lactic acidosis.

Both lactate and acetate are vasodilatators. Rapid administration aggravates the reduction of the systemic vascular resistance that normally occurs in response to volume loading. Both lactate and acetate are also fuels, although the calorific content in 1 l of any Ringer's solution is quite low (approximately 5 kcal).

Although the differences between lactate and acetate are usually negligible, several factors suggest that acetate is the better buffer in the presence of a compromised circulation and in shock.

Pharmacokinetics

During intravenous infusion the Ringer's solutions distribute from the plasma to the interstitial fluid space in a process that requires 25–30 min for completion. The distribution half-life is approximately 8 min [5,9].

The elimination (by voiding) in volunteers is so rapid that the fluid may exhibit one-compartment kinetics, which has been interpreted to imply that the fluid is distributed from the plasma to well-perfused areas of the interstitial fluid space only. In contrast, elimination is greatly retarded during surgery where Ringer's always exhibits two-compartment kinetics [10] (see Chapter 15 – Body volumes and fluid kinetics). Infusion of 2 l of Ringer's in volunteers is followed by elimination of 50–80% of the fluid within 2 h, whereas the corresponding figure in anesthetized patients is only 10–20%. Lowered blood pressure, vasodilatation and activation of the renin–aldosterone axis are factors thought to be responsible for the slow turnover of Ringer's during anesthesia and surgery [11]. Naturally, the retarded elimination makes it easier to cause edema by overhydration in a patient than in a volunteer.

For the infusion rates normally used during surgery, the ratio of the plasma to the expandable parts of the interstitial fluid space is 1:3, which means that 30% of the infused fluid is retained in the plasma (if we disregard elimination) [9]. However, one can count on the effect of distribution resulting in much stronger plasma volume expansion than offered by this relationship as long as the infusion continues (see Chapter 15).

The fluid distributed to the interstitial fluid space in the course of crystalloid volume loading is bound in the interstitial gel. However, free fluid can accumulate rapidly in the tissue spaces if an infusion of crystalloid fluid is provided so fast that the normally negative interstitial fluid pressure becomes positive [1]. This creates *pitting edema*, by which we can expect that the ratio of 1:2 has been abruptly reduced.

Clinical use

The pharmacodynamics of the Ringer's solutions is strongly related to their capacity to expand the ECF volume.

These fluids may be used to replace preoperative losses of fluid due to diarrhea. In contrast, vomiting should be replaced by normal saline.

The Ringer's solutions are commonly used (in a volume of approximately 500 ml) to compensate the blood volume for the expansion of the vascular tree that occurs from induction of both regional and general anesthesia.

The Ringer's solutions reverse the compensatory changes in blood pressure and sympathetic tone resulting from hypovolemia. There are numerous reports confirming that rapid infusion of Ringer's is a life-saving treatment in excessive hemorrhage due to the resulting expansion of the plasma volume.

In contrast, crystalloid fluid cannot reverse drug-induced hypotension [11]. If a crystalloid bolus has no effect in reversing hypotension during surgery, the anesthetist should change strategy and lighten the anesthesia, or else institute treatment with an adrenergic drug, rather than providing several liters of crystalloid fluid.

As crystalloids are inexpensive and carry no risk of allergic reactions, a Ringer's solution is often used to replace smaller blood losses while colloids are withheld until 10–15% of the blood volume has been lost. The commonly recommended dosage is to infuse three times as much Ringer's as the amount of blood lost (3:1 principle). If the patient's legs are placed in stirrups, a 2:1 replacement scheme can be used, with the last third given as a bolus infusion when the legs are lowered from the stirrups [12].

Dosing

The rate and volume of infused Ringer's solutions vary considerably during surgery.

In healthy adult females very rapid infusions of Ringer's (2 l over 15 min) caused swelling sensations, dyspnea and headache [13]. No symptoms were observed after infusing the same volume more slowly. This rate (133 ml/min) should not be exceeded in the absence of blunt hypovolemia.

In elderly and debilitated patients the rate of infusion of crystalloid fluid should be further reduced and adjusted according to the patient´s *cardiovascular status*.

Too rapid volume loading might be complicated by instant *pulmonary edema*. Both the dilution of the plasma proteins and the increased cardiac pressures promote such edema, which should be treated with acute vasodilatation, administration of loop diuretics and application of continuous positive airway pressure (or positive end-expiratory pressure if the patient is mechanically ventilated).

There is a risk of pulmonary edema developing also in the postoperative period if the total volume infused during the day of surgery amounts to 10 l or more. Arieff [14] reported development of pulmonary edema in 7.6% of 8195 patients who underwent major surgery. The mortality in this group was 11.9%.

Volume loading with 3 l of lactated Ringer's in volunteers (mean age 63 years) reduced the forced expiratory capacity and the peak flow rate [15].

Outcome studies using prospective registration of postoperative adverse events have demonstrated that crystalloid fluid administration during colonic surgery should be closer to 4 ml/(kg h) than 12 ml/(kg h) [16]. Many similar outcome studies will be discussed later in this book that advise the anesthestist about the optimal infusion rates during various surgeries.

There are concerns about the use of Ringer's in *brain injury*, because the fluid is slightly hypotonic (270 mosmol/kg) and increases brain cell mass when the central nervous system is traumatized. Normal saline is likely to be a better choice during neurosurgery. However, in volunteers acetated Ringer's did not increase the ICF volume because the urinary sodium concentration was only half as high as that of the plasma [16].

All Ringer's should also be infused cautiously in patients with *renal insufficiency* since these patients may not be able to excrete an excess amount of crystalloid fluid.

Plasma-Lyte

The infusion fluid Plasma-Lyte A is constructed to further refine the "balanced" composition of acetated Ringer's solution. Here, the sodium and chloride concentrations are virtually identical to those of human plasma (Table 1.1).

To make up for the increase in cation and decrease of anion concentration the solution also contains the negatively charged ion gluconate, which is also metabolized to carbon dioxide and water but still has only a weak alkalinizing effect.

Glucose solutions

Glucose (dextrose) solutions are used to administer calories to prevent starvation, and also to provide body water. They are the only available infusion fluids that add volume to both the ECF and the ICF volumes. However, the volume component of the glucose solutions is distributed throughout the total body water only after the glucose added to the sterile water has been metabolized to carbon dioxide, which needs to be removed by ventilation, and water.

Pharmacokinetics

Infused *glucose* distributes rapidly over two-thirds of the expected ECF space. Elimination occurs by insulin-dependent uptake by the body cells. The half-life is approximately 15 min in healthy volunteers [17] but twice as long during laparoscopic cholecystectomy [18]. Elimination apparently occurs even more slowly in the presence of diabetes.

The *volume* component of isotonic glucose 2.5% with electrolytes and plain glucose 5% (the latter fluid is sometimes abbreviated to D5W) initially expands the plasma volume as effectively as acetated Ringer's solution [17]. The fluids show no distribution phase, which means that they do not significantly expand the interstitial fluid space. Instead, fluid leaving the plasma volume enters the ICF space due to the osmotic strength of the "eliminated" glucose molecules. Hence, the kinetics of the fluid component of glucose solutions is coupled with the glucose metabolism. A slow redistribution of volume to the total body water then begins because the osmotic strength of glucose fades away when being incorporated into large glycogen molecules, and later when being the subject of metabolism.

Glucose 2.5% with electrolytes and plain glucose 5% are almost entirely eliminated within 2.5 h in volunteers (which is faster than Ringer's) [17]. Some of the volume component of glucose 5% still resides in the ICF space at that time.

Glucose solutions of 10% and 20% are hypertonic and withdraw fluid from the ICF to the ECF by virtue of osmosis. This volume returns to the cells when the glucose is metabolized.

Clinical use

Glucose solutions are widely used to treat debilitated hospital patients. Besides preventing starvation, glucose solutions hydrate the ICF volume in those who cannot be fed orally.

In the perioperative period, infusing a glucose solution with little or no electrolytes is the most logical way to provide free water to compensate for vaporization from airways and surgical wounds.

The glucose component of the fluid is indicated in patients at risk of developing hypoglycemia, such as in diabetes, alcohol dependency, hepatomas and pancreatic islet cell tumors. Certain drugs, like propranolol, increase the risk of hypoglycemia.

Alternatively, there seems to be little reason to routinely administer glucose perioperatively. In the vast majority of patients hormonal changes associated with surgery raise the blood glucose level sufficiently (by stimulating glycogenolysis and gluconeogenesis) to maintain normoglycemia, or even to reach mild hyperglycemia. The stress response, in turn, makes it difficult for the body to adequately use exogenous glucose to limit gluconeogenesis and protein catabolism ("protein-sparing effect").

Another argument to refrain from glucose administration perioperatively is that a very high glucose concentration worsens the *cerebral damage* that develops in association with cardiac arrest [19,20]. Therefore, glucose solution is contraindicated in acute stroke and not recommended in operations associated with a high risk of perioperative cerebral ischema, such as carotid artery and cardiopulmonary bypass surgery.

If used, plain glucose must be infused quite slowly (alongside other fluids) as there is otherwise a risk of blunt hyperglycemia developing [21].

Hypertonic glucose solutions (10% and 20%) must be monitored by measurements of the plasma glucose concentration. These fluids are used for more ambitious supplementation of calories in postoperative care and also in the intensive care unit.

In the past decade, modifying the plasma glucose level by glucose infusions and insulin has become a tool to reduce complications and improve survival after intensive care and cardiac surgery [22,23]. Cardiac function may even be improved in patients undergoing cardiac surgery by infusing a solution containing glucose, insulin and potassium [24].

In Europe "glucose loading" by mouth is sometimes performed in the evening and morning before abdominal operations, the purpose being to reduce nausea and insulin resistance [25].

Dosing

The basic need for glucose in an adult corresponds to 4 l of glucose 5% per 24 h (800 kcal), which prevents blunt starvation while not providing adequate nutrition. However, the amount administered to hospital patients is more often guided by the need for "free" body water, which is 2–3 l per 24 h. Although the commonly infused amount provides less glucose than the body utilizes, the glucose supplementation reduces muscle wasting [21]. As stated previously, this "nitrogen-sparing effect" of glucose is poorer in association with surgery due to the accompanying physiological stress response.

The rate of glucose infusion should not increase plasma glucose concentrations above the *renal threshold*, which is 12–15 mmol/l. Higher levels induce *osmotic diuresis* in which water and electrolytes losses are poorly controlled. This limit is reached by infusing 1 l of glucose 5% over 1 h in healthy volunteers [17].

Due to the ease by which plasma glucose becomes elevated during surgery, most anesthetists prefer to use glucose 2.5% with electrolytes in the perioperative setting. During laparoscopic cholecystectomy 1.4 l of glucose 2.5% with electrolytes over 60 min raised plasma glucose from normal to the renal threshold for osmotic diuresis (16 mmol/l) [18]. The limitations set to the infusion rate due to the risk of hyperglycemia make both glucose 2.5% and 5% unsuitable for use as plasma volume expanders.

Glucose metabolism yields CO_2, and the accompanying increased breathing might be a problem in debilitated patients with impaired lung function.

Hyponatremia

Repeated infusion of electrolyte-free glucose solution (usually plain 5%) might induce *subacute hyponatremia* [26]. This complication usually develops 2–3 days after surgery and is characterized by neurological disturbances, nausea and vomiting [27]. When symptoms appear, serum sodium is usually between 120 and 130 mmol/l (normal level 138–140 mmol/l).

Hyponatremia might cause permanent brain damage if left untreated. Menstruating women are most prone to develop such sequelae [28]. The surgery might be trivial but has often (at some stage) been complicated by sudden hypotension, which boosts the vasopressin concentration. Impaired renal function and liberal postoperative ingestion of soft juice drinks devoid of salt are other risk factors [26,29].

Treatment in symptomatic patients consists of hypertonic saline, which should be monitored so as to increase serum sodium no faster than 1–2 mmol/(l h). If hyponatremia has not appeared after surgery the development has probably been more gradual, and serum sodium in such *chronic hyponatremia* should be raised even more slowly (0.5 mmol/[l h]). The reason for the caution is that the brain gradually adapts to the lower osmolality and damage might occur if the normal concentration is attained fast.

Subacaute hyponatremia can be prevented by limiting the amount of plain glucose 5% to 1 l only. All other glucose solutions should contain sodium.

Rebound hypoglycemia

Moderate hypoglycemia and hypovolemia are likely to develop 30 min after a glucose infusion has been stopped abruptly in subjects with a strong insulin response to glucose, or when glucose is infused together with insulin [30]. This complication is called "rebound hypoglycemia" and is an issue when, for example, parenteral nutrition is turned off.

This complication may also occur during *labor*. Glucose from the mother passes the placenta and induces an insulin response in the fetus. At birth a strong insulin effect remains in the newborn, whose capacity to increase endogenous glucose production is limited [31]. Dangerous hypoglycemia develops, which might result in convulsions and brain damage. The "rebound" effect can be avoided by infusing the glucose no faster than required to prevent blunt starvation, which is 1 l glucose 5% over 6 h. A practical rule is to slow the rate of infusion of the glucose solution at the end of delivery.

The same critical situation for the newborn might develop if maternal volume loading is provided with glucose-containing fluid just before Cesarean section [32].

Mannitol

Mannitol is an isomer of glucose that is not metabolized in the body but is eliminated by renal excretion. The molecule remains essentially in the ECF fluid. The half-life is approximately 130 min but can be twice as long in the presence of impaired kidney function [33].

The isotonic concentration of mannitol is the same as for 5% glucose, which is sometimes used as an irrigating solution in endoscopic surgery. The clinical use of mannitol for intravenous administration is restricted to a plain 10% or 20% solution (in some countries only 15%), which induces diuresis in failing, oliguric kidneys. The mechanism is that the renal excretion of mannitol occurs by virtue of osmotic diuresis, by which the body loses water.

The hypertonic nature of 15% mannitol has made it a means of acutely reducing the intracranial pressure in patients with head trauma. The volume used is then 500–750 ml, of which half is given as a bolus infusion. Despite a long history, mannitol treatment remains poorly evaluated in outcome studies. As the fluid contains no electrolytes, users should be aware the osmotic diuresis creates an absolute loss of sodium and other electrolytes from the body that may need to be replaced.

The marked increase in ECF volume makes infusion of hypertonic mannitol contraindicated in congestive heart failure.

Like all hypertonic fluids, mannitol 15% should not be administered together with erythrocyte transfusions.

References

1. Guyton AC, Hall JE. *Textbook of Medical Physiology*, 9th edn. Philadelphia: WB Saunders Company, 1996; 185–6, 298–313.

2. Scheingraber S, Rehm M, Sehmisch C, Finisterer U. Rapid saline infusion produces hyperchloremic acidocis in patients undergoing gynecologic surgery. *Anesthesiology* 1999; **90**: 1265–70.

3. Williams EL, Hildebrand KL, McCormick SA, Bedel MJ. The effect of intravenous lactated Ringer´s solution vs. 0.9% sodium chloride solution on serum osmolality in human volunteers. *Anesth Analg* 1999; **88**: 999–1003.

4. Wilkes NJ, Woolf R, Mutch M, *et al.* The effects of balanced versus saline-based hetastarch and crystalloid solutions on acid-base and electrolyte status and gastric mucosal perfusion in elderly surgical patients. *Anesth Analg* 2001; **93**: 811–16.

5. Drobin D, Hahn RG. Kinetics of isotonic and hypertonic plasma volume expanders. *Anesthesiology* 2002; **96**: 1371–80.

6. Reid F, Lobo DN, Williams RN, Rowlands BJ, Allison SP. (Ab)normal saline and physiological Hartmann's solution: a randomized double-blind crossover study. *Clin Sci* 2003; **104**: 17–24.

7. Ahlborg G, Hagenfeldt L, Wahren J. Influence of lactate infusion on glucose and FFA metabolism in man. *Scand J Clin Lab Invest* 1976; **36**: 193–201.

8. Thomas DJB, Albertini KGMM. Hyperglycaemic effects of Hartmann's solution during surgery in patients with maturity onset diabetes. *Br J Anaesth* 1978; **50**: 185–8.

9. Ewaldsson C-A, Hahn RG. Kinetics and extravascular retention of acetated Ringer's solution during isoflurane and propofol anesthesia for thyroid surgery. *Anesthesiology* 2005; **103**: 460–9.

10. Hahn RG. Volume kinetics of infusion fluids (review). *Anesthesiology* 2010; **113**: 470–81.

11. Norberg Å, Hahn RG, Husong Li, *et al.*, Population volume kinetics predicts retention of 0.9% saline infused in awake and isoflurane-anesthetized volunteers. *Anesthesiology* 2007; **107**: 24–32.

12. Hahn RG. Blood volume at the onset of hypotension in TURP performed during epidural anaesthesia. *Eur J Anaesth* 1993; **10**: 219–25.

13. Hahn RG, Drobin D, Ståhle L. Volume kinetics of Ringer´s solution in female volunteers. *Br J Anaesth* 1997; **78**: 144–8.

14. Arieff AI. Fatal postoperative pulmonary edema. Pathogenesis and literature review. *Chest* 1999; **115**: 1371–7.

15. Holte K, Jensen P, Kehlet H. Physiologic effects of intravenous fluid administration in healthy volunteers. *Anesth Analg* 2003; **96**: 1504–9.

16. Hahn RG, Drobin D. Rapid water and slow sodium excretion of Ringer´s solution dehydrates cells. *Anesth Analg* 2003; **97**: 1590–4.

17. Sjöstrand F, Edsberg L, Hahn RG. Volume kinetics of glucose solutions given by intravenous infusion. *Br J Anaesth* 2001; **87**: 834–43.

18. Sjöstrand F, Hahn RG. Volume kinetics of 2.5% glucose solution during laparoscopic cholecystectomy. *Br J Anaesth* 2004; **92**: 485–92.

19. Myers RE, Yamaguchi S. Nervous system effects of cardiac arrest in monkeys. *Arch Neurol* 1977; **34**: 65–74.

20. Siemkowicz E. The effect of glucose upon restitution after transient cerebral ischemia: a summary. *Acta Neurol Scand* 1985; **71**: 417–27.

21. Sieber FE, Smith DS, Traystman RJ, Wollman H. Glucose: a reevaluation of its intraoperative use (review). *Anesthesiology* 1987; **67**: 72–81.

22. Van der Berghe G, Wouters P, Weekers F, *et al.* Intensive insulin therapy in critically ill patients. *New Engl J Med* 2001; **345**: 1359–67.

23. Lebowitz G, Raizman E, Brezis M, *et al.* Effects of moderate intensity glycemic control after cardiac surgery. *Ann Thorac Surg* 2010; **90**: 1825–32.

24. Gradinac S, Coleman GM, Taegtmeyer H, Sweeney MS, Frazier OH. Improved cardiac function with glucose-insulin-potassium after aortocoronary bypass grafting. *Ann Thorac Surg* 1989; **48**: 484–9.

25. Nygren J, Soop M, Thorell A, *et al.* Preoperative oral carbohydrate administration reduces postoperative insulin resistance. *Clin Nutr* 1998; **17**: 65–71.

26. Chung HM, Kluge R, Schrier RH, Anderson RJ. Postoperative hyponatremia: A prospective study. *Arch Intern Med* 1986; **146**: 333–6.

27. Arieff AI. Hyponatremia, convulsions, respiratory arrest, and permanent brain damage after elective surgery in healthy women. *New Engl J Med* 1986; **314**: 1529–35.

28. Ayus JC, Wheeler JM, Arieff AI. Postoperative hyponatremic encephalopathy in menstruant women. *Ann Intern Med* 1992; **117**: 891–7.

29. Häggström J, Hedlund M, Hahn RG. Subacute hyponatraemia after transurethral resection of the prostate. *Scand J Urol Nephrol* 2001; **35**: 250–1.

30. Berndtson D, Olsson J, Hahn RG. Hypovolaemia after glucose-insulin infusions in volunteers. *Clin Sci* 2008; **115**: 371–8.

31. Philipson EH, Kalham SC, Riha MM, Pimentel R. Effects of maternal glucose infusion on fetal acid-base status in human pregnancy. *Am J Obstet Gynecol* 1987; **157**: 866–73.

32. Kenepp NB, Shelley WC, Gabbe SG, *et al.* Neonatal hazards of maternal hydration with 5% dextrose before caesarean section. *Lancet* 1982; **1**: 1150–2.

33. Anderson P, Boréus L, Gordon E, *et al.* Use of mannitol during neurosurgery: interpatient variability in the plasma and CSF levels. *Eur J Clin Pharmacol* 1988; **35**: 643–9.

Chapter 2

Colloid fluids

Robert G. Hahn

The term *colloid fluid* refers to a sterile water solution with added macromolecules that pass through the capillary wall only with great difficulty. The osmotic strength of macromolecules is not great, so a colloid fluid must also contain electrolytes to be non-hemolytic. As long as macromolecules reside within the capillary walls their contribution to the total osmolality (the *colloid osmotic pressure*) is still sufficient to distribute a large proportion of the infused fluid volume inside the bloodstream.

Colloid fluids are used as plasma volume expanders and have more long-lasting effect than crystalloid fluids. They carry a risk of allergic reactions not shared by crystalloid fluids (see Chapter 16 – Adverse reactions). Therefore, one usually replaces smaller blood losses by crystalloid fluid, while colloids are withheld until 10–15% of the blood volume has been lost. The recommended use of colloid fluids in more specific clinical situations is further explained in many chapters in this book.

There is a current trend to provide colloids in balanced electrolyte solutions instead of in normal saline. The reason for this is the metabolic acidosis induced by normal saline, but the changeover is important only if 2–3 l of the colloid is administered.

Albumin

Albumin is the most abundant protein in plasma and, therefore, has an important role in maintaining the intravascular colloid osmotic pressure. Albumin has a molecular weight of 70 kD. Albumin solutions are prepared from blood donors and have a strength of 3.5%, 4% or 5%, and are even available as a hyperoncotic 20% preparation.

Pharmacokinetics

Albumin 5% expands the plasma volume by 80% of the infused volume. In healthy volunteers, the plasma volume expansion fades away slowly according to a mono-exponential function, the half-life being 2.5 h [1].

An infusion of 10 ml/kg of albumin 5% increases the serum albumin concentration by 10%, which remains unchanged for more than 8 h. Restoration of normal blood volume is governed by translocation of albumin molecules from the plasma to the interstitial fluid space. Moreover, the plasma volume expansion per se has a diuretic effect. The albumin is gradually transported back to the plasma via lymphatic pathways, and the half-life in the

---

Clinical Fluid Therapy in the Perioperative Setting, ed. Robert G. Hahn. Published by Cambridge University Press. © Cambridge University Press 2011.

body is much longer (approximately 16 h) than the half-life of the plasma volume expansion when albumin solution is infused.

Clinical use

Albumin is a "natural" colloid and remains an effective means of restoring the plasma volume and normal hemodynamics in hypovolemic shock.

Albumin is still the most commonly used plasma volume expander in children. In adults the high cost and the risk of allergic reactions have limited the clinical importance of albumin in favor of artificial colloids. Moreover, albumin seems to have no clinical benefit over synthetic colloids in intensive care [2,3].

Acute reduction of serum albumin is a sign of *capillary leak* in inflammatory disorders, such as sepsis. The use of albumin as a plasma volume expander is then a double-edged sword. The solution expands the plasma volume transiently, but the infused albumin will create peripheral edema later on, as the lymphatic drainage might not be able to catch up with the increased loss of protein from the plasma. In these situations, one should select colloids based on macromolecules that are eliminated from the blood by metabolism or renal excretion rather than by capillary leak.

In intensive care, albumin infusions have been used to treat *hypoalbuminemia*. This therapy has gradually been taken out of practice as low serum albumin is a sign of severe disease rather than a problem in itself. The added albumin will soon be subject to catabolism and used in the same way as amino acids in the body.

Albumin may be used to replace excessive albumin losses in special medical conditions, such as nephritis.

The "albumin debate"

In 1998, the Cochrane Library published a meta-analysis of 1419 patients from 30 studies in which albumin was used. The results were surprising since albumin treatment seemed to increase the mortality. The relative risk of death was 1.46 when albumin was given to treat hypovolemia, 1.69 if the indication was hypoalbuminemia and 2.40 when albumin was given for burns [4]. In the United Kingdom, the use of albumin decreased by 40% during the months following publication of the meta-analysis [5].

A later review of the same topic indicated that the risk of death associated with the use of albumin appeared to be lower the better a study was conducted. The best studies did not support that albumin increases the risk of death [6].

These meta-analyses were followed by a randomized study (the SAFE study) that compared albumin 4% with normal saline [7]. No difference in outcome was found in 7000 intensive care patients depending on the choice of infusion fluid. The mortality after 28 days was virtually identical in the groups (726 vs. 729).

However, a subgroup analysis of the SAFE study comprising the 460 patients with *head injury* showed that albumin 4% was followed by a higher mortality than normal saline (33% vs. 20%). The difference was greatest in the most severe cases [8].

Dextran

Long chains of glucose molecules (polysaccharides) are synthesized by bacteria to serve as macromolecules in the group of infusion fluids called the *dextrans* (sometimes abbreviated to DEX). As with albumin, the osmolality of a water solution containing only the macro-molecules is quite low and necessitates that electrolytes are added as well.

Commercially available dextran solutions have an average molecular weight of 70 kD (dextran 70) or 40 kD (dextran 40) and concentrations used are 3%, 6% or 10%. The most widely used, 6% dextran 70, expands the plasma volume with the same volume as the infused amount, while initially being somewhat stronger. The plasma volume expansion subsides with a half-life of approximately 3–4 h [9].

A solution of 10% dextran 40 expands the plasma volume by twice the infused volume. The half-life is shorter than for dextran 70.

The dextran molecules are either excreted by the kidneys or metabolized by an endogenous hydrolase (dextranase) to carbon dioxide and water.

The dextrans decrease blood viscosity and improve microcirculatory blood flow. This can sometimes be noted by visual inspection of the cut surface in a surgical wound as oozing, small vessels seem to open and bleed more. This might be disturbing to the surgeon but is not dangerous, as the total blood loss during a surgical operation will not be increased provided that the infused volume is limited to 500–1000 ml [10].

Dextran in hypertonic (7.5%) saline is available in some countries as an effective plasma volume expander in emergencies and pre-hospital care (see Chapter 9 – Hypertonic fluids). In volunteers, the effectiveness of this solution to expand the plasma volume is six to seven times stronger than for normal saline [11].

Clinical use

Dextran 70 is used to expand the plasma volume and/or to prevent thromboembolism.

Dextran 40 is used to improve the microcirculation after vascular surgery.

The maximum dose is 1.5 g/(kg day), which corresponds to 1.5–2.0 l of 6% dextran 70 in an adult. Hemorrhagic complications may ensue if larger amounts are given.

There is a risk of *anaphylaxis* developing in patients having irregular antibodies to dextran. This complication is prevented by pre-treatment with dextran molecules of very small size (1 kD) which should be injected intravenously just before dextran 40 or 70 is infused (see Chapter 16 – Adverse effects). Dextran 1 is less essential when treating pre-hospital trauma victims, as the associated stress response prevents anaphylaxis.

Starch

Hydroxyethyl starch (HES) also consists of polysaccharides and is prepared from plants such as grain or maize.

Several different formulations are marketed. They vary in concentration, usually being 6% or 10%. They also vary in chemical composition with respect to molecular weight, the number of hydroxyethyl groups per unit of glucose (substitution), and the placement of these hydroxyethyl groups on the carbon atoms of the glucose molecules (C2/C6 ratio).

The variability in chemical composition determines the differences in clinical effect between the solutions. Over the past decades, the trend has been to use molecules of smaller size to reduce the half-life and the risk of hemorrhagic complications. *Hetastarch* contains the largest molecules (450 kD) and *pentastarch* contains intermediate-sized molecules (260 kD). The most recently developed HES preparations have an even lower molecular size, on average 130 kD. The degree of substitution may be low (0.45–0.60) or high (0.62–0.70) and the C2/C6 ratio is low if less than eight.

The preparations are usually described with the key characteristics of molecular size and substitution, with or without being followed by the C2/C6 ratio. Hence, currently the most widely promoted HES preparations are denoted HES 130/0.4/9:1 (Voluven from Fresenius-Kabi) and HES 130/0.62/6:1 (Venofundin from B. B. Braun).

The degree of substitution is the key determinant for half-life. The risk of adverse effects in the form of anaphylactoid reactions, coagulopathy and postoperative itching increases with the molecular size (see Chapter 16 – Adverse effects).

As with dextran, 6% HES mixed in hypertonic (7.5%) saline is also marketed for emergency and trauma situations. Such a solution expands the plasma by much more than the infused volume, by virtue of osmotic volume transfer from the ICF space.

Pharmacokinetics

A 6% HES solution in iso-osmotic saline or balanced electrolytes expands the plasma volume by almost as much as the infused volume. Considerable variability in this respect may be encountered when administered to intensive care patients [12].

The *elimination* of HES is a complex issue. The solutions contain molecules with a spectrum of sizes of which the smallest (< 60–70 kD) are quickly eliminated by renal excretion. Larger molecules first need to be cleaved by endogenous alpha-amylase into smaller fragments before being excreted, a process that increases the osmotic strength per gram of polysaccharide. The HES molecules are also subjected to phagocytosis by the reticuloendothelial system, and remnants may be found in the liver and spleen even after several years. Hence, the half-life of the HES molecules might not correspond closely with the plasma volume expansion over time.

The half-life of the HES molecules in Venofundin was 3.8 h when administered to volunteers [13]. The half-life of the HES molecules of Voluven from plasma is said to be shorter, 1.4 h, although the terminal half-life is 12 h. After 72 h, approximately 60% of the HES molecules can be recovered in the urine [14].

The highest recommended dose of Voluven to be given during 24 h is 3.5 l in an adult of 70 kg. Only half as much should be allowed for dextran and HES preparations that contain larger molecules.

Clinical use

Hydroxyethyl starch is indicated solely for plasma volume expansion.

Although small-sized HES (130 kD) preparations have a shorter persistence in the blood they have the same clinical efficacy as median-sized HES preparations while being safer [15].

The first 10–20 ml should be infused slowly and the patient closely observed with respect to allergic reactions, which are rare and less severe than for dextran.

Treatment with large amounts of HES should be avoided in *septic patients* One study found a smaller change in creatinine concentration in patients treated with 3% gelatin as compared with 6% HES 200/0.60–0.66 [16] (Elohes, Fresenius-Laboratories), and a second study reported lactated Ringer's to be superior to 10% HES 200/0.5 (Hemohes, Fresenius Kabi) [17]. In a small study of burn patients the latter hyperoncotic HES preparation also seemed to promote renal failure and even death [18].

These studies may in part reflect the fact that all hyperoncotic colloid solutions carry a risk of inducing renal failure, particularly in dehydrated patients.

Gelatin

Gelatin solutions consist of polypeptides from bovine raw material. These colloids are considered to have a fairly good plasma volume expanding effect. The duration is short (approximately 2 h) due to the relatively small size of the molecules, which makes them excretable by the kidneys. Mild anaphylactoid reactions occur at a frequency of 0.3%, but severe reactions are rare [19].

Plasma

Human plasma should be used to administer coagulation factors and only as a last resort as a plasma volume expander. However, plasma volume expansion is much more variable with plasma than with albumin 5% [1]. The difference is probably due to increased capillary leak due to occasional cross-reactions with the recipient's immunological system.

Other drawbacks with the use of human plasma include the high occurrence of fever reactions (3–4%), the risk of anaphylaxis in patients with hereditary IgA deficiency, and the rare but dangerous complication called "transfusion-related acute lung injury" (TRALI).

Miscellaneous effects

Colloid fluids have a number of medical effects beyond their ability to expand the plasma volume. These include improvement of microcirculation, antioxidant effects (albumin) and suppression of trauma-induced immune activation (dextran, HES). Most of these characteristics are laboratory findings with unclear clinical relevance.

The only miscellaneous effect that is used clinically is the rheological effect of dextran, which effectively improves microcirculatory blood flow and also prevents thromboembolism.

All colloid fluids affect coagulation in a dose-dependent manner, although there are differences between the intensity of the changes (see Chapter 16 – Adverse reactions). It is important to be aware of the maximum doses to limit the risk of hemorrhage. These limits are of particular importance when infusing dextran and HES.

The elimination of crystalloid fluid is known to be greatly retarded by anesthesia and surgery [20]. Unfortunately, there are virtually no data on the distribution and elimination of colloid fluids in the perioperative setting.

Crystalloid or colloid?

Whether crystalloid or colloid fluid should be preferred was debated lively in the 1980s. The choice between crystalloid and colloid fluids should probably *not* be addressed as a general preference issue but rather governed by the specific clinical situation. Nevertheless, three meta-analyses have been performed to elucidate whether crystalloid or colloid fluids result in better survival.

The oldest of these meta-analyses, based on only eight studies, indicated that crystalloid fluid should be preferred in trauma as it was associated with a 12.3% lower mortality than colloids. When non-trauma patients were studied, however, there was a 7.8% difference in favor of *colloid* therapy. The overall result showed a 5.7% relative difference in mortality rate in favor of crystalloid therapy [21].

A decade later, in 1998, a meta-analysis comprised 1622 patients from 37 studies treated for surgery, trauma or burns. The data showed an overall risk of death of 24% in the colloid group but only 20% in the crystalloid group, giving a relative risk of 1.29 for death by treatment with a colloid (95% confidence interval 0.94–1.77) [22].

Another meta-analysis evaluated 814 patients from 17 studies. Here, there was no difference in overall mortality between the two types of fluid, but the relative risk of death was only 0.39 when crystalloid fluid was used in trauma patients [23].

Since these studies were published there has been a strong trend towards using avoidable surgical complications as a more refined outcome measure. Survival is undoubtedly of great interest to the patient but, scientifically, it is a rough measure that is prone to be truly multifactorial. In contrast, the past decade has demonstrated that fluid therapy greatly affects the incidence of many surgical complications, and more clearly so in debilitated and poor-risk patients than in healthy youngsters.

References

1. Hedin A, Hahn RG. Volume expansion and plasma protein clearance during intravenous infusion of 5% albumin and autologous plasma. *Clin Sci* 2005; **106**: 217–24.

2. Marik PE. The treatment of hypoalbuminemia in the critically ill patient. *Heart Lung* 1993; **22**: 166–70.

3. Guthrie RD, Hines C. Use of intravenous albumin in the critically ill patient. *Am J Gastroenterol* 1991; **86**: 255–63.

4. Cochrane Injuries Group Albumin Reviewers. Human albumin administration in critically ill patients: systematic review of randomised trials. *BMJ* 1998; **317**: 235–40.

5. Roberts I, Edwards P, McLelland B. More on albumin. Use of human albumin in UK fell substantially when systematic review was published (letter). *BMJ* 1999; **318**: 1214–15.

6. Wilkes MM, Navickis RJ. Patient survival after human albumin administration. A meta-analysis of randomized, controlled trials. *Ann Intern Med* 2001; **135**: 149–64.

7. The SAFE Study Investigators. A comparison of albumin and saline for fluid resuscitation in the intensive care unit. *New Engl J Med* 2004; **350**: 2247–56.

8. The SAFE Study Investigators. Saline or albumin for fluid resuscitation in patients with traumatic brain injury. *New Engl J Med* 2007; **357**: 874–84.

9. Svensén C, Hahn RG. Volume kinetics of Ringer solution, dextran 70 and hypertonic saline in male volunteers. *Anesthesiology* 1997; **87**: 204–12.

10. Hahn RG. Dextran 70 and the blood loss during transurethral resection of the prostate. *Acta Anaesthesiol Scand* 1996; **40**: 820–4.

11. Drobin D, Hahn RG. Kinetics of isotonic and hypertonic plasma volume expanders. *Anesthesiology* 2002; **96**: 1371–80.

12. Christensen P, Andersson J, Rasmussen SE, Andersen PK, Henneberg SW. Changes in circulating blood volume after infusion of hydroxyethyl starch 6% in critically ill patients. *Acta Anaesthesiol Scand* 2001; **45**: 414–20.

13. Lehmann GB, Asskali F, Boll M, *et al.* HES 130/0.42 shows less alteration of pharmacokinetics than HES 200/0.5 when dosed repeatedly. *Br J Anaesth* 2007; **98**: 635–44.

14. Voluven 6% hydroxyethyl starch 130/0.4 product monograph. Bad Homburg (Germany), Fresenius Kabi, 2007.

15. Ickx BE, Bepperling F, Melot C, Schulman C, van der Linden PJ. Plasma substitution effects of a new hydroxyethyl starch HES 130/0.4 compared with HES 200/0.5 during and after extended acute normovolaemic haemodilution. *Br J Anaesth* 2003; **91**: 196–202

16. Schortgen F, Lacherade LC, Bruneel F, *et al.* Effects of hydroxyethyl starch and gelatin on renal function in severe sepsis: a multicentre randomised study. *Lancet* 2001; **357**: 911–16.

17. Brunkhorst FM, Engel C, Bloos F, *et al.* Intensive insulin therapy and pentastarch resuscitation in severe sepsis. *N Engl J Med* 2008; **358**: 125–38.

18. Béchir M, Puhan MA, Neff SB, *et al.* Early fluid resuscitation with hyperoncotic hydroxyethyl starch 200/0.5 (10%) in severe burn injury. *Crit Care* 2010; **14**: R123.

19. Laxenaire MC, Charpentier C, Feldman L. Anaphylactoid reactions to colloid plasma substitutes: incidence risk factor mechanisms. A French multicenter prospective study. *Ann Fr Anesth Reanimat* 1994; **13**: 301–10.

20. Hahn RG. Volume kinetics of infusion fluids (review). *Anesthesiology* 2010; **113**: 470–81.

21. Velanovich V. Crystalloid versus colloid fluid resuscitation: a meta-analysis of mortality. *Surgery* 1989; **105**: 65–71.

22. Schierhout G, Roberts I. Fluid resuscitation with colloid or crystalloid solutions in critically ill patients: a systematic review of randomised trials. *BMJ* 1998; **316**: 961–4.

23. Choi PT, Yip G, Quinonez LG, Cook DJ. Crystalloids vs. colloids in fluid resuscitation: a systemtic review. *Crit Care Med* 1999; **27**: 200–10.

Rules of thumb

Hengo Haljamäe

The choice of an optimal perioperative fluid strategy may be of major importance for the clinical outcome of a surgical patient. However, the characterization of the "most optimal fluid strategy" is still a matter of dispute as "restrictive," "balanced" as well as "liberal" fluid therapies have been advocated as the most favourable [1]. Therefore no evidence-based standardized perioperative surgical procedure-specific guidelines for fluid therapy have so far been agreed upon.

Most clinicians feel that it is essential in the perioperative period to achieve and maintain an acceptable fluid balance whereby adequate tissue perfusion and oxygenation of vital organs is guaranteed. In case fluid imbalance occurs this could result in an obvious risk of impaired postoperative recovery, increased morbidity and prolonged hospital stay [2, 3].

A strategy for optimization of perioperative fluid management could be to include a combination of rather fixed crystalloid administration to replace basal fluid requirements and extravascular losses, together with more individualized goal-directed colloid administration to maintain an adequate intravascular volume and thereby a maximal cardiac stroke volume and favorable tissue perfusion [1].

In the present survey basal principles of perioperative fluid requirements of adult patients will be presented together with suggestions on acceptable types of standardized fluid treatment routines, as a rule of thumb, in connection with different types of non-cardiac surgical procedures.

General aspects of perioperative fluid therapy

The different challenges included in well-balanced perioperative fluid therapy management are summarized in Table 3.1 and commented on below.

Provide basal fluid requirements

The daily basal fluid requirements (to compensate *perspiratio insensibilis* and urinary and fecal fluid losses) for elderly patients are 25–30 ml/kg (70 kg = 1750–2100 ml/24 h; = 1.04–1.25 ml/[kg h]) and for young adults are about 40 ml/kg (70 kg = 2800 ml/24 h; = 1.67 ml/[kg h]).

It should be remembered that the fluid content of males (55–65%) is generally higher than that of females (45–55%) due to a higher proportion of body fat in females, and that the fluid content of all elderly patients decreases with advancing age. However, a routine of

Clinical Fluid Therapy in the Perioperative Setting, ed. Robert G. Hahn. Published by Cambridge University Press. © Cambridge University Press 2011.

Table 3.1. Basal principles of perioperative fluid therapy.

Provide daily basal fluid requirements
Rehydrate fluid-deficient patients
Maintain normovolemia and hemodynamic stability
Enhance microvascular blood flow
Maintain adequate plasma COP to avoid tissue edema formation
Prevent/moderate trauma induced activation of cascade systems and enhancement of coagulation
Guarantee adequate transport of oxygen to tissue cells
Promote/monitor diuresis

COP, colloid osmotic pressure

1.5 ml/(kg h) is an acceptable perioperative fluid routine for elderly as well as young adults irrespective of gender.

Therefore, use the principle of infusing 1.5 ml/(kg h) throughout the perioperative period including also the hours of actual preoperative fluid restriction. At anesthesia induction, a rather high initial fluid infusion rate is favorable to counteract the negative effects of anesthetic agents on cardiovascular stability.

Rehydrate fluid-deficient patients

In case of suspected preoperative fluid derangements, these should be assessed and compensated for preoperatively or, if less pronounced, in the early intraoperative phase (immediately before or at anesthesia induction). It should be noted that functional intravascular volume deficit seems to be common in patients before surgery [4]. Although the deficit in general is rather minor, some patients may still present a deficit of clinical relevance. Therefore, in case of signs of hemodynamic instability at anesthesia induction, infuse more fluid and in case of more pronounced reaction consider inclusion of a colloid [4]. Even patients having fasted for minor surgical procedures seem to benefit from administration of about 1 l of fluid pre- or intraoperatively [5].

Maintain normovolemia and hemodynamic stability

Proper monitoring of hemodynamics is always essential for safe patient care. Monitoring should always include blood pressure (BP), heart rate, electrocardiogram and pulse oximetry. In high-risk patients, one may add central venous pressure, arterial line-derived BP, cardiac output monitoring and measurement of urinary output. Signs of hypovolemia should be corrected swiftly by infusion of, preferably, a colloid (rather than crystalloid), if necessary in combination with vasopressors, since prolonged intraoperative hypotension seems associated with increased postoperative mortality [6].

Enhance microvascular blood flow

Hemorheologic factors influencing microvascular blood flow are: microvascular dimensions, blood and plasma viscosities, red blood cell deformability and aggregability, endothelial cell function and endothelial–white blood cell interactions [7]. Crystalloid-based fluid therapy may impair capillary blood flow due to leakage of crystalloid out into the interstitial space, whereby capillaries are compressed.

A much better enhancement of microvascular blood flow will be achieved by infusion of a colloid that remains mainly in the intravascular compartment [7,8]. Therefore, it is not surprising that colloid-based fluid regimens have been shown to enhance tissue blood flow and oxygen tension while crystalloid-based fluids will rather impair tissue perfusion and oxygenation [9]. The anti-inflammatory characteristics of modern hydroxyethyl starch (HES 130/0.4) preparations may be an additional factor enhancing microvascular blood flow by reducing endothelial–white blood cell interactions [10].

Maintain adequate plasma colloid osmotic pressure to avoid tissue edema formation

The transcapillary fluid exchange is, as given in Starling's equilibrium, dependent on hydrostatic as well as colloid osmotic pressure (COP) differences in addition to available capillary surface area for fluid exchange and the reflection coefficient for macromolecules. There is a non-linear relationship between serum oncotic pressure and interstitial edema, i.e., edema becomes progressively greater per unit decrease of oncotic pressure. Therefore, in case of massive fluid requirements in the perioperative period, a colloid should be preferred to crystalloid to avoid tissue edema formation that might impair organ function.

Prevent/moderate trauma-induced activation of cascade systems and coagulation

It is well-known that surgical trauma will activate a multitude of inflammatory mediators that will negatively affect tissue homeostasis [11]. In addition to perioperative use of anti-inflammatory drugs it is also well known that some modern colloids (e.g., HES 130/0.4 but not gelatin) will moderate the inflammatory reaction induced by surgical trauma [12]. Early infusion of such a colloid with anti-inflammatory properties will diminish the inflammatory response and protect vital organ function without negative effects on blood coagulation.

Guarantee adequate transport of oxygen to tissue cells

Preoperative anemia, defined as a blood hemoglobin (Hb) level < 120 g/l in females and < 130 g/l in males, seems common and is associated with increased mortality [13]. During surgery, however, much lower Hb levels are commonly accepted.

Data from randomized controlled trials suggest that hemodynamic, pulmonary and oxygen transport variables, as well as overall morbidity and mortality, are not different between restrictive (Hb transfusion threshold between 70 and 80 g/l) and liberal transfusion strategies (Hb ≥ 100 g/l), and that a restrictive transfusion strategy is not associated with increased adverse outcomes [14]. In fact, a restrictive strategy may be associated with decreased adverse outcomes in younger and less sick critical care patients.

The majority of existing guidelines conclude that transfusion is rarely indicated when the Hb concentration is greater than 100 g/l and is almost always indicated when it falls below a threshold of 60 g/l in healthy, stable patients.

In older, sicker patients a Hb level of 80–100 g/l is recommended [14]. Another important role of red blood cells (RBCs) relates to primary hemostasis and a higher trigger level of Hb may be appropriate in coagulopathic patients. Frequent intraoperative assessment of blood loss and check of the actual Hb level is essential to guarantee adequate tissue oxygenation.

Promote/monitor diuresis

In major surgery the maintenance of an adequate urine output (usually defined as > 0.5 ml/ [kg h]) is essential and justifies an indwelling urinary catheter for continuous monitoring. Urine output is promoted by combined infusion of crystalloid fluid as well as colloid for intravascular plasma volume support and thereby renal perfusion.

Guidelines for routine fluid management

Standard "rules of thumb" for perioperative fluid administration are suggested below.

1. Before anesthesia induction, set 1 l of crystalloid – preferably Ringer's.
2a. At induction of general anesthesia (GA) infuse 200–400 ml.
2b. When using spinal/epidural anesthesia – use crystalloid as above, and in case of hypotension preferably a vasopressor; if more pronounced hypotension infuse 300–500 ml of colloid.
3. Intraoperatively – basal 1.5 ml/(kg h) plus procedure-dependent 2–5 ml/(kg h).
4. Blood loss – compensate by infusion of equal volume of colloid. If cell saver is used (should be favored whenever possible) support the regained RBC volume by infusion of colloid.
5. Postoperatively – infuse crystalloid to cope with basal fluid requirements and compensate ongoing fluid/blood losses as needed (crystalloid, colloid, RBC).

Ad 1. One liter of a crystalloid, preferably a Ringer's type of balanced electrolyte solution, is set after the establishment of an iv line.

Ad 2a. When GA is used, 200–400 ml of fluid should be infused at anesthesia induction to minimize the local vascular pain induced by some iv anesthetics and also to counteract the depressive effects of anesthetic drugs on the cardiovascular system. In case more pronounced hypotension occurs the alternative is more fluid, crystalloid up to 500–600 ml followed by 200–400 ml of colloid. If hypotension persists in spite of these measures, consider administration of a vasopressor.

Ad 2b. In case spinal or epidural block is used, the sympathetic nerve block will rather frequently be accompanied by more pronounced hypotension which might justify an iv volume preload. A crystalloid-based preload of 500 ml does not seem to prevent hypotension and decreased CO, unless combined with infusing 500 ml of colloid [15].

If it is felt essential to reduce the crystalloid fluid load to the patient, the most justified initial approach to cope with the regional block-induced hypotension is to combine administration of 500 ml of colloid with a vasopressor [16].

Ad 3. In the intraoperative period, a continuous infusion of basal fluid requirements should be combined with additional procedure-specific infusions of fluid, which may vary between 2 and 5 ml/(kg h) (see procedure-specific management below). The procedure-specific losses consist of fluid as well as of blood plasma due to exudation from the surgical area. Balanced crystalloid is an adequate choice to compensate these losses.

Ad 4. Measured/estimated blood loss should be compensated for by infusion of an iso-oncotic colloid. In case a cell saver is used then the reinfusion of the washed RBC concentrate should be combined with infusion of equal amount of colloid to compensate for the loss of plasma proteins at the washing procedure.

Ad 5. In the postoperative phase a close assessment of ongoing fluid and blood losses is essential and these should continuously be compensated for. At the same time hourly basal fluid requirements should be provided. For this purpose a glucose-containing fluid should be considered to also cover some of the energy requirements of the patient. For each individual patient it is also of importance to decide the lowest acceptable Hb level so that unnecessary blood transfusions can be avoided.

Procedure-specific fluid management

Here fluid management in connection with some types of common major surgical procedures (orthopedic, gastrointestinal, peripheral vascular) is commented on in more detail.

Orthopedic surgery

Minor orthopedic surgery carried out under local anesthesia, nerve blocks or GA does not include any concerns related to fluid therapy. Fluid (0.5 or 1.0 l) is usually set to guarantee open venous access and, when the fluid has been infused, postoperative oral fluid intake is usually possible.

More extensive orthopedic procedures often dealt with in clinical routine practice are *knee* and *hip replacement* surgery (arthroplasty) and *hip fracture* surgery. The preoperative characteristics of patients are usually advanced age and the presence of a number of disease conditions, such as cardiovascular, cerebrovascular, renal and mental disorders.

Regional anesthesia is mostly preferred for these patients. A common concern at the onset of the spinal or epidural block is interference with the hemodynamic stability. Sometimes a practice of routine prehydration of patients by infusion of a crystalloid solution (up to 15 ml/kg) for prevention of spinal anesthesia-induced hypotension is used. Such an approach increases cardiovascular stability by compensating for the regional block-induced reduction in systemic vascular resistance. In spite of this a BP reduction may still occur. Therefore, the previously suggested more moderate approach consisting of crystalloid-based preload with about 500 ml combined with infusion of 250–500 ml of colloid and, if clinically indicated, addition of a vasopressor seems a more justified routine [15,16].

Intraoperatively the basal fluid requirement (1.5 ml/[kg h]) should be satisfied. In hip surgery, even minor procedure-specific losses should be compensated for. A total crystalloid infusion of about 4 ml/(kg h) seems to be sufficient. The fluid used to rinse the wound area should be documented, and the measured difference to regained fluid should be considered to represent exudation and bleeding, and be compensated for by infusion of equal volume of colloid. When the predetermined safe lowest Hb level for the patient has been reached, available blood should be infused (cell-saver derived, predonated autologous, heterologous). In the postoperative phase basal fluid requirements have to be provided and measured fluid and blood losses compensated for.

For **hip surgery** the following "rule of thumb" for perioperative fluid therapy seems advantageous.

1. Before and during induction of neuroaxial block – infuse about 500 ml crystalloid combined with 250–500 ml of colloid. Add a vasopressor if hemodynamically indicated.
2. Intraoperatively – infuse 4 ml/(kg h) of crystalloid and compensate measured exudation and blood loss with equal volume of colloid.
3. Postoperatively – provide basal fluid requirements 1.5 ml/(kg h) and compensate measured ongoing losses (mainly bleeding) with colloid.
4. Blood should be transfused when predetermined critical Hb level is reached.

Knee surgery is mostly carried out under spinal/epidural anesthesia and tourniquet ischemia. At the induction of the tourniquet ischemia an endogenous transfusion of up to 0.5 l of blood from the leg will reach the central vascular compartment. Therefore, a more moderated compensation for the regional block-induced hemodynamic effects is justified and an intraoperative crystalloid fluid infusion of 2–4 ml/(kg h) in total is sufficient.

Prior to the release of the tourniquet, however, a *bolus* of at least 500 ml of colloid should be infused and, at release, the leg should be *raised* to decrease the systemic effects of the local hyperemic reperfusion response in the leg. The blood loss should be assessed and initially compensated for by infusion of an equal volume of colloid. When the predetermined safe lowest Hb level has been reached blood should be infused as indicated above.

For **knee prosthesis surgery** the following "rule of thumb" for perioperative fluid therapy seems advantageous.

1. Before and during induction of neuroaxial block – infuse about 500 ml crystalloid in combination with vasopressor if hemodynamically indicated.
2. Intraoperatively – infuse 2–4 ml/(kg h) of crystalloid. Prior to release of tourniquet infuse 500 ml of colloid.
3. Postoperatively – provide basal fluid requirements 1.5 ml/(kg h) and compensate measured ongoing losses (mainly bleeding) with colloid.
4. Blood should be transfused when predetermined critical Hb level is reached.

Gastrointestinal surgery (GIS)

Optimal fluid therapy for *open abdominal surgery* has remained a matter of controversy. Too liberal a fluid strategy may include a risk of GI edema and impaired postoperative recovery of GI function, while a too restrictive strategy may instead cause splanchnic hypoperfusion and tissue hypoxia, which also may impair postoperative recovery of GI function.

A recent assessment of seven randomized clinical trials reveals that there is still a lack of well-defined evidence-based procedure-specific fluid treatment recommendations for GIS [1]. Using predetermined clinical endpoints for crystalloid-based compared with colloid-based fluid strategy in connection with major abdominal surgery, it has been possible to show that the former strategy results in reduction of tissue oxygen tension while the colloid-based one markedly improves tissue oxygenation [9].

In the planning of perioperative fluid therapy for GIS it should also be remembered that before surgery the patient is quite often subjected to bowel preparation with hyperosmolar solutions that will enhance any preoperative fluid deficit [17]. Preoperative fluid restriction will further add to the fluid deficit. Therefore a rather liberal initial fluid administration is usually recommended. However, crystalloid fluid administration to maintain left ventricular end diastolic volume index and cardiac index during open abdominal surgery seems to be in the range of 6 ± 2 ml/(kg h) (about 400–600 ml/h for an 80 kg adult patient) [18]. A more liberal crystalloid-based fluid strategy (intraoperatively ~ 4.2 l; postoperative during 24 h ~ 6.3 l) will result in a positive fluid balance and a high incidence of complications (57%) [19].

It has been suggested that the evaporative loss from the abdominal cavity is highly overestimated and the non-anatomical third space loss is based on flawed methodology and most probably does not exist [20]. Furthermore, the fluid volume accumulated in traumatized tissue is small. Therefore, a more moderated strategy including a combination of crystalloid administration to replace basal fluid requirements and extravascular losses, together with colloid administration to maintain an adequate intravascular volume and favourable tissue perfusion, has been suggested as a more optimal approach [1,9].

Colloid administration (goal-directed) markedly increases microcirculatory blood flow in the small intestine and thereby intestinal tissue oxygen tension after abdominal surgery. In contrast, goal-directed crystalloid and restricted crystalloid administrations were found not to include such beneficial effects [21].

These results consequently support the idea that perioperative fluid therapy, including colloids, might be the most beneficial approach to maintain an adequate fluid balance during major open abdominal surgery.

For **open gastrointestinal surgery** the following "rule of thumb" for perioperative fluid therapy seems advantageous.

1. Before and during anesthesia induction infuse about 500 ml of balanced (Ringer's) crystalloid (to compensate for bowel preparation and preoperative fluid restriction).
2. Intraoperatively – infuse 4 ml/(kg h) of crystalloid + 4 ml/(kg h) of colloid.
3. Measured blood loss should be compensated with equal volume of colloid until predetermined critical Hb level for blood transfusion is reached.
4. Postoperatively – provide basal fluid requirements 1.5 ml/(kg h) and compensate measured ongoing losses with a mixture of crystalloid and colloid.
5. Blood transfusion when indicated.

Laparoscopic GI surgery (LGIS) is becoming an increasingly common alternative to open abdominal surgery since the small incision will reduce blood loss, postoperative pain and thereby shorten the recovery. It seems reasonable to assume that the fluid therapy chosen may be less important in this situation. The crystalloid fluid load to maintain left ventricular end diastolic volume index and cardiac index for laparoscopic surgery seems to be only about 60% of that needed during open abdominal surgery [18]. However, the abdomen is usually insufflated with carbon dioxide gas which, together with necessary positioning maneuvers, will influence intra-abdominal pressure and thereby venous return, tissue hydration (stasis-induced tissue edema) and hemodynamic stability. These factors may contribute to the fact that *postoperative nausea and vomiting* (PONV) is a rather common problem after LGIS.

Following laparoscopic cholecystectomy, PONV is more effectively moderated by intraoperative infusion of a large volume of lactated Ringer's solution (40 ml/kg) than by smaller amounts (15 ml/kg) [22]. The higher volume load was found to lead to significant improvements in postoperative pulmonary function, exercise capacity and a reduced stress response (aldosterone, antidiuretic hormone and angiotensin II). Nausea, general well-being, thirst, dizziness, drowsiness, fatigue and balance function were also significantly improved, and significantly more patients fulfilled discharge criteria and were discharged on the day of surgery with the high-volume fluid substitution [22].

It seems obvious that perioperative administration of a sufficient volume of intravenous fluids to correct the fasting hours fluid deficit and intraoperative fluid shifts may effectively prevent PONV, without the expense or the potential for side effects seen with pharmacological approaches. Comparison of preloading with either crystalloid or colloids on the incidence of PONV following laparoscopic cholecystectomy under general anesthesia has shown that preloading with crystalloid (10 ml/kg) results in a lower incidence of PONV than preloading with colloid (10 ml/kg) [23]. Considering the available data, it seems that a total volume load of at least 15–20 ml/kg of balanced electrolyte solution (Ringer's type) is to be recommended during laparoscopic cholecystectomy.

> For **laparoscopic cholecystectomy** the following "rule of thumb" for perioperative fluid therapy seems advantageous.
>
> 1. Before anesthesia/regional block induction preload with at least 10 ml/kg followed by an additional 10–15 ml/kg during the laparoscopic procedure, which usually lasts about 1 h.
> 2. Postoperatively – basal fluid requirements + crystalloid-based compensation of ongoing fluid losses.

In connection with *laparoscopic gastric, colonic* and *rectal* surgery it is important to establish a well-functioning gastrointestinal anastomosis. In this situation liberal crystalloid administration may cause edema and impair tissue oxygenation and thereby the functional healing of the anastomosis.

Recent experimental studies clearly indicate that perianastomotic tissue oxygen tension will markedly benefit from infusion of colloid (preferably 6% HES 130/0.4, which also possesses anti-inflammatory properties) [24]. It seems obvious that GI anastomotic procedures will benefit from a combination of crystalloid (to replace basal fluid requirements and extravascular losses) and colloid to maintain an adequate intravascular volume and microcirculatory tissue perfusion [1].

> For **laparoscopic gastric, colonic and rectal surgery** the following "rule of thumb" for perioperative fluid therapy seems advantageous.
>
> 1. Before anesthesia/regional block induction preload with 5 ml/kg of colloid followed intraoperatively by 3 ml/(kg h) of crystalloid + 3 ml/(kg h) of colloid.
> 2. Measured blood loss should be compensated with equal volume of colloid until predetermined critical Hb level for blood transfusion is reached.
> 3. Postoperatively – basal fluid requirements + crystalloid and colloid-based compensation of ongoing fluid losses.

Vascular surgery

Patients scheduled for vascular reconstructions of the *lower limb* or *abdominal aortic surgery* constitute a high-risk population. Most patients are elderly, quite often also diabetic, suffering from atherosclerotic disease affecting cardiovascular as well as renal function. Therefore non-traumatic procedures are quite often chosen.

Revascularization of the lower limb can sometimes be achieved by the use of endovascular approaches for which local anesthesia at the site of incision is sufficient. In these cases crystalloid fluid to keep an iv line open is sufficient. Addition of colloid (HES 130/0.4 with anti-inflammatory properties) to enhance tissue perfusion and prevent endothelial injury following reflow may sometimes be indicated.

More extensive revascularization procedures of the lower limb as well as abdominal aortic aneurysm (AAA) repairs are carried out under either GA, spinal or epidural block. GA as well as neuroaxial block are safe approaches, but the latter approach seems to reduce the risk of postoperative cardiac complications and pneumonia [25,26].

The perioperative fluid therapy of patients undergoing major vascular surgery should be rather *restrictive* since liberal fluid therapy (> 3 l perioperatively) seems to impair clinical outcome [27] and a positive fluid balance in AAA surgery predicts major adverse events [28]. A recent study shows that a restricted perioperative fluid regimen prevents major complications and significantly reduces overall hospital stay following AAA repair [29]. Therefore, at the induction of of neuroaxial block only about 0.5 l of crystalloid should be infused, and vasopressors used if indicated to raise BP.

Current aspects of perioperative fluid handling in vascular surgery favor the concept that normovolemia should be maintained by protocol-based replacement of extracellular losses (urinary output plus insensible perspiration) with isotonic balanced crystalloid, and blood volume should be optimized by using iso-oncotic colloids [30]. The choice of a balanced HES solution (130/0.4) with anti-inflammatory properties seems to have a protective effect on kidney integrity in major surgery [31].

For major **vascular surgery** the following "rule of thumb" for perioperative fluid therapy seems advantageous.

1. Before and during onset of GA/neuroaxial block infuse about 4 ml/kg of balanced (Ringer's type) crystalloid and treat hypotension with vasopressors or a bolus of 250 ml of iso-oncotic colloid (preferably HES 130/0.4)
2. Intraoperatively – infuse 2 ml/(kg h) of crystalloid + 2 ml/(kg h) of colloid.
3. Measured blood loss should be compensated with equal volume of colloid until predetermined critical Hb level for blood transfusion is reached.
4. Postoperatively – provide basal fluid requirements 1.5 ml/(kg h) and compensate measured ongoing losses with a mixture of crystalloid and colloid.
5. Blood transfusion when indicated.

Summary

The optimal perioperative fluid strategy is still a matter of dispute and no evidence-based standardized perioperative surgical procedure-specific guidelines for fluid therapy have so far been agreed upon. In the perioperative period it is of importance to achieve and maintain an acceptable fluid balance and hemodynamic stability whereby adequate tissue perfusion and oxygenation is guaranteed. In the present survey "rule of thumb" approaches, based mainly on recently presented research data, are suggested for perioperative fluid therapy in connection with orthopedic, gastrointestinal and vascular surgery.

References

1. Bundgaard-Nielsen M, Secher NH, Kehlet H. "Liberal" vs. "restrictive" perioperative fluid therapy – a critical assessment of the evidence. *Acta Anaesthesiol Scand* 2009; **53**: 843–51.

2. Varadhan KK, D.N. Lobo DN. A meta-analysis of randomised controlled trials of intravenous fluid therapy in major elective open abdominal surgery: getting the balance right. *Proc Nutr Soc* 2010; **2**: 1–11.

3. Haljamäe H. Use of fluids in trauma. *Int J Intensive Care* 1999; **6**: 20-30.

4. Bundgaard-Nielsen M, Jörgensen CC, Secher NH, Kehlet H. Functional intravascular volume deficit in patients before surgery. *Acta Anaesthesiol Scand* 2010; **54**: 464–9.

5. Holte K, Kehlet H. Compensatory fluid administration for preoperative dehydration – does it improve outcome? *Acta Anaesthesiol Scand* 2002; **46**: 1089–93.

6. Bijker JB, van Klei WA, Vergouwe Y, *et al.* Intraoperative hypotension and 1-year mortality after noncardiac surgery. *Anesthesiology* 2009; **111**: 1217–26.

7. Haljamäe H (ed.). Plasma volume support. *Baillière's Clin Anaesthesiol* 1997; **11**: 1–184.

8. Haljamäe H. Adverse reactions to infusion fluids. In: Hahn RG, Prough DS, Svensen CH, eds. *Perioperative Fluid Therapy*. New York: Informa Healthcare, 2006; pp. 459–75.

9. Lang K, Boldt J, Suttner S, *et al.* Colloids versus crystalloids and tissue oxygen tension in patients undergoing major abdominal surgery. *Anesth Analg* 2001; **93**: 405–9.

10. Wang P, Li Y, Li J. Protective roles of hydroxyethyl starch 130/0.4 in intestinal inflammatory response and oxidative stress after hemorrhagic shock and resuscitation in rats. *Inflammation* 2009; **32**: 71–82.

11. Bengtson A, Haljamäe H. Complement activation and organ function in critically ill surgical patients. *Acute Care* 1988–89; **14–15**: 111–37.

12. Boldt J, Brosch Ch, Röhm K, *et al.* Comparison of the effects of gelatin and a modern hydroxyethyl starch solution on renal function and inflammatory response in elderly cardiac surgery patients. *Br J Anaesth* 2008; **100**: 457–64.

13. Beattie WS, Karkouti K, Wijeysundera DN, *et al.* Risk with preoperative anemia in noncardiac surgery: a single-center cohort study. *Anesthesiology* 2009; **110**: 574–81.

14. Hardy JF. Current status of transfusion triggers for red blood cell concentrates. *Transfus Apher Sci* 2004; **31**: 55–66.

15. Riesmeier A, Schellhaass, Boldt J, *et al.* Crystalloid/colloid versus crystalloid intravascular volume administration before spinal anesthesia in elderly patients: the influence of cardiac output and stroke volume. *Anesth Analg* 2009; **108**: 650–4.

16. Morgan P. The role of vasopressors in the management of hypotension induced by spinal and epidural anaesthesia. *Can J Anaesth* 1994; **41**: 404–13.

17. Holte K, Nielsen KG, Madsen JL, *et al.* Physiological effects of bowel preparation. *Dis Colon Rectum* 2004; **47**: 1397–402.

18. Concha MR, Mertz VF, Cortinez LI, *et al.* The volume of lactated Ringer's solution required to maintain preload and cardiac index during open and laparoscopic surgery. *Anesth Analg* 2009; **108**: 616–22.

19. Warrillow SJ, Weinberg L, Parker F, *et al.* Perioperative fluid prescription, complications and outcomes in major elective open gastrointestinal surgery. *Anaesth Intensive Care* 2010; **38**: 259–65.

20. Brandstrup B. Fluid therapy for the surgical patient. *Best Pract Res Clin Anaesthesiol* 2006; **20**: 265–83.

21. Hiltebrand LB, Kinberger O, Arnberger M, *et al.* Crystalloids versus colloids for goal-directed fluid therapy in major surgery. *Crit Care* 2009; **13**: R 40.

22. Holte K, Klarskov B, Christensen DS, *et al.* Liberal versus restrictive fluid administration to improve recovery after laparoscopic cholecystectomy: a randomized, double-blind study. *Ann Surg* 2004; **240**: 892–9.

23. Turkistani A, Abdullah K, Manaa E, *et al.* Effect of fluid preloading on postoperative nausea and vomiting following laparoscopic cholecystectomy. *Saudi J Anaesth* 2009; **3**: 48–52.

24. Kimberger O, Arnberger M, Brandt S, *et al.* Goal-directed colloid administration improves the microcirculation of healthy and perianastomotic colon. *Anesthesiology* 2009; **110**: 496–504.

25. Barbosa FT, Cavalcante JC, Juca MJ, *et al.* Neuroaxial anaesthesia for lower limb revascularization. *Cochrane Database Syst Rev* 2010; CD007083.

26. Singh N, Sidawy AN, Dezee K, *et al.* The effects of the type of anesthesia on outcomes of lower extremity infrainguinal bypass. *J Vasc Surg* 2006; **44**: 964–8.

27. Adesanya A, Rosero E, Timaran C, *et al.* Intraoperative fluid restriction predicts improved outcomes in major vascular surgery. *Vasc Endovascular Surg* 2008; **42**: 531–6.

28. McArdle GT, Price G, Lewis A, *et al.*, Positive fluid balance is associated with complications ofter elective open infrarenal abdominal aortic aneurysm repair. *Eur J Endovasc Surg* 2007; **34**: 522–7.

29. McArdle GT, McAuley DF, McKinley A, *et al.* Preliminary results of a prospective randomized trial of restrictive versus standard fluid regime in elective open abdominal aneurysm repair. *Ann Surg* 2009; **250**; 28–34.

30. Jacob M, Chappell D, Hollmann MW. Current aspects of perioperative fluid handling in vascular surgery. *Curr Opin Anaesthesiol* 2009; **22**: 100–8.

31. Rittoo D, Gosling P, Simms MH, *et al.* The effects of hydroxyethyl starch compared with gelofusine on activated endothelium and the systemic inflammatory response following aortic aneurysm repair. *Eur J Vasc Endovasc Surg* 2005; **30**: 520–4.

Chapter

4

Intra-abdominal surgery

Yifat Klein and Idit Matot

Current practice of perioperative fluid administration remains controversial with regard to how much to infuse [1–9]. Although fluid restriction is accepted in thoracic surgery [4,10,11], the situation differs in the general surgical population.

Abdominal surgery has been traditionally associated with dehydration. The etiology is multifactorial and includes preoperative fasting, bowel preparation, underlying illness, perioperative fluid and electrolyte deficits due to blood and insensible loss and fluid shifts between physiological compartments ("third spacing") [4,12–14]. Current practice of intraoperative fluid administration is still guided by algorithms based on the assumption that these deficits are to be replaced by crystalloids using a "ml/(kg h)" formula [15]. Accordingly, patients undergoing major intra-abdominal procedures should be administered with 10–15 ml/(kg h) of fluids [16,17]. However, the bases of such formulas are being questioned [1,18–22]. For example, substitution for third space losses [19] and replacement of blood loss by three times the amount of crystalloid [23] may be flawed. In fact, blood volume after fasting is normal, and a fluid-consuming third space has never been reliably shown [20–22].

Moreover, recent accelerated care protocols for gastrointestinal surgery have significantly affected the volume status of the surgical patient: bowel preparation is less often required, thus preoperative salt and water depletion is less frequent; re-institution of oral fluids in the immediate postoperative phase further diminishes the propensity for iatrogenic dehydration; and the use of laparoscopic instead of open techniques may also reduce fluid loss as well as the need for epidural analgesia (which is often accompanied by an "epidural preload") [24]. Altogether such perioperative management reduces the need for liberal hydration.

Finally, several reports of significant deleterious effects of overhydration with crystalloids question this practice [18,25,26]. Perioperative liberal fluid administration often leads to overhydration and weight gain in the range of 3–10 kg. The latter has been associated with higher postoperative morbidity and mortality rates, and a longer length of stay (LOS) in the intensive care (ICU) [27]. In healthy volunteers, infusion of 40 ml/kg of lactated Ringer's solution over 3 h caused significant increases in body weight and poor pulmonary function compared with infusions of 5 ml/kg [18]. Additionally, Arieff presented 13 fatal cases of postoperative pulmonary edema in healthy individuals that may have been secondary to excessive fluid administration [25].

The hypothesis that liberal use of fluids should significantly increase tissue oxygenation and therefore decrease the incidence of postoperative wound infection was disproved by Kabon et al. who demonstrated that supplemental hydration does not reduce the rate of

Clinical Fluid Therapy in the Perioperative Setting, ed. Robert G. Hahn. Published by Cambridge University Press. © Cambridge University Press 2011.

wound infection in a cohort of colonic surgical patients [28]. On the contrary, positive post-operative fluid balance may result in gut edema that contributes to intestinal dysfunction [4,29]. Back in the 1930s, Mecray et al. found that modest positive salt and water balance caused weight gain after elective colectomy and was associated with delayed recovery of gastrointestinal function, increased complication rate and extended hospital stays [30].

The abovementioned data, in addition to the expansion of monitoring tools that guide fluid therapy, have led to the growing interest in relating various fluid strategies to patient outcome. This is reflected by the rising number of publications in the last decade [24]. The studies have reached conflicting conclusions (Tables 4.1 and 4.2). In this chapter we wish to provide a comprehensive review of the literature, discuss the evidence presented herein, and highlight critical considerations in fluid therapy that clinicians may wish to address in order to improve patient outcomes following abdominal surgery.

Clinical trials comparing the effect of two "fixed" fluid volumes on outcome

Nine randomized clinical trials (RCTs) compared the effect of two different "fixed" fluid volumes on postoperative outcome in adults undergoing major abdominal surgery. Intra-abdominal procedures included colorectal surgery [1,5,28,31–38] or various abdominal procedures [7,34,35] (Table 4.1). The fluid regimens included, in addition to the "fixed" volume, supplementary intravenous fluid boluses administered according to an algorithm based on hemodynamic parameters and/or urine output.

Studies with improved outcome following a restricted fluid regimen

Five studies found that a restrictive fluid regimen improves outcome after major abdominal surgery [1,5,7,31,35].

Lobo et al. focused on the postoperative fluid management of 20 adults after elective colonic resection [5]. Intraoperative fluid application was relatively liberal in all patients, but postoperatively, patients were randomly assigned to either a restrictive ($\leq$ 2 l and 77 mmol sodium per day) or a standard ($\geq$ 3 l and 154 mmol sodium per day) protocol. The latter caused a significant weight gain, a delayed return of bowel function and a prolonged hospital stay [5]. In a randomized, controlled trial, Brandstrup et al. investigated 141 patients undergoing major colorectal surgery [1]. Unlike the liberal group, the restrictive group received no fluids before administration of an epidural, neither was there a replacement for third space loss. Intra- and postoperative fluid restriction (mean ~2.7 vs. ~5.4 l per day) significantly reduced the incidence of major and minor complications, such as anastomotic leakage, pulmonary edema, pneumonia and wound infection, without compromising renal function [1]. It is noteworthy that the two groups received different types of fluids (more colloids in the restrictive group vs. normal saline in the liberal group) and that the restrictive group included more proximal anastomoses and more smokers.

Nisanevich et al. applied intraoperative restrictive or liberal fluid regimens in 152 patients undergoing various major intra-abdominal procedures. Decreased postoperative morbidity and a shortened hospital stay were documented in the restrictive group [7]. Holte et al. compared restrictive (~1.6 l) vs. a liberal (~5 l) intraoperative fluid strategy in a small group of patients (n = 23) undergoing fast-track colon surgery. They found an improvement

Table 4.1. Perioperative methodology and outcomes of "fixed" volume randomized clinical trials.

Procedure / patients (n)	ASA (%) I/II/ III/IV	Volume administered (median [range])		Primary endpoint	Result[a]	Reference
		Liberal	Restrictive			
Hemicolectomy / 20	—	18.0 l (16.4–19.3)[b] cumulative over days 0–4 (iv + oral)	11.6 l (10.4–12.2)[b] cumulative over days 0–4 (iv + oral)	gastric emptying time	**pro restriction:** ↑GI recovery ↓hospital stay (9 vs. 6 days)	Lobo et al. 2005[5]
Colorectal resection / 140	47/51/2/0	5.4 l (2.7–11)[c] on day of surgery	2.7 l (1.1–8)[c] on day of surgery	complications	**pro restriction:** ↓complications	Brandstrup et al. 2003[1]
Major abdominal surgery / 142	22/52/26/0	3.7 l (1.9–8.8) intraoperatively	1.2 l (0.5–7.8) intraoperatively	complications and mortality	**pro restriction:** ↑GI recovery ↓complications, hospital stay (9 vs. 8 days) →death	Nisanevich et al. 2005[7]
Major abdominal surgery / 60	—	intraoperative: 1 l/h[d] postoperative: 2–3 l/24 h	intraoperative: nil postoperative: only oral intake	coagulation	**pro restriction:** ↓thrombosis, DVT	Janvrin et al. 1980[35]
Colonic surgery / 32 (fast-track)	22/25/53/0	5 l (3.6–8) intraoperatively	1.6 l (0.94–2.3) intraoperatively	pulmonary function and hypoxemia	**pro restriction:** ↑pulmonary function, oxygenation **against restriction:** ↑vasoactive hormones, length of hospital stay	Holte et al. 2007[31]
Colon resection / 253	10/75/15/0	5.7 ± 2 l[d] intraoperatively + the first postoperative hour	3.1 ± 1.5 l[d] intraoperatively + the first postoperative hour	wound infection	**inconclusive:** →wound infection	Kabon et al. 2005[28]

Table 4.1. (cont.)

Procedure / patients (n)	ASA (%) I/II/ III/IV	Volume administered (median [range])		Primary endpoint	Result[a]	Reference
		Liberal	Restrictive			
Colorectal resection / 69	5/70/24/1	8.75 l (8.00–9.80) cumulative iv fluids over days 0–4	4.50 l (4.00–5.62) cumulative iv fluids over days 0–4	length of hospital stay	**inconclusive:** → length of hospital stay, GI recovery, complications	Mackay et al. 2006[32]
Colon resection / 56	11/82/7/0	intraoperative: 3.8 ± 1.9 l[d] postoperative: 1.2 ± 0.3 l[d]	intraoperative: 2.2 ± 0.97 l[d] postoperative: 0.65 ± 0.3 l[d]	tissue perfusion and tissue oxygen pressure	**against restriction:** ↓ tissue perfusion, tissue oxygen pressure	Arkilic et al. 2003[33]
Major abdominal surgery / 62	14/73/13/0	2.5 l during 24 h postoperatively	1.5 l during 24 h postoperatively	length of hospital stay	**against restriction:** length of hospital stay, complications	Vermeulen et al. 2009[34]
Laparoscopic cholecystectomy / 48	88/12/0/0	2.9 l (1.95–3.9) intraoperatively	0.99 l (0.72–1.45) intraoperatively	physiological recovery	**against restriction:** ↓ pulmonary function, recovery ↑ hospital stay → exercise capacity	Holte et al. 2004[38]

[a.] Results refer to the restrictive group. ↑, increased/improved; ↓, decreased; →, no change/significant difference.

[b.] Liberal group received ≥ 3 l water and 154 mmol sodium per day; restrictive group received ≤ 2 l water and 77 mmol sodium per day.

[c.] Liberal group received preloading of epidural analgesia with 500 ml HAES 6%, and 0.9% saline replacement of third space loss.

[d.] Average values (median values were not mentioned).

DVT, deep vein thrombosis; GI, gastrointestinal

Table 4.2. Perioperative methodology and outcomes of goal-directed randomized clinical trials.

Procedure / patients (n)	Infusion strategy	Timing & means	Volume infused	Endpoints	Result[a]	Reference
Major bowel resection / 55	ED; SV optimization with FTc > 0.35 s	intraoperative fluids	control vs. GDT: total: 55.2 vs. 64.6 ml/kg coll: 19.4 vs. 28.0 ml/kg	hemodynamic performance hospital stay postoperative complications	↑SV and CO (↑) hospital stay (↓) postoperative complications ↓ critical care admissions	Conway et al. 2002[40]
Major bowel surgery / 128	ED; SV optimization and increase in CVP < 3 mmHg	intraoperative fluids	control vs. GDT: cryst: same (3000 ml) coll[c]: 1500 vs. 2000 ml	hospital stay gut function	↓ hospital stay ↑ gut function recovery ↓ gastrointestinal and overall morbidity	Wakeling et al. 2005[43]
Colorectal resection / 108	ED; SV optimization with FTc of 0.35–0.40 s	intraoperative fluids & inotropes	control vs. GDT[b.]: cryst: 2625 vs. 2298 ml coll: 1209 vs. 1340 ml inotrope: 50% vs. 31%	hospital stay	↓ hospital stay ↓ complications ↑ gut recovery	Noblett et al. 2006[42]
Major general, urologic or gynecologic surgery / 98	ED; SV optimization with FTc of 0.35–0.40 s	intraoperative fluids	control vs. GDT[b.]: coll: 282 vs. 847 ml cryst: 4375 vs. 4405 ml blood: 118 vs. 168 ml	hospital stay GI and renal function	↓ hospital stay ↓ PONV ↑ gut recovery	Gan et al. 2002[41]

Table 4.2. (cont.)

Procedure / patients (n)	Infusion strategy	Timing & means	Volume infused	Endpoints	Result[a]	Reference
Upper GI surgery / 40	ITBV of 850–950 ml/m²	intraoperative fluids	control vs. GDT[b]: cryst: 4043 vs. 4047 ml coll: 1255 vs. 1411 ml	inflammatory response: serum PCT, CRP, TNFα	→ PCT, CRP, TNF-α	Szakmany et al. 2005[50]
Major abdominal surgery / 80	radial artery line, PiCCOplus monitor; SPV < 10%	intraoperative fluids	control vs. GDT: cryst: 4250 vs. 4500 ml coll: 1000 vs. 1500 ml	organ function & perfusion	→ oxygen transport and organ function → ICU stay, mortality → length of mechanical ventilation	Buettner et al. 2008[48]
Elective abdominal[c] / 33	radial artery line; ΔPOP ≤ 10%	intraoperative fluids	control vs. GDT[b]: cryst: 1,563 vs. 2,176 ml coll[d]: 0 vs. 2247 ml	hospital stay	↓ hospital stay ↓ ICU stay ↓ complications ↓ length of mechanical ventilation	Lopes et al. 2007[47]

| Major abdominal surgery[c] / 60 | radial artery line, FloTrac/Vigileo device; CI ≥ 2.5 l/(min/m²) | intraoperative fluids & inotropes | control vs. GDT[b]: cryst[d]: 3153 vs. 2489 ml coll[d]: 817 vs. 1188 ml dobu[d]: 30.4 vs. 4.1 $\mu g\ kg^{-1}\ h^{-2}$ | hospital stay postoperative complications | ↓ hospital stay ↓ complications | Mayer et al. 2010[49] |

[a.] Results refer to the intervention group. ↑, increased/improved ($p < 0.05$); (↑), $p > 0.05$; ↓, decreased/reduced ($p < 0.05$); (↓), $p > 0.05$; → unchanged

[b.] Average values (median values were not mentioned)

[c.] High-risk surgery;

[d.] $p < 0.05$. All but two inconclusive trials (Szakmany et al. 2005; Buettner et al. 2008) were pro-GDT approach.

CI, cardiac index; CO, cardiac output; Coll, colloids; CRP, creactive protein; Cryst., crystalloids; CVP, central venous pressure; ED, esophageal Doppler; FTc, corrected flow time; GDT, goal-directed fluid therapy; ICU, intensive care unit; ITBV, intrathoracic blood volume; PCT, procalcitonin; PONV, postoperative nausea and vomiting; ΔPOP, plethysmographic waveform; SV, Stroke volume; TNFα, tumor necrosis factor α in pulmonary function and postoperative hypoxemia with the restrictive regimen [31]. This group, however, also endured significantly higher concentrations of cardiovascular active hormones (renin, aldosterone and angiotensin II) [31]. In one of the earlier RCT studies, Janvrin *et al.* demonstrated an association between intravenous fluids and venous thrombosis [35]. They randomized 60 patients undergoing mixed abdominal surgery into receiving either "wet" or "dry" postoperative fluid therapy (~2–3 l per day vs. no iv fluids). The "wet" patients were significantly more hemodiluted and hypercoagulable than the "dry" ones, and had a significantly higher incidence of deep vein thrombosis [35].

When attempting to deduce conclusions based on these trials, one should be aware of the major differences between them with regard to the definitions (i.e., liberal vs. restrictive regimens), methodology (i.e., inclusion and exclusion criteria; perioperative period studied; type of fluids administered; standardized anesthesia and analgesia; timing of intervention) and defined outcome parameters. Nevertheless, the outcome data were similar, highlighting the beneficial effect of a relatively restricted approach to fluid therapy in this surgical setting.

Studies with no difference in outcome

Two studies reported no difference between the liberal and the restrictive fluid regimens [28,32].

In a study of 80 patients undergoing mixed abdominal surgery, with a third of the procedures being laparoscopic, MacKay *et al.* found no statistical difference in the time of return of gastrointestinal function and length of hospital stay between the two regimens [32]. However, both groups were treated rather restrictively (mean 2.6 vs. 2.0 l per day) and no patient received more than 3 l of fluid a day. Therefore, most likely even their standard group was treated too restrictively to cause a potentially harmful effect [32].

Kabon *et al.* investigated a homogenous collective of 253 patients admitted for an elective colon resection with an anticipated duration of surgery > 2 h. They disproved the theory that supplemental hydration reduces wound infection rate [28].

Studies with improved outcome following a liberal fluid regimen

Two studies indicated that a liberal fluid regimen improves outcomes after major abdominal surgery, including a shortened hospital stay, fewer postoperative complications and increased tissue oxygenation [24,33,34].

Arkilic *et al.* reported that liberal fluid administration (~2.1 vs. 3.8 l perioperatively) increased tissue oxygenation (measured subcutaneously via a polarographic tissue oxygen sensor positioned in patients' upper arms after induction of anesthesia) in 56 patients undergoing colon resection [33], suggesting a lower risk for surgical wound infection [36,37]. However, tissue oxygenation was the only reported outcome parameter. Weight gain, edema formation, anastomosis healing, coagulation factors, length of hospital stay, bowel function and cardiopulmonary complications – all well-known effects of excessive fluid overload [1,5,7] – were not measured. Moreover, in a subsequent study the same authors failed to show that this increase in tissue oxygenation with liberal fluid administration can be translated into a lower wound infection rate [28].

In a double-blinded randomized trial, Vermeulen *et al.* randomized 62 patients undergoing major abdominal surgical procedures (primarily of the biliary and pancreatic regions) to restrictive or standard fluid management in the postoperative period (1.5 vs. 2.5 l for 24 h postoperatively) [34]. This study had several flaws. The protocol did not include a clinical relevant algorithm for supplementary fluid bolus administration, and there were many post-randomization dropouts due to severe bleeding, need for reoperation or infusion pump failure. When analyzing the data per intention to treat the authors found a significantly longer hospital stay and more major complications in the restrictive group. However, no significant differences were found in the per-protocol analysis.

Accumulating evidence suggest that higher fluid volumes have beneficial effects in minor procedures. In laparoscopic cholecystectomy, a very liberal vs. liberal fluid handling (40 vs. 15 ml/kg of lactated Ringer's intraoperatively; median duration of surgery ~1 h) reduced postoperative nausea and vomiting and hormonal vasoactive stress, improved lung function, general well-being and exercise capacity, and led to a shortened hospital stay [38].

In accord, Tatara *et al.* developed a mathematical model in order to analyze how duration of surgery affects fluid balance during abdominal surgery [39]. Their model was based on segmental bioelectrical impedence measurements from 30 patients undergoing elective abdominal surgery [8,39]. According to this model, abdominal procedures shorter than 3 h allow a wide range of fluid infusion rates (2.0–18.5 ml/[kg h]) without causing significant interstitial edema. In contrast, surgery with a duration of > 6 h requires a narrow range (5–8 ml/[kg h]) of infusion rates in order to maintain intravascular and interstitial volumes within critical values, thus dictating restrictive fluid regimens in major procedures [39].

Clinical trials assessing the effect of goal-directed fluid volumes on outcome

Attempts to optimize perioperative fluid management have led clinicians to the concept of goal-directed therapy (GDT). This is a tailored individualized technique that utilizes either a relatively noninvasive (continuous esophageal Doppler cardiac output monitoring) or invasive enhanced hemodynamic monitoring (via arterial and central lines) to guide fluid titration in order to optimize oxygen delivery. Most studies involve high-risk patients undergoing a variety of intra-abdominal procedures (including vascular surgery) and the optimization strategy included, in addition to fluids, the administration of inotropes (i.e., dopexamine/dobutamine/norepinephrine/epinephrine). In the following we provide a brief review of RCTs consisting of non-vascular intra-abdominal procedures and in which fluid optimization was the key method to improve oxygen delivery.

Four RCTs have attempted to determine the effects of Doppler-guided intraoperative fluid management on outcome after major abdominal surgery [40–43].

In these trials patients were randomized to receive iv fluid treatment guided by either Doppler-monitored ventricular filling or conventional parameters including heart rate, blood pressure, central venous pressure (CVP) and urine output (Table 4.2). Intra-abdominal procedures included colorectal resection [40,42,43] or mixed general, urologic and gynecologic procedures [41]. Meta-analyses of these trials found an overall reduction of the length of hospital stay, significantly fewer complications (both minor and major) and admissions to the ICU, fewer requirements for inotropes and faster return of gut function in patients who received esophageal Doppler-guided hemodynamic management [44–46]. There was no evidence of a significant difference in intraoperative crystalloid administration between the Doppler and control arms [45]; however, three trials reported significantly more colloid in the Doppler group [40,41,43].

In yet another randomized double-blinded clinical multicenter trial of 150 patients undergoing elective colorectal surgery, Brandstrup et al. compared GDT to near maximal stroke volume guided by esophageal Doppler to goal-directed fluid therapy to normal body weight and zero fluid balance, i.e., restrictive fluid regimen (personal communication). An intention-to-treat analysis of the results found comparable postoperative morbidity, mortality and hospital between the groups. These findings suggest that restrictive fluid management is not inferior to GDT strategy in which higher cardiac outputs and stroke volumes were achieved.

Five RCTs utilized other monitoring techniques and flow-related hemodynamic parameters to guide fluid administration in intra-abdominal (non vascular) surgery, i.e., pulse pressure variation [47], systolic pressure variation [48], cardiac index based on FloTrac/ Vigileo device [49], intrathoracic blood volume [50] and serum lactate levels [51]. Two of these trials included high-risk patients [47,49]. Importantly, all of these trials concluded that starting GDT at any time during the perioperative period has shown benefit compared with standard fluid regimes.

In a small randomized trial of 33 high-risk patients, Lopes and colleagues [47] analyzed the effect of intraoperative fluid optimization of pulse pressure variation. The intervention group received more fluids (both groups received relatively restricted fluid volumes) and exhibited a significant reduction in LOS, postoperative complications, median duration of mechanical ventilation and stay in the ICU.

Buettner et al. studied the effect of systolic pressure variation-guided intraoperative fluid management on organ function and perfusion in 80 patients admitted for major abdominal surgery [48]. Although at 3 and 6 h systolic pressure variation was significantly higher in the control group, all outcome measures – i.e., oxygen transport, organ function, length of mechanical ventilation, ICU stay and mortality – were comparable.

In a very recent randomized controlled trial, Mayer et al. investigated the influence of an optimization protocol that included fluids and inotropes on outcome in 60 high-risk patients scheduled for major abdominal surgery [49]. The GDT-group patients received enhanced hemodynamic monitoring via the FloTrac/Vigileo device and an attempted cardiac index of at least 2.5 $l/(min\ m^2)$. The GDT protocol consisted of dobutamine, norepinephrine and colloid boluses, and resulted in a significant reduction of the length of hospital stay and perioperative complications compared with a standard management with pressure-based goals.

Szakmany et al. compared intrathoracic blood volume (IBV)-guided fluid management and CVP-based titration, in affecting the early systemic inflammatory response in 40 patients who underwent esophageal, gastric and pancreatic surgery [50]. The intervention and control groups received fluids to maintain the IBV index between 850 and 950 ml/m^2, and the CVP between 8 and 12 mmHg, respectively. Serial measurements of inflammatory parameters were performed and included serum tumor necrosis factor α (TNF-α), C-reactive protein and procalcitonin; this showed no significant difference in the inflammatory response between the intervention and control groups [50].

In a randomized, observer-blinded, single-center trial, Wenkui et al. compared the effect of a restricted intravenous fluid regimen adjusted by serum lactate levels with a standard restricted regimen on complication rate after major elective surgery for gastrointestinal malignancy [51]. All patients ($n = 214$) received a "restricted intravenous fluid regimen" according to "fast-track" protocols (well-defined multimodal programs aimed at earlier ambulation and oral nutrition and thereby reduced postoperative length of hospital stay). In addition, the treatment group received fluid adjustments according to blood lactate levels, intraoperatively and in the early postoperative period. The regimen guided by serum lactate decreased systemic postoperative complications but not overall total complications.

Fluid management in hepatic surgery

Bleeding during hepatic surgery has been recognized as a significant factor adversely affecting postoperative outcome [52]. Therefore, strategies to prevent intraoperative hemorrhage were sought. During liver resection, low CVP seems to play a prominent role in reducing blood loss [53–57]. A CVP of 1–5 mmHg is considered as an optimal target. Several studies reported that low CVP during liver resection significantly reduced intraoperative blood loss and transfusions, decreased the incidence of postoperative complications and shortened hospital stay [56–58]. Therefore, fluid restriction, as a means of maintaining low CVP during the resection phase of the operation, is recommended [53–57, 59].

The same principle applies for liver transplantation, where blood transfusions and total intraoperative fluids were found as predictors of adverse postoperative outcome [60], though data are less clear. In the setting of liver transplantation, transfusion of plasma, or > 4 units of red blood cells has shown correlation with decreased one-year survival rate [61]. Reyle-Hahn and Rossaint had long ago advocated "volume restrictive substitution therapy" during the dissection phase to decrease venous pressure in the surgical field and intravascular volume in portosystemic collaterals [62]. Massicotte *et al.* described a regimen based on fluid restriction, phlebotomy (during the transplantation), vasopressors and strict, protocol-guided product replacement associated with very low blood product use [59]. In contrast, a retrospective comparison between low vs. normal CVP in patients undergoing liver transplantation indicated that even though low CVP reduced blood transfusions, it was also associated with increased rates of postoperative renal failure and 30-day mortality [63].

Conclusions and perspectives

Research on perioperative fluid therapy in intra-abdominal surgery has recently focused on two strategies, "fixed" high- versus low-volume regimens and individualized optimization strategies, so-called goal-directed therapy [64]. To this end there is an increasing amount of data to support the notion that perioperative fluid restriction yields positive postoperative outcome in elective abdominal surgery and thus should be favored, with the exception of minor procedures, where liberal administration of fluids may be applied.

The differential terminology of "fixed" vs. goal-directed fluid therapy is misleading. Both approaches are "goal directed." The first treats the patient with crystalloids according to standard parameters (blood pressure, heart rate, urine output, blood loss, etc.), while the latter utilizes a battery of tools (i.e., administration of colloids, crystalloids, inotropes and blood products) to optimize measurements indicative of stroke volume, cardiac output and oxygen delivery. Hence, the focus of debate should be, rather than restrictive vs. liberal, whether all patients undergoing elective abdominal surgery will benefit from a goal directed approach that is not just cost and time consuming but may also cause harm via various etiologies (including misinterpretations of the data, inherited risks and limitations of each monitor and drug administered, etc.).

Of importance is the fact that most studies showing benefit with a goal-directed approach have used an esophageal Doppler to guide therapy. Despite its obvious advantages, the esophageal Doppler monitor has several limitations. Certain conditions might introduce inaccuracies when translating the descending aortic blood flow velocity into cardiac output

(CO): for example, states of acute illness causing redistribution of the CO, general anesthetics that alter vascular tone and thereby CO distribution, or aortic plaque burden in the elderly which often decreases aortic compliance thereby affecting aortic flow dynamics [65]. Esophageal Doppler is contraindicated in conditions that restrict free access to the patient's head, and in any pathology that predisposes the patient to an increased risk of injury or bleeding. Finally, although proven to be valuable in the anesthetized patient, esophageal Doppler is not optimal in the conscious patient, nor in an anesthetized patient who needs frequent repositioning (such as left/right tilt, Trendelenburg/reverse Trendelenburg etc.) and is therefore not applicable for the entire perioperative period.

Others use a variety of approaches that estimate cardiac output and/or oxygen delivery assuming that optimization will result in better tissue oxygenation with a consequent improved outcome. This point is yet to be proven in a large multicenter trial.

Most GDT trials have utilized colloid boluses to adjust flow-related measures, which raised the possibility that it is the colloid itself rather than the timed administration that led to the observed outcomes. Kimberger et al. confirmed this theory by showing that colloid-based GDT significantly increased microcirculatory blood flow and tissue oxygen tension in healthy and perianastomotic colon compared with goal-directed crystalloid fluid therapy in a porcine model of abdominal surgery [66]. Interestingly, there were no significant differences in any of the measured parameters, i.e., heart rate, mean arterial pressure, CVP, cardiac index, pulmonary capillary wedge pressure and arterial lactate among the treatment groups. This study adds important new knowledge to the understanding of the apparent beneficial effects of colloid administration in surgical patients.

Another question that remains unresolved is the preferred timing of intervention. Flooding the patient with liters of fluids in order to optimize cardiac output and organ perfusion in a short period of time, i.e., during the perioperative period, may be harmful. Achievement of optimal fluid status is not just a matter of fluid substitution per se. It should take into account the pathophysiology of the surgery, the trauma caused by the surgery and the body response to trauma as well as the injury initiated by manual handling of the organs – all of which are at their peak during the perioperative period. This period, which comprises only a very small fraction of the hospitalization period, might not be the right time for liberal fluid administration (as shown by Tartara et al. [39]) but rather attention should be given to the pre- and mostly to the postoperative period.

A predefined strategy to fluid management may be inadequate for some surgical patients, such as those at high risk or those who have long been hospitalized before surgery and in whom hypovolemia is suspected. As standard monitored parameters do not accurately reflect perioperative perfusion status, in a subgroup of high-risk patients, advanced monitoring and GDT may be preferred. The type of intervention and the optimal algorithm to be used (colloids, vasopressors, inotropes, etc.) is yet to be defined.

References

1. Brandstrup B, Tonnesen H, Beier-Holgersen R, et al. Effects of intravenous fluid restriction on postoperative complications: comparison of two perioperative fluid regimens: a randomized assessor-blinded multicenter trial. *Ann Surg* 2003; **238**: 641–8.

2. Bundgaard-Nielsen M, Secher NH, Kehlet H. 'Liberal' vs. 'restrictive' perioperative fluid therapy – a critical assessment of the evidence. *Acta Anaesthesiol Scand* 2009; **53**: 843–51.

3. Holte K, Kehlet H. Fluid therapy and surgical outcomes in elective surgery: a need for reassessment in fast-track surgery. *J Am Coll Surg* 2006; **202**: 971–89.

4. Holte K, Sharrock NE, Kehlet H. Pathophysiology and clinical implications of perioperative fluid excess. *Br J Anaesth* 2002; **89**: 622–32.

5. Lobo DN, Bostock KA, Neal KR, Perkins AC, Rowlands BJ, Allison SP. Effect of salt and water balance on recovery of gastrointestinal function after elective colonic resection: a randomised controlled trial. *Lancet* 2002; **359**: 1812–18.

6. Lobo DN, Macafee DA, Allison SP. How perioperative fluid balance influences postoperative outcomes. *Best Pract Res Clin Anaesthesiol* 2006; **20**: 439–55.

7. Nisanevich V, Felsenstein I, Almogy G, Weissman C, Einav S, Matot I. Effect of intraoperative fluid management on outcome after intraabdominal surgery. *Anesthesiology* 2005; **103**: 25–32.

8. Tatara T, Tashiro C. Quantitative analysis of fluid balance during abdominal surgery. *Anesth Analg* 2007; **104**: 347–54.

9. Wiedemann HP, Wheeler AP, Bernard GR, *et al.* Comparison of two fluid-management strategies in acute lung injury. *N Engl J Med* 2006; **354**: 2564–75.

10. Parquin F, Marchal M, Mehiri S, Herve P, Lescot B. Post-pneumonectomy pulmonary edema: analysis and risk factors. *Eur J Cardiothorac Surg* 1996; **10**: 929–32; discussion 33.

11. Slinger PD. Perioperative fluid management for thoracic surgery: the puzzle of postpneumonectomy pulmonary edema. *J Cardiothorac Vasc Anesth* 1995; **9**: 442–51.

12. Shires T, Williams J, Brown F. Acute change in extracellular fluids associated with major surgical procedures. *Ann Surg* 1961; **154**: 803–10.

13. Carrico CJ, Canizaro PC, Shires GT. Fluid resuscitation following injury: rationale for the use of balanced salt solutions. *Crit Care Med* 1976; **4**: 46–54.

14. Woerlee GM, *Common perioperative problems and the anaesthetist.* Dordrecht, Netherlands: Kluwer Academic Publishers, 1988.

15. Kaye AD KI. Intravascular fluid and electrolyte physiology. In: Miller R, ed. *Miller's anesthesia.* Philadelphia, PA: Elsevier, 2005, pp. 1763–98.

16. Hwang G MJ. Anesthesia for abdominal surgery. In: Hurford WEBM, Davison JK, Haspel KL, Rosow C, eds. *Clinical Anesthesia Procedures of the Massachusetts General Hospital.* Philadelphia, PA: Lippincott-Raven, 1997, pp. 330–46.

17. Sendak M. Monitoring and management of perioperative fluid and electrolyte therapy. In: Rogers MC Longnecker DETJ, eds *Principles and Practice of Anesthesiology.* New York: Mosby-Year Book, 1993.

18. Holte K, Jensen P, Kehlet H. Physiologic effects of intravenous fluid administration in healthy volunteers. *Anesth Analg* 2003; **96**: 1504–9.

19. Twigley AJ, Hillman KM. The end of the crystalloid era? A new approach to peri-operative fluid administration. *Anaesthesia* 1985; **40**: 860–71.

20. Brandstrup B. Fluid therapy for the surgical patient. *Best Pract Res Clin Anaesthesiol* 2006; **20**: 265–83.

21. Doty DB, Hufnagel HV, Moseley RV. The distribution of body fluids following hemorrhage and resuscitation in combat casualties. *Surg Gynecol Obstet* 1970; **130**: 453–8.

22. Nielsen OM. Extracellular fluid and colloid osmotic pressure in abdominal vascular surgery. A study of volume changes. *Dan Med Bull* 1991; **38**: 9–21.

23. Michalski AH, Lowenstein E, Austen WG, Buckley MJ, Laver MB. Patterns of oxygenation and cardiovascular adjustment of acute, transient normovolemic anemia. *Ann Surg* 1968; **168**: 946–56.

24. Shields CJ. Towards a new standard of perioperative fluid management. *Ther Clin Risk Manag* 2008; **4**: 569–71.

25. Arieff AI. Fatal postoperative pulmonary edema: pathogenesis and literature review. *Chest* 1999; **115**: 1371–7.

26. Moller AM, Pedersen T, Svendsen PE, Engquist A. Perioperative risk factors in elective pneumonectomy: the impact of excess fluid balance. *Eur J Anaesthesiol* 2002; **19**: 57–62.

27. Lowell JA, Schifferdecker C, Driscoll DF, Benotti PN, Bistrian BR. Postoperative fluid overload: not a benign problem. *Crit Care Med* 1990; **18**: 728–33.

28. Kabon B, Akca O, Taguchi A, *et al.* Supplemental intravenous crystalloid administration does not reduce the risk of surgical wound infection. *Anesth Analg* 2005; **101**: 1546–53.

29. Moretti EW, Robertson KM, El-Moalem H, Gan TJ. Intraoperative colloid administration reduces postoperative nausea and vomiting and improves postoperative outcomes compared with crystalloid administration. *Anesth Analg* 2003; **96**: 611–17.

30. Mecray PM, Barden RP, Ravdin IS. Nutritional edema: its effect on the gastric emptying time before and after gastric operations. 1937. *Nutrition* 1990; **6**: 278–89.

31. Holte K, Foss NB, Andersen J, *et al.* Liberal or restrictive fluid administration in fast-track colonic surgery: a randomized, double-blind study. *Br J Anaesth* 2007; **99**: 500–8.

32. MacKay G, Fearon K, McConnachie A, *et al.* Randomized clinical trial of the effect of postoperative intravenous fluid restriction on recovery after elective colorectal surgery. *Br J Surg* 2006; **93**: 1469–74.

33. Arkilic CF, Taguchi A, Sharma N, *et al.* Supplemental perioperative fluid administration increases tissue oxygen pressure. *Surgery* 2003; **133**: 49–55.

34. Vermeulen H, Hofland J, Legemate DA, Ubbink DT. Intravenous fluid restriction after major abdominal surgery: a randomized blinded clinical trial. *Trials* 2009; **10**: 50.

35. Janvrin SB, Davies G, Greenhalgh RM. Postoperative deep vein thrombosis caused by intravenous fluids during surgery. *Br J Surg* 1980; **67**: 690–3.

36. Greif R, Akca O, Horn EP, Kurz A, Sessler DI. Supplemental perioperative oxygen to reduce the incidence of surgical-wound infection. Outcomes Research Group. *N Engl J Med* 2000; **342**: 161–7.

37. Gottrup F, Firmin R, Rabkin J, Halliday BJ, Hunt TK. Directly measured tissue oxygen tension and arterial oxygen tension assess tissue perfusion. *Crit Care Med* 1987; **15**: 1030–6.

38. Holte K, Klarskov B, Christensen DS, *et al.* Liberal versus restrictive fluid administration to improve recovery after laparoscopic cholecystectomy: a randomized, double-blind study. *Ann Surg* 2004; **240**: 892–9.

39. Tatara T, Nagao Y, Tashiro C. The effect of duration of surgery on fluid balance during abdominal surgery: a mathematical model. *Anesth Analg* 2009; **109**: 211–16.

40. Conway DH, Mayall R, Abdul-Latif MS, Gilligan S, Tackaberry C. Randomised controlled trial investigating the influence of intravenous fluid titration using oesophageal Doppler monitoring during bowel surgery. *Anaesthesia* 2002; **57**: 845–9.

41. Gan TJ, Soppitt A, Maroof M, *et al.* Goal-directed intraoperative fluid administration reduces length of hospital stay after major surgery. *Anesthesiology* 2002; **97**: 820–6.

42. Noblett SE, Snowden CP, Shenton BK, Horgan AF. Randomized clinical trial assessing the effect of Doppler-optimized fluid management on outcome after elective colorectal resection. *Br J Surg* 2006; **93**: 1069–76.

43. Wakeling HG, McFall MR, Jenkins CS, *et al.* Intraoperative oesophageal Doppler guided fluid management shortens postoperative hospital stay after major bowel surgery. *Br J Anaesth* 2005; **95**: 634–42.

44. Abbas SM, Hill AG. Systematic review of the literature for the use of oesophageal Doppler monitor for fluid replacement in major abdominal surgery. *Anaesthesia* 2008; **63**: 44–51.

45. Walsh SR, Tang T, Bass S, Gaunt ME. Doppler-guided intraoperative fluid management during major abdominal surgery: systematic review and meta-analysis. *Int J Clin Pract* 2008; **62**: 466–70.

46. Giglio MT, Marucci M, Testini M, Brienza N. Goal-directed haemodynamic therapy and gastrointestinal complications in major surgery: a meta-analysis of randomized controlled trials. *Br J Anaesth* 2009; **103**: 637–46.

47. Lopes MR, Oliveira MA, Pereira VO, Lemos IP, Auler JO, Jr., Michard F. Goal-directed fluid management based on pulse pressure variation monitoring during high-risk surgery: a pilot randomized controlled trial. *Crit Care* 2007; **11**: R100.

48. Buettner M, Schummer W, Huettemann E, Schenke S, van Hout N, Sakka SG. Influence of systolic-pressure-variation-guided intraoperative fluid management on organ function and oxygen transport. *Br J Anaesth* 2008; **101**: 194–9.

49. Mayer J, Boldt J, Mengistu AM, Rohm KD, Suttner S. Goal-directed intraoperative therapy based on autocalibrated arterial pressure waveform analysis reduces hospital stay in high-risk surgical patients: a randomized, controlled trial. *Crit Care* 2010; **14**: R18.

50. Szakmany T, Toth I, Kovacs Z, et al. Effects of volumetric vs. pressure-guided fluid therapy on postoperative inflammatory response: a prospective, randomized clinical trial. *Intensive Care Med* 2005; **31**: 656–63.

51. Wenkui Y, Ning L, Jianfeng G, et al. Restricted perioperative fluid administration adjusted by serum lactate level improved outcome after major elective surgery for gastrointestinal malignancy. *Surgery* 2010; **147**: 542–52.

52. Scheele J, Stang R, Altendorf-Hofmann A, Paul M. Resection of colorectal liver metastases. *World J Surg* 1995; **19**: 59–71.

53. Jarnagin WR, Gonen M, Fong Y, et al. Improvement in perioperative outcome after hepatic resection: analysis of 1,803 consecutive cases over the past decade. *Ann Surg* 2002; **236**: 397–406; discussion -7.

54. Jones RM, Moulton CE, Hardy KJ. Central venous pressure and its effect on blood loss during liver resection. *Br J Surg* 1998; **85**: 1058–60.

55. Melendez JA, Arslan V, Fischer ME, et al. Perioperative outcomes of major hepatic resections under low central venous pressure anesthesia: blood loss, blood transfusion, and the risk of postoperative renal dysfunction. *J Am Coll Surg* 1998; **187**: 620–5.

56. Smyrniotis V, Kostopanagiotou G, Theodoraki K, Tsantoulas D, Contis JC. The role of central venous pressure and type of vascular control in blood loss during major liver resections. *Am J Surg* 2004; **187**: 398–402.

57. Wang WD, Liang LJ, Huang XQ, Yin XY. Low central venous pressure reduces blood loss in hepatectomy. *World J Gastroenterol* 2006; **12**: 935–9.

58. Johnson M, Mannar R, Wu AV. Correlation between blood loss and inferior vena caval pressure during liver resection. *Br J Surg* 1998; **85**: 188–90.

59. Massicotte L, Lenis S, Thibeault L, Sassine MP, Seal RF, Roy A. Effect of low central venous pressure and phlebotomy on blood product transfusion requirements during liver transplantations. *Liver Transpl* 2006; **12**: 117–23.

60. Bennett-Guerrero E, Feierman DE, Barclay GR, et al. Preoperative and intraoperative predictors of postoperative morbidity, poor graft function, and early rejection in 190 patients undergoing liver transplantation. *Arch Surg* 2001; **136**: 1177–83.

61. Massicotte L, Sassine MP, Lenis S, Seal RF, Roy A. Survival rate changes with transfusion of blood products during liver transplantation. *Can J Anaesth* 2005; **52**: 148–55.

62. Reyle-Hahn M, Rossaint R. Coagulation techniques are not important in directing blood product transfusion during liver transplantation. *Liver Transpl Surg* 1997; **3**: 659–63.

63. Schroeder RA, Collins BH, Tuttle-Newhall E, et al. Intraoperative fluid management during orthotopic liver transplantation. *J Cardiothorac Vasc Anesth* 2004; **18**: 438–41.

64. Grocott MP, Mythen MG, Gan TJ. Perioperative fluid management and clinical outcomes in adults. *Anesth Analg* 2005; **100**: 1093–1106.

65. Schober P, Loer SA, Schwarte LA. Perioperative hemodynamic monitoring with transesophageal Doppler technology. *Anesth Analg* 2009; **109**: 340–53.

66. Kimberger O, Arnberger M, Brandt S, *et al.* Goal-directed colloid administration improves the microcirculation of healthy and perianastomotic colon. *Anesthesiology* 2009; **110**: 496–504.

Chapter

5

Spinal anesthesia

Michael F.M. James and Robert A. Dyer

Spinal anesthesia is inevitably associated with some degree of hypotension as a result of the combined effects of reductions of sympathetic tone, peripheral fluid pooling and falling venous return. Estimates of the incidence of clinically relevant hypotension vary from 25% to over 80% depending on the criteria used to identify clinically relevant decreases in blood pressure and on the population group studied.

Two groups of patients have been extensively studied. The first is the obstetric population, in whom hypotension has implications for the fetus (reduction in placental perfusion) and for the mother (cardiovascular collapse and unpleasant side effects of nausea and vomiting). The other patient population of concern is comprised of elderly patients undergoing a variety of surgical procedures for which spinal anesthesia is appropriate, including bladder and prostate procedures and lower limb surgery, particularly joint replacements.

A variety of causative factors have been suggested to explain the hypotension following spinal anesthesia, including diminished cardiac output as a result of a reduction in venous return, arteriolar capillary dilatation and paralysis of the sympathetic nerve supply to the heart and adrenal glands resulting in reduced catecholamine responsiveness and unmasking of hypovolemia. In the pregnant patient these may be complicated by aorto-caval compression. Preexisting hypertension may increase the risk of spinal anesthesia-associated hypotension in older patients [1]. Older texts referred to the value of electrolyte solutions in minimizing the hypotensive response and suggest that volumes of 2 l may be adequate. These assumptions have been challenged by a substantial body of research over the last 20 years.

Obstetric spinal anesthesia

In obstetric patients, an early study showed that the administration of a 20 ml/kg crystalloid preload failed to prevent significant hypotension whether the load was given rapidly over 10 min or more slowly over 20 min. However, in the rapid preload group, three patients were found to have a marked rise in central venous pressure. The authors queried the role of isotonic crystalloid preload in the management of spinal anesthesia for elective Cesarean section [2], and the same group recommended that there should be no delays for the administration of a crystalloid preload prior to spinal anesthesia for elective Cesarean section [3].

Jackson and colleagues evaluated the use of a preload of 1000 ml prior to spinal anesthesia for Cesarean section and were unable to demonstrate any advantage over a preload of 200 ml. They also concluded that crystalloid preload was not of value [4].

Clinical Fluid Therapy in the Perioperative Setting, ed. Robert G. Hahn. Published by Cambridge University Press. © Cambridge University Press 2011.

A study in pre-eclamptic patients has also failed to demonstrate significant benefit from a preload of 1000 ml crystalloid, although the authors commented that changes in uterine artery velocity waveforms were minimal and there was no adverse effect on the neonate [5]. There have been a number of concerns regarding the possible adverse consequences of saline-based solutions given in large volumes in terms of generating hyperchloremic metabolic acidosis, but this does not seem to be of particular consequence to either mother or child when saline solution is compared with lactated Ringer's for preload [6].

Non-obstetric spinals

In a study conducted in elderly patients aged 60 years or over, the overall incidence of arterial hypotension during spinal anesthesia was 27%, rising to 60% when temperature sensation was blocked to T7. If the block reached T4, all patients required vasopressor therapy. Patients were divided into three groups receiving 16 ml/kg, 8 ml/kg or zero acetated Ringer's solution as a preload; crystalloid preloading had no effect on the incidence of hypotension [7]. However, a relatively small preload (7 ml/kg) of 3% hypertonic saline was significantly better than 0.9% saline at reducing the requirement for vasopressor support in patients undergoing prostatectomy [8].

In a review of spinal anesthesia in elderly patients, Critchley concluded that an adequate venous preload was necessary, but any fluid loading should be ideally administered as the block is developing (subsequently termed *coload* in an obstetric anesthesia study [9]), rather than as a preload [10]. In an early study of volume kinetics during epidural anesthesia, it was shown that a crystalloid coload of 15 ml/kg was better retained within the circulation in those patients who showed a substantial decrease in systolic pressure. Nevertheless, despite volume loading, there was a relative hypovolemia, as evidenced by hemodilution, in all patients throughout the development of hypotension [11].

Crystalloid vs. colloid

The relative lack of efficacy of crystalloid loading prior to spinal anesthesia can be explained by a number of factors including the physiological responses of patients with normal fluid balance status to a rapid fluid load, and the volume kinetics of crystalloid solutions. Pouta and colleagues demonstrated a significant increase in the release of atrial natriuretic peptide, and a lesser effect on endothelin-1, following crystalloid loading in healthy parturients following a crystalloid load of 2000 ml lactated Ringer's solution. They concluded that this could offset the effects of volume load on blood pressure during Cesarean delivery [12]. This release of hormone was correlated significantly with the increase in atrial stretch as indicated by an increase in central venous pressure. Pre-eclamptic patients showed a greater response, possibly in line with reduced diastolic function in these patients [13].

Studies on the effects of spinal anesthesia on cardiac output suggested that volume preloading had to be sufficient to produce a significant increase in cardiac output if hypotension was to be minimized [14]. These authors showed that colloid preload was more effective than crystalloid in enhancing cardiac output and, consequently, in reducing spinal hypotension during elective Cesarean section. Lactated Ringer's was shown to sustain, but not increase cardiac output in healthy patients undergoing lower extremity surgery [15].

In older patients, cardiac output was shown to diminish in patients who received no preload, or only 500 ml saline as a preload, whereas 500 ml colloid sustained cardiac output, but did not significantly reduce the incidence of hypotension [16], possibly because the volumes used were too small.

Fluid kinetics modeling has shown that crystalloids rapidly redistribute away from the central compartment, and tend to enhance the second compartment. The redistribution time constants of crystalloid are quite rapid [17] and these kinetics may contribute to the relative lack of efficacy of crystalloid solutions in preventing spinal anesthesia-associated hypotension. Volunteer studies have shown that an infusion rate of 50 ml/min is required to yield an increase in blood volume of approximately 10% and that this would need be maintained for at least 40 min to produce the required volume expansion; this volume load rapidly dissipates [18].

In terms of mechanisms, therefore, it appears that *crystalloid preloading is relatively ineffective* since it is rapidly redistributed and has limited ability to increase cardiac output during spinal anesthesia. The increase of vasodilator peptides induced by a rapid increase in atrial stretch may also contribute to the lack of efficacy of fluid loading in preventing spinal hypotension. Important considerations thus appear to be the appropriate volume and timing of any fluid load, since the administration of a fluid load during the onset of spinal anesthesia could be more effective than preloading. The final issue to be resolved is whether the use of colloid solutions would be advantageous by virtue of their retention in the circulating blood volume for a longer period than crystalloids.

Whilst logic would suggest that colloid preloading would be advantageous compared with crystalloid loading, the data on this topic are inconsistent. Riley and colleagues suggested that a preload of 500 ml hydroxyethyl starch (HES) together with 1 l lactated Ringer's was superior to 2 l lactated Ringer's in terms of reductions in the incidence of hypotension and requirements for ephedrine in obstetric patients [19]. However, a study found that 500 ml of gelatin colloid preload was not superior to a similar volume of crystalloid or no preload at all in parturients [20]. The same group also failed to show a benefit of a combination of 500 ml each of HES and crystalloid in elderly patients receiving spinal anesthesia [21].

Obstetrics studies using 1 l colloid showed significantly less hypotension than no preload [22], or preloading with either 1.5 l lactated Ringer's or 500 ml HES [14]. A systematic review at this time concluded that crystalloid preload was inconsistent in preventing hypotension, whereas colloid was generally effective in minimizing hypotension, but neither was effective in minimizing maternal nausea, and there were few differences in neonatal outcomes [23]. Dahlgren and colleagues confirmed that 1 l colloid was more effective than an equivalent volume of crystalloid for the prevention of hypotension [24] and subsequently demonstrated that supine stress testing could accurately predict those patients in whom a colloid preload would likely be beneficial [25]. Davies and colleagues demonstrated that 10 ml/kg of colloid was more effective than 5 ml/kg at minimizing obstetric spinal hypotension [26].

A comparison between combinations of 1 l each of lactated Ringer's combined with gelatin or HES-based colloids demonstrated that the HES-lactated Ringer's was superior to either the gelatin combination or 1 l HES alone [27]. A recent Cochrane review concluded that crystalloids were more effective than no fluids (relative risk [RR] 0.78, 95% confidence interval [CI] 0.60–1.00; one trial, 140 women, sequential analysis) and colloids were more effective than crystalloids (RR 0.68, 95% CI 0.52–0.89; 11 trials, 698 women) in preventing hypotension following spinal anesthesia at Cesarean section [28]. Although no differences were detected for different doses, rates or methods of administering colloids or crystalloids, the literature review presented above suggests that at least 1 l of colloid appears to be required to produce a significant reduction in the incidence of hypotension in healthy patients.

Timing

As the administration of crystalloids to healthy, volume-replete subjects is likely to trigger off physiological responses such as secretion of atrial natriuretic peptide and increased renal excretion of the fluid, and volume kinetics suggest very rapid redistribution of fluid loads in the absence of a hypovolemic state, the administration of fluids as a coload at the time of onset of spinal anesthesia might be more efficacious than administering a preload. Initial studies using 20 ml/kg of crystalloid as a rapid bolus at the time of the performance of spinal anesthesia suggested that a significant reduction in ephedrine requirements could be achieved by this method [9].

A meta-analysis of preload vs. coload failed to confirm the advantage of coload, although the authors commented that the only study in which coload was effective was the one that used the highest infusion volume, i.e., 20 ml/kg [29]. Fluid kinetic studies have shown that the distribution of crystalloids from the plasma to the interstitium is markedly delayed during the onset of spinal, epidural and general anesthesia [30] and this lends support to the concept that coload with crystalloids may be more effective than preload, but definitive data are lacking.

A recent study using either crystalloid (1000 ml) or colloid (500 ml) coload in older patients showed that both forms of fluid therapy sustained cardiac output above baseline values for 30 min, but the effect of crystalloids waned after 20 min [31]. There is no evidence that colloid coload is more effective than colloid preload [32].

Conclusions

Current data suggest that crystalloids are only minimally effective at limiting hypotension and then only if given in doses of 20 ml/kg or greater, preferably as a rapid coload immediately after induction of spinal anesthesia. Such a large fluid bolus may be disadvantageous in elderly patients with limited cardiac reserve and in pre-eclamptic patients in whom diastolic dysfunction may predispose to the development of pulmonary edema.

Colloid fluid loading given as either a coload or preload appears to be more successful as a preventative strategy and the weight of evidence appears to suggest that a volume of 15 ml/kg may be optimal in the normal pregnant patient.

A smaller volume load of colloid may be appropriate in older patients undergoing spinal anaesthesia and similar conditions may apply in pre-eclampsia, although firm data in this area are lacking. The height of the block required for surgery may also be important as most elderly patients require a much lower block than do Cesarean section patients and may thus require a smaller fluid load (Table 5.1).

The use of fluids to manage hypotension during spinal anesthesia is, at best, only moderately effective and early intervention with vasopressors will be required in many patients regardless of the fluid strategy adopted, if hypotension is to be minimized. The best that can be achieved with optimal fluid therapy is an overall reduction in the total dosage of vasopressor required. However, this endpoint is worth achieving since vasopressors may have adverse consequences in both obstetric and non-obstetric patients undergoing spinal anesthesia.

The best possible management of spinal hypotension would appear to be optimal fluid therapy combined with early, carefully graded management of subsequent hypotension with the appropriate vasopressor, dependent on cardiovascular status. Newer techniques involving analysis of cardiac performance, using the response of dynamic indices to a fluid

Table 5.1. Suggested fluid options in spinal anesthesia. These volumes represent the best guidelines that can currently be obtained from the literature, but conclusive evidence for these suggestions is lacking.

Patient	Fluid type	Volume (ml/kg)	Timing
Healthy obstetrics	crystalloid	20	coload
Healthy obstetrics	colloid	15	preload or coload
Pre-eclamptics	colloid (?)	5–7	preload or coload
Older patients block *below* T10	no fluid load	replacement and maintenance fluids only	
Older patients block *above* T10	colloid	5–7	coload

challenge, may give better guidelines than currently available for the administration of the appropriate volume of fluid in association with spinal anesthesia.

References

1. Critchley LA, Stuart JC, Short TG, *et al.* Haemodynamic effects of subarachnoid block in elderly patients. *Br J Anaesth* 1994; **73**: 464–70.

2. Rout CC, Akoojee SS, Rocke DA, *et al.* Rapid administration of crystalloid preload does not decrease the incidence of hypotension after spinal anaesthesia for elective caesarean section. *Br J Anaesth* 1992; **68**: 394–7.

3. Rout CC, Rocke DA, Levin J, *et al.* A reevaluation of the role of crystalloid preload in the prevention of hypotension associated with spinal anesthesia for elective cesarean section. *Anesthesiology* 1993; **79**: 262–9.

4. Jackson R, Reid JA, Thorburn J. Volume preloading is not essential to prevent spinal-induced hypotension at caesarean section. *Br J Anaesth* 1995; **75**: 262–5.

5. Karinen J, Rasanen J, Alahuhta S, *et al.* Maternal and uteroplacental haemodynamic state in pre-eclamptic patients during spinal anaesthesia for Caesarean section. *Br J Anaesth* 1996; **76**: 616–20.

6. Chanimov M, Gershfeld S, Cohen ML, *et al.* Fluid preload before spinal anaesthesia in Caesarean section: the effect on neonatal acid-base status. *Eur J Anaesthesiol* 2006; **23**: 676–9.

7. Coe AJ, Revanas B. Is crystalloid preloading useful in spinal anaesthesia in the elderly? *Anaesthesia* 1990; **45**: 241–3.

8. Baraka A, Taha S, Ghabach M, *et al.* Hypertonic saline prehydration in patients undergoing transurethral resection of the prostate under spinal anaesthesia. *Br J Anaesth* 1994; **72**: 227–8.

9. Dyer RA, Farina Z, Joubert IA, *et al.* Crystalloid preload versus rapid crystalloid administration after induction of spinal anaesthesia (coload) for elective caesarean section. *Anaesth Intensive Care* 2004; **32**: 351–7.

10. Critchley LA. Hypotension, subarachnoid block and the elderly patient. *Anaesthesia* 1996; **51**: 1139–43.

11. Drobin D, Hahn RG. Time course of increased haemodilution in hypotension induced by extradural anaesthesia. *Br J Anaesth* 1996; **77**: 223–6.

12. Pouta AM, Karinen J, Vuolteenaho OJ, *et al.* Effect of intravenous fluid preload on vasoactive peptide secretion during Caesarean section under spinal anaesthesia. *Anaesthesia* 1996; **51**: 128–32.

13. Pouta A, Karinen J, Vuolteenaho O, *et al.* Pre-eclampsia: the effect of intravenous fluid preload on atrial natriuretic peptide secretion during caesarean section under spinal anaesthesia. *Acta Anaesthesiol Scand* 1996; **40**: 1203–9.

14. Ueyama H, He YL, Tanigami H, *et al.* Effects of crystalloid and colloid preload on blood volume in the parturient undergoing spinal anesthesia for elective Cesarean section [see comments]. *Anesthesiology* 1999; **91**: 1571–6.

15. Kamenik M, Paver-Erzen V. The effects of lactated Ringer's solution infusion on cardiac output changes after spinal anesthesia. *Anesth Analg* 2001; **92**: 710–14.

16. Riesmeier A, Schellhaass A, Boldt J, *et al.* Crystalloid/colloid versus crystalloid intravascular volume administration before spinal anesthesia in elderly patients: the influence on cardiac output and stroke volume. *Anesth Analg* 2009; **108**: 650–4.

17. Svensen CH, Rodhe PM, Prough DS. Pharmacokinetic aspects of fluid therapy. *Best Pract Res Clin Anaesthesiol* 2009; **23**: 213–24.

18. Hahn RG, Svensen C. Plasma dilution and the rate of infusion of Ringer's solution. *Br J Anaesth* 1997; **79**: 64–7.

19. Riley ET, Cohen SE, Rubenstein AJ, *et al.* Prevention of hypotension after spinal anesthesia for cesarean section: six percent hetastarch versus lactated Ringer's solution. *Anesth Analg* 1995; **81**: 838–42.

20. Buggy D, Higgins P, Moran C, *et al.* Prevention of spinal anesthesia-induced hypotension in the elderly: comparison between preanesthetic administration of crystalloids, colloids, and no prehydration. *Anesth Analg* 1997; **84**: 106–10.

21. Buggy D, Fitzpatrick G. Intravascular volume optimisation during repair of proximal femoral fracture. Regional anaesthesia is usually technique of choice. *BMJ* 1998; **316**: 1090.

22. Ngan Kee WD, Khaw KS, Lee BB, *et al.* Randomized controlled study of colloid preload before spinal anaesthesia for caesarean section. *Br J Anaesth* 2001; **87**: 772–4.

23. Morgan PJ, Halpern SH, Tarshis J. The effects of an increase of central blood volume before spinal anesthesia for cesarean delivery: a qualitative systematic review. *Anesth Analg* 2001; **92**: 997–1005.

24. Dahlgren G, Granath F, Pregner K, *et al.* Colloid vs. crystalloid preloading to prevent maternal hypotension during spinal anesthesia for elective cesarean section. *Acta Anaesthesiol Scand* 2005; **49**: 1200–6.

25. Dahlgren G, Granath F, Wessel H, *et al.* Prediction of hypotension during spinal anesthesia for Cesarean section and its relation to the effect of crystalloid or colloid preload. *Int J Obstet Anesth* 2007; **16**: 128–34.

26. Davies P, French GW. A randomised trial comparing 5 mL/kg and 10 mL/kg of pentastarch as a volume preload before spinal anaesthesia for elective caesarean section. *Int J Obstet Anesth* 2006; **15**: 279–83.

27. Vercauteren MP, Hoffmann V, Coppejans HC, *et al.* Hydroxyethylstarch compared with modified gelatin as volume preload before spinal anaesthesia for Caesarean section. *Br J Anaesth* 1996; **76**: 731–3.

28. Cyna AM, Andrew M, Emmett RS, *et al.* Techniques for preventing hypotension during spinal anaesthesia for caesarean section. *Cochrane Database Syst Rev* 2006; CD002251.

29. Banerjee A, Stocche RM, Angle P, *et al.* Preload or coload for spinal anesthesia for elective Cesarean delivery: a meta-analysis. *Can J Anaesth* 2010; **57**: 24–31.

30. Hahn RG. Volume kinetics for infusion fluids. *Anesthesiology* 2010; **113**: 470–81.

31. Zorko N, Kamenik M, Starc V. The effect of Trendelenburg position, lactated Ringer's solution and 6% hydroxyethyl starch solution on cardiac output after spinal anesthesia. *Anesth Analg* 2009; **108**: 655–9.

32. Siddik-Sayyid SM, Nasr VG, Taha SK, *et al.* A randomized trial comparing colloid preload to coload during spinal anesthesia for elective cesarean delivery. *Anesth Analg* 2009; **109**: 1219–24.

Geriatric, obstetric and pulmonary surgery

Kathrine Holte

The limited knowledge of both pathophysiology and clinical outcomes of perioperative fluid management has precluded formation of evidence-based, rational guidelines. While plenty of studies have focused on fluid therapy in critically ill patients, clinical research into fluid administration in elective (or emergency) surgical procedures has, until recently, largely been absent [1]. However, the past decade has seen a growing interest in perioperative fluid management, shifting focus from the (still unresolved) question of *which type* of fluid to administer to *which amount* of fluid to be administered. Attention is now focused on the avoidance of fluid overload, i.e., avoidance of large positive perioperative fluid balances.

The perioperative patient is predisposed to fluid retention and thus potential postoperative fluid overload, as sodium and water are retained as a consequence of the physiologic stress response to surgery as well as fluid accumulation in peripheral tissues [2]. Historically, this saline conservation has been essential to survival and only recent practices of intravenous saline administration have made the capacity to excrete saline important. Thus, even healthy, non-operated volunteers may not readily excrete 1–3 l intravenous crystalloid.

Currently, no available technique may reliably determine perioperative fluid status, a fact no doubt contributing greatly to the controversy of which amounts of fluid to be administered perioperatively [3,4]. While weighing the patient may reflect on overall fluid status, weight gain, the essential parameter, may easily exist in the presence of hypovolemia. It is well known that pressure-guided cardiovascular monitoring methods (such as blood pressure and central venous pressures) are not adequate determinants of intravascular volume and have generally been disappointing when applied to guide fluid administration in clinical trials [5].

In contrast, guiding intraoperative fluid administration by individual flow-directed cardiovascular monitoring (so-called "goal-directed fluid therapy") has been shown to improve outcome in some, but not all studies [6]. Although other techniques are available, the only goal-directed fluid administration strategy sufficiently evaluated in clinical trials consists of colloid infusions guided by cardiac filling pressures obtained via a transesophageal Doppler device [5]. Both hypovolemia and fluid overload may obviously lead to impaired outcomes; however, these issues have not been systematically investigated.

Regarding the type of fluid to administer, a systematic review of all 80 randomized clinical trials in elective, non-cardiac surgery concluded that available data offered no conclusions on the choice of fluid to administer, mainly due to most studies being underpowered (very few studies with > 100 patients) as well as the failure to report relevant outcomes [7].

Perioperative fluid management – current controversial issues

Geriatric surgery
    similar issues as in non-geriatric surgery:
        "liberal" vs. "restrictive" vs. goal-directed fluid administration
        which type of fluid to administer

Pulmonary surgery
    role of fluid administration in post-pneumonectomy pulmonary edema

Obstetrics
    preload to alleviate hypotension in regional analgesia for labour

Figure 6.1. The terms "liberal" vs. "restrictive" or "high" vs. "low" fluid (internationally accepted in the medical literature) simply describe two different levels of fluid administration and do not infer conclusions regarding the suitability of either regimen. However, these terms have contributed to confusion in the literature and whenever possible, the actual amounts of fluid administered are mentioned. The term "fluid administration" refers to intravenous crystalloid administration unless stated otherwise.

Furthermore, perioperative care was generally not standardized and the follow-up period tended not to include the postoperative period (see Figure 6.1).

A multimodal revision of the principles of perioperative care (so-called "fast-track surgery") has been found to shorten hospital stay and improve convalescence in various surgical procedures [8]. Core components of this concept are opioid-sparing analgesia, early enteral feeding, mobilization as well as preoperative patient education and standardized postoperative care protocols. As early oral intake without restrictions combined with intravenous fluid therapy being applied only on specific indications, the result is an overall decrease in intravenous fluid administration within fast-track protocols.

Geriatric surgery

Despite an increasing number of surgical procedures being performed in the elderly population, few studies have been specifically concerned with the elderly. Furthermore elderly patients are often excluded from investigational trials, leaving very little specific evidence on the care of the elderly surgical patient. There is no general consensus on the exact definition of the elderly patient, who often is defined as a patient > 65 years. The age-related impairment of various organ systems and general implications for perioperative management are reviewed in detail elsewhere [9].

The propensity for fluid retention described above applies for elderly patients as well, as infusion of ~3 l of crystalloids results in a significant although small (~5–7%) decrease in pulmonary function in addition to a significant weight gain over 24 h in non-operated elderly (median 63 years) volunteers [10].

Preoperative fluid management

Preoperative bowel preparation decreases the functional cardiovascular capacity in the elderly (median 63 years) despite a daily oral fluid intake in excess of 2.5 l [11]. As this functional impairment presumably is caused by dehydration, it may very well be even more pronounced in older patients because they have a decreased capacity for oral intake due to reduced sensation of thirst [12]. Thus, in elderly patients undergoing preoperative bowel preparation, 2–3 l supplemental intravenous crystalloid infusion may be administered with the bowel preparation.

Perioperative fluid management

As mentioned previously, very few studies have specifically investigated elderly patients. Nevertheless, in many of the available studies, which mostly have been conducted in the area of abdominal and/or colorectal surgery, a major proportion of the participants, despite the lack of a formal age limit, may be considered elderly (> 65 years).

In abdominal surgery, one randomized, double-blind study in 32 patients, median age 75 years and no patient below 50 years of age, was conducted within a setting of fast-track colonic surgery [13]. A "liberal" (total ~6 l on the day of surgery including oral intake) crystalloid-based fluid regiment was compared with a "restrictive" (~2.6 l) regimen, and no differences in main outcomes were seen between groups. However, three patients receiving "restrictive" fluid vs. none receiving the "liberal" fluid regimen had anastomotic leaks, and though not significant, this warrants caution that without a sufficient pre- and early intra-operative volume load, so-called "restrictive" fluid regimens may theoretically predispose to increased morbidity.

This hypothesis is confirmed by a recent randomized study in 299 patients finding a pure "restricted" fluid regiment to cause increased morbidity compared with a "restricted" fluid regimen with added fluid infusions guided by the serum lactate level [14]. Several other recent randomized, clinical trials of fluid management in elective abdominal surgery conclude that avoidance of perioperative fluid overload may improve outcome [7,15,16]. In summary, it would seem that both fluid overload and a too restrictive perioperative fluid regimen worsen the outcome.

In elective orthopedic surgery, a randomized study in knee replacement surgery (fast-track), found "liberal" (4250 ml) vs. "restrictive" (1740 ml) intraoperative crystalloid-based fluid administration to result in significant hypercoagulability (confirming previous reports in healthy volunteers) though with no differences in morbidity or recovery [17]. Following proximal femoral fracture, a disease typical of the elderly population, a Cochrane review of two randomized, clinical studies with 130 patients found goal-directed fluid administration to shorten hospital stay [18].

A systematic review of various types of fluids administered in a general (not age-restricted) surgical population fails to find differences between the various types of fluid because the available studies are of insufficient volume and/or quality to draw firm conclusions [7].

Postoperative fluid management

No studies have specifically targeted the elderly population postoperatively, and generally, the literature on postoperative fluid management is very sparse.

In the context of fast-track surgery, an early start of normal food intake (in the absence of ileus) greatly diminishes the need for postoperative intravenous fluid administration. Less than 10% of patients undergoing fast-track colonic surgery receive a postoperative intravenous fluid supplement [8].

Obstetric surgery

The debate on fluid management in obstetrics largely centers on the relevance of fluid infusions to counteract hypotension in conjunction with regional anesthesia administered for pain relief during labor. The theory is that regional anesthesia (spinal, epidural or combined spinal–epidural) may induce hypotension, which again may cause fetal heart rate abnormalities due to a decrease in intrauterine blood flow. However, both the underlying mechanism and the clinical significance of these heart rate abnormalities are unclear.

A Cochrane review from 2004 included six trials with 473 patients in which 0.5–1.0 l of crystalloid vs. none was administered for preload before regional analgesia in labor [19]. The authors concluded that the overall effects of preloading were questionable. In one (of two) studies, in which high-dose local anesthetics were given, preload reduced maternal hypotension and fetal heart rate abnormalities. No effects of preload were seen in the other trial applying high-dose local anesthetic or in the remaining four trials of low-dose local anesthetics or combined spinal–epidural anesthesia [19].

For Cesarean section performed under spinal anesthesia, a Cochrane review from 2006 concluded preload with colloids to be more efficient than crystalloids, which again were more effective than placebo in preventing maternal hypotension [20]. Ephedrine and phenylephrine also were effective in this context. Even though both colloids and sympatomimetics reduced maternal hypotension, no intervention has been found to alleviate it. The lack of fluid efficacy may be attributed to the relatively short volume expansion and a possibly concomitant increase in ANP secretion [2] (for a detailed discussion see Chapter 5 – Spinal anesthesia).

A recent review has provided a general overview of fluid and blood management in the obstetric patient [21].

Pulmonary surgery

The obligatory decrease in pulmonary function after surgery may theoretically be amplified by fluid overload predisposing to pneumonia and respiratory failure [2]. A well-known complication to pulmonary surgery is pulmonary edema, with reported frequencies of 10–15%, though the pathophysiology is complex including multiple factors such as impaired lymphatic drainage and ischemia/reperfusion injury [22]. Thus, theoretically, patients subjected to lung surgery may be at particular risk of complications related to fluid overload. However, no randomized clinical trials have been performed in pulmonary surgery investigating the influence of perioperative fluid administration.

Several retrospective studies do find a correlation between the amounts of administered fluid (mainly crystalloids) and pulmonary edema, indicating a greater risk with a 24 h crystalloid administration > 3 l, or intraoperative administration > 2 l [2]. Moreover, general postoperative complications have been found to correlate with a positive fluid balance of > 4 l [7,23].

References

1. Holte K. Pathophysiology and clinical implications of peroperative fluid management in elective surgery. *Dan Med Bull* 2010; **57**: B4156.

2. Holte K, Sharrock NE, Kehlet H. Pathophysiology and clinical implications of perioperative fluid excess. *Br J Anaesth* 2002; **89**: 622–32.

3. Johnston WE. PRO: Fluid restriction in cardiac patients for noncardiac surgery is beneficial. *Anesth Analg* 2006; **102**: 340–3.

4. Spahn DR. CON: Fluid restriction for cardiac patients during major noncardiac surgery should be replaced by goal-directed intravascular fluid administration. *Anesth Analg* 2006; **102**: 344–6.

5. Bundgaard-Nielsen M, Holte K, Secher NH *et al*. Monitoring of perioperative fluid administration by individualized goal-directed therapy. *Acta Anaesthesiol Scand* 2007; **51**: 331–40.

6. Grocott MP, Mythen MG, Gan TJ. Perioperative fluid management and clinical outcomes in adults. *Anesth Analg* 2005; **100**: 1093–106.

7. Holte K, Kehlet H. Fluid therapy and surgical outcomes in elective surgery: a need for reassessment in fast-track surgery. *J Am Coll Surg* 2006; **202**: 971–89.

8. Kehlet H, Wilmore DW. Evidence-based surgical care and the evolution of fast-track surgery. *Ann Surg* 2008; **248**: 189–98.

9. Jin F, Chung F. Minimizing perioperative adverse events in the elderly. *Br J Anaesth* 2001; **87**: 608–24.

10. Holte K, Jensen P, Kehlet H. Physiologic effects of intravenous fluid administration in healthy volunteers. *Anesth Analg* 2003; **96**: 1504–9.

11. Holte K, Nielsen KG, Madsen JL, *et al*. Physiologic effects of bowel preparation. *Dis Colon Rectum* 2004; **47**: 1397–1402.

12. Phillips PA, Rolls BJ, Ledingham JG, *et al*. Reduced thirst after water deprivation in healthy elderly men. *N Engl J Med* 1984; **311**: 753–9.

13. Holte K, Foss NB, Andersen J, *et al*. Liberal or restrictive fluid administration in fast-track colonic surgery: a randomized, double-blind study. *Br J Anaesth* 2007; **99**: 500–8.

14. Wenkui Y, Ning L, Jianfeng G *et al*. Restricted perioperative fluid administration adjusted by serum lactate level improved outcome after major elective surgery for gastrointestinal malignancy. *Surgery* 2010; **147**: 542–52.

15. Brandstrup B, Tonnesen H, Beier-Holgersen R, *et al*. Effects of intravenous fluid restriction on postoperative complications: comparison of two perioperative fluid regimens: a randomized assessor-blinded multicenter trial. *Ann Surg* 2003; **238**: 641–8.

16. Nisanevich V, Felsenstein I, Almogy G, *et al*. Effect of intraoperative fluid management on outcome after intraabdominal surgery. *Anesthesiology* 2005; **103**: 25–32.

17. Holte K, Kristensen BB, Valentiner L, *et al*. Liberal versus restrictive fluid management in knee arthroplasty: a randomized, double-blind study. *Anesth Analg* 2007; **105**: 465–74.

18. Price JD, Sear JW, Venn RM. Perioperative fluid volume optimization following proximal femoral fracture. *Cochrane Database Syst Rev* 2004; CD003004.

19. Hofmeyr G, Cyna A, Middleton P. Prophylactic intravenous preloading for regional analgesia in labour. *Cochrane Database Syst Rev* 2004; CD000175.

20. Cyna AM, Andrew M, Emmett RS, *et al*. Techniques for preventing hypotension during spinal anaesthesia for caesarean section. *Cochrane Database Syst Rev* 2006; CD002251.

21. Ickx BE. Fluid and blood transfusion management in obstetrics. *Eur J Anaesthesiol* 2010; **27**: 1031–5.

22. Jordan S, Mitchell JA, Quinlan G, J *et al*. The pathogenesis of lung injury following pulmonary resection. *Eur Respir J* 2000; **15**: 790–9.

23. Moller AM, Pedersen T, Svendsen PE, *et al*. Perioperative risk factors in elective pneumonectomy: the impact of excess fluid balance. *Eur J Anaesthesiol* 2002; **19**: 57–62.

Day surgery

Jan Jakobsson

Day surgery is expanding. More patients and procedures are transferred from traditional in-hospital care to day-case or short-stay logistics. This trend – to shorten the hospital stay – affects the preparation and planning of patient care. The concept of fast tracking has become well established in a variety of surgical settings and is a most fundamental part of day surgery [1]. Rapid recovery and a minimum of residual effects are factors of upmost importance for the handling of the day-case patient. Resumption of oral intake, drinking and eating are traditional variables for the assessment of eligibility for discharge and thus an essential part of day surgery.

Most surgical specialities are today performing day-case surgery and the proportion of traditional in-hospital vs. day surgery is, in many disciplines, much in favor of the day cases. However, the proportion of day-case surgery for one and the same procedure varies considerably between countries and may also vary considerably within nations between different institutions. Explanations for these differences include tradition and economical factors.

Day surgery calls for vigilant assessment and preparation. Patient, procedure, institutional resources, anesthesia and a structured and quality-assured plan are needs to be considered. A structured anesthesia and analgesia protocol is fundamental. Multimodal analgesia should include a combination of local anesthesia and non-opioid analgesics (paracetamol and nonsteroidal anti-inflammatory drugs [NSAIDs]), then add on a weak opioid and, as further rescue, oral strong opioids in an escalating fashion. These factors are cornerstones in the widely accepted standard of care [1].

The adoption of day surgery must not jeopardize safety. However, the experience of day surgery as of today is reassuring. The outcomes at 30 days in large patient cohorts show very low mortality and incidences of major morbidity. Classical follow-up studies, such as the ones by Warner et al. [2], Mezei and Chung [3] and the 60-day follow up of day surgery in Copenhagen [4], have all documented most reassuring safety. On the other hand, the increasing numbers of more complex procedures and acceptance of patients with more extensive medical history for day-case surgery must be acknowledged, and surveillance of outcome is of upmost importance in order to evaluate the maintenance of safe practice.

More elderly patients

The number of elderly patients undergoing day surgery increases. A positive result of this trend is that avoidance of hospitalization and change in environment reduces the risk of

Clinical Fluid Therapy in the Perioperative Setting, ed. Robert G. Hahn. Published by Cambridge University Press. © Cambridge University Press 2011.

postoperative cognitive impairment. However, further effort to evaluate the outcome of day surgery in the growing elderly population is warranted. Alternatively, the experience from cataract surgery in office-based or day-surgery practice is most reassuring and has gained wide acceptance as a cost-effective approach with high patient satisfaction.

Elderly patients are also, in increasing numbers, scheduled for day surgery that requires general anesthesia. The elderly are prone to have somewhat more minor perioperative cardiovascular events, the most frequent being hypertension and dysrythmia. Hypotension and hypovolemia are relatively less frequent compared with patients of all ages; hypotension constitutes about one tenth of all cardiovascular events seen [5].

Preoperative fasting routines

One important part of patient care is proper preparation with regard to intake of food and fluid in order to minimize the risk of regurgitation and aspiration in conjunction with the anesthesia.

Many countries have adopted revised *fasting guidelines* that allow patients without risk factors to eat a light meal up to 6 h and to ingest clear fluids up to 2 h prior to the induction of anesthesia [6]. The safety of a more liberal fasting regime in patients without obvious risk factors for delayed gastric emptying receives support by a recent Cochrane systematic meta-analysis review [7]. The acceptable safety of intake of clear fluid up to 2 h prior to surgery has also been shown in obese patients and in children [8–10].

Avoiding prolonged fasting and fluid restriction have beneficial effects on patient satisfaction, and may also have positive effects on outcome, reduced fatigue, postoperative nausea and vomiting (PONV) and glucose intolerance [11].

Adherence to the new more physiological fasting guidelines is not yet well adopted. For simplicity it may be easier to inform a patient not to take food or fluids after midnight.

Elective day-case surgery should allow proper planning and timing and, thus, information about intake of clear fluids up to 2–3 h prior to anesthesia should be promoted in patients without risk factors. Shortening the preoperative fasting and promoting intake of clear liquid for up to 2 h prior to anesthesia is today considered to be well established and evidence based.

The authors' conclusion in the Cochrane meta-analysis is clear; there was no evidence to suggest a shortened fluid fast results in an increased risk of aspiration, regurgitation or related morbidity compared with the standard "nil by mouth from midnight" fasting policy. Permitting patients to drink water preoperatively resulted in significantly smaller gastric volumes.

Clinicians should be encouraged to appraise this evidence for themselves and, when necessary, adjust any remaining standard fasting policies (nil-by-mouth from midnight) for patients that are not considered "at risk" during anesthesia [7].

Preoperative nutrition, correction of deficits

Correction of malnutrition and specific nutritional or vitamin deficits should always be assessed before elective surgery and, as far as possible, substituted. The typical day-surgery patients are rarely those exhibiting a more extensive degree of malnourishment but, if present, it should be handled in accordance with general nutritional routines.

Preoperative testing of the clinically healthy patient has recently been questioned [12]. Patients showing signs or symptoms of being malnourished should be identified and possibly supported in order to restore proper nutritional status before surgery. Likewise, in patients with severe obesity, proper preoperative diet preparations have become standard care in most bariatric centers. Fluid deficits, low plasma/blood volume and/or a low hematocrit should be evaluated and corrected whenever there are any signs, symptoms or history raising suspicion about its occurrence.

Preoperative nutrition, "energy loading"

There are reports from studies evaluating the effects of preoperative nutritive fluid intake suggesting potential benefits without risk [13]. An increasing amount of evidence indicates that instead of being operated on in the traditional overnight fasted state, undergoing surgery in the carbohydrate-fed state has many clinical benefits. Many of these clinical effects can be related to the reduced postoperative insulin resistance by preoperative carbohydrate loading.

In many centers preoperative carbohydrates have become established for use before major surgery. Those who advocate preoperative energy support suggest that carbohydrate loading should be considered for all patients scheduled for elective surgery and are allowed to drink clear fluid [14]. The value of such efforts in minor intermediate elective day surgery in ASA 1–2 patients may be debated.

Perioperative fluid therapy – anesthetic considerations

Perioperative fluid therapy in day surgery should be instituted on the basis of the case profile.

The benefit of fluid therapy can be questioned in minor surgical procedures of short duration (less than 15–20 min) and without any substantial fluid losses during the procedure.

Fluid therapy is more clearly beneficial in intermediate surgery, and administration of more liberal volumes probably leads to better recovery compared with lower volumes. Study design, fluid administered and variables used for evaluation of effects vary between studies, and thus it is hard to provide clear, explicit guidelines (Table 7.1). The administered fluid has, in most studies, consisted of crystalloid fluid solutions such as lactated Ringer's solution.

Administration of about 1 l isotonic electrolyte solution to compensate for the fasting, and a further 1 l during surgery seems to improve the postoperative course of laparoscopic cholecystectomy. The group of Holte et al. has conducted several studies of the effects of perioperative fluid on outcome. They showed that administration of 30–40 ml/kg compared with 10–15 ml/kg lactated Ringer's solution for laparoscopic cholecystectomy improves recovery of organ functions and reduces hospital stay [17]. In contrast, a benefit from using a liberal fluid regime during thyroid surgery was not supported in a study of similar design [18].

The effects of high volume (30–40 ml/kg) perioperatively should also be put into perspective. Infusion of 40 ml/kg of lactated Ringer's solution in volunteers decreased pulmonary function for 8 h and also resulted in a significant weight gain which lasted for 24 h [19]. Therefore, a more restricted fluid therapy should be adopted in the elderly. The risk of reduced lung function and edema must be acknowledged in the elderly, and fluid volume be adjusted accordingly.

Large volumes of crystalloid and colloid fluid has been compared in one study showing no difference in outcome with regard to the variables studied [15].

Table 7.1. Clinical trials of fluid therapy in intermediate-sized day surgery.

Reference	Surgery	Active	Control	Fluid	No. patients	Results
Yogendran et al., 1995 [21]	ambulatory surgery	20 ml/kg	2 ml/kg	isotonic electrolyte solution	2 × 100	significant positive thirst, drowsiness and dizziness
Elhakim et al., 1998 [22]	termination of pregnancy	1000 ml	0	sodium lactate	2 × 50	significant positive PONV
Bennett et al., 1999 [23]	dental surgery	17 ml/kg	2 ml/kg	isotonic solution	2 × 77	significant positive feelings of well-being
McCaul et al., 2003 [19]	gynecological laparoscopy	1.5 ml/kg ± glucose		sodium lactate ± glucose	3 × 40	glucose; higher blood glucose and more thirst
Ali et al., 2003 [24]	laparoscopic cholecystectomy /gynecological surgery	15 ml/kg	2 ml/kg	Hartmann's solution	2 × 40	significant positive PONV
Holte et al., 2004 [15]	laparoscopic cholecystectomy	40 ml/kg	15 ml/kg	lactated Ringer's	2 × 24	significant positive pulmonary function, dizziness, drowsiness and fatigue
Magner et al., 2004 [25]	gynecological laparoscopy	30 ml/kg	10 ml/(kg h)	sodium lactate	2 × 70	significant positive PONV
Maharaj et al., 2005 [26]	gynecological laparoscopy	2 ml/(kg h)	3 ml/kg	sodium lactate	2 × 40	significant positive PONV and pain
Chohedri et al., 2006 [27]	ambulatory surgery	20 ml/kg	2 ml/kg	isotonic electrolyte solution	2 × 100	significant positive PONV and thirst

Table 7.1. (cont.)

Reference	Surgery	Active	Control	Fluid	No. patients	Results
Goodarzi et al., 2006 [28]	strabism	30 ml/(k h)	10 ml/(kg h)	lactated Ringer's	2 × 50	significant positive PONV and thirst
Chaudhary et al., 2008 [18]	open cholecystectomy	12 ml/kg	2 ml/kg	lactated Ringer's hetastarch	2 × 30	significant positive PONV, no diff crystalloid vs. colloid
Dagher et al., 2009 [16]	thyroid surgery	30 ml/kg	1 ml/kg	sodium lactate	2 × 50	no effect
Lambert et al., 2009 [29]	gynecological laparoscopy	1000 ml	2 ml/kg		2 × 23	significant positive PONV

PONV, postoperative nausea and vomiting

The independent effect of adding glucose to the infused fluid has been studied by McCaul et al. [16]. They could see no major benefit in adding glucose, which rather increased thirst and the incidence of pain besides elevating the blood glucose concentration.

The expansion of day-case surgery is moving rapidly and there are reports of successful bariatric surgery performed on an ambulatory basis. Some institutions perform transurethral prostatectomy in day-case practice. The fluid management in association to these special procedures is addressed in other chapters. Procedure-specific fluid protocols should be used regardless of whether the patient is operated in ambulatory practice or as an in-patient.

Postoperative fluids

Rapid recovery, which allows the patient to possibly bypass the conventional recovery room stay, is a common goal in minor day-case procedures. Rapid regain of vital function and thus capacity to drink is also part of the management of intermediate day cases. Traditional discharge criteria include drinking, although the necessity of oral intake has been questioned in later versions [20].

Allowing and supporting patients to drink clear fluids up to 2 h before induction of anesthesia and promoting early postoperative intake reduce the need for administration of intravenous fluids. Hence, intravenous fluids may be used only to maintain venous access, which is a prerequisite for the rapid administration of anesthetics and analgesics.

Adjunct medications with impact on fluid balance

Steroids have become increasingly popular as part of the anesthetic management for day-case surgery in order to reduce pain, emesis and fatigue. However, the impact of 4–8 mg dexamethasone or bethametasone on fluid balance is not well studied.

The potential effect of NSAIDs on renal function and subsequent risk of fluid retention should also be acknowledged. NSAIDs have become a key part of pain management in day-case surgery. Renal impairment has been described, associated to the use of ketorolac.

Outcome

Major morbidity is most rarely seen in conjunction with day surgery. Several major follow-up studies have documented good safety associated to elective day surgery [2–4]. For example, a huge 60-day follow-up after day surgery study in Copenhagen revealed a very low incidence of adverse events. Wound-related complications, hematoma and infection were the most commonly seen [4]. Minor perioperative cardiovascular events, dysrhythmia and hypertensive episodes are not uncommon, but signs of hypovolemia are rare [5].

Rapid return of vital functions is an important goal in day surgery. However, fatigue, dizziness and nausea are often reported during the early postoperative period. The independent effects of preoperative and perioperative fluid administration on quality of recovery have been evaluated to some extent, while the effects of postoperative fluid therapy (parenteral or oral) are not well studied.

Fatigue can be reduced by supporting fluid intake up to 2–3 h prior to surgery. Administration of intravenous fluid during minor surgery may not exert a major effect, but during intermediate surgery such as laparoscopic cholecystectomy a liberal fluid program has been shown to improve recovery and reduce postoperative fatigue.

Postoperative nausea and vomiting, the "little big problem," is still a major concern in day-case anesthesia and surgery. The independent effects of liberal fluid administration on PONV are not consistent but the risk vs. benefit seems to be in favour for its routine use in ASA 1–2 patients.

Efforts to minimize postoperative pain is of huge importance in day surgery and all opioid-sparing techniques should be acknowledged. Some studies evaluating the effects of liberal fluid administration have shown positive effects, including a reduction of post-operative pain.

Adequate hydration is needed when NSAID analgesics are used in order to minimize the risk of renal impairment.

Conclusions

Day surgery is growing in importance. More patients and procedures are transferred from traditional in-hospital care to day surgery. A number of factors have contributed to the growth of day-case surgery; these include the development of minimally invasive techniques and better understanding of the surgical trauma and how the surgical stress response can be reduced. Introduction of new anesthetics with rapid onset and offset of action after cessation of administration have also contributed. Better use of the multi-modal approach to reduce pain and pain-associated distress is also of huge importance.

Day surgery includes minor and intermediate surgery and is not commonly associated to major perioperative fluid losses. The anesthetist should still strive to maintain normal physiology by avoiding fluid and energy depletion.

Efforts to avoid fluid shifts and circulatory disturbances during the entire perioperative period improve the postoperative course. They promote rapid recovery and combat adverse effects such as fatigue, nausea and vomiting and may also have effects on pain, thus improving well-being and satisfaction.

Key messages

Follow updated preoperative fasting guidelines, support intake of clear fluids up to 2 h prior to elective day-case surgery in non-risk patients.

In intermediate day-case surgery a more liberal fluid administration – 30–40 ml/kg of lactated Ringer's solution perioperatively – is associated to improved quality of recovery in ASA 1–2 patients.

There is no need for patients to drink before discharge; intake of fluid and food should be recommended but not pushed.

References

1. Jakobsson J. *Day Case Anaesthesia.* Oxford, UK: Oxford Library Press 2009.

2. Warner MA, Shields SE, Chute CG. Major morbidity and mortality within 1 month of ambulatory surgery and anesthesia. *JAMA* 1993; **270**: 1437–41.

3. Mezei G, Chung F. Return hospital visits and hospital readmissions after ambulatory surgery. *Ann Surg* 1999; **230**: 721–7.

4. Engbaek J, Bartholdy J, Hjortsø NC. Return hospital visits and morbidity within 60 days after day surgery: a retrospective study of 18,736 day surgical procedures. *Acta Anaesthesiol Scand* 2006; **50**: 911–19.

5. Chung F, Mezei G, Tong D. Adverse events in ambulatory surgery. A comparison between elderly and younger patients. *Can J Anaesth* 1999; **46**: 309–21.

6. Søreide E, Eriksson LI, Hirlekar G, Eriksson H, Henneberg SW, Sandin R, *et al.* (Task

Force on Scandinavian Pre-operative Fasting Guidelines, Clinical Practice Committee Scandinavian Society of Anaesthesiology and Intensive Care Medicine). Pre-operative fasting guidelines: an update. *Acta Anaesthesiol Scand* 2005; **49**: 1041–7.

7. Brady M, Kinn S, Stuart P. Preoperative fasting for adults to prevent perioperative complications. *Cochrane Database Syst Rev* 2003: CD004423.

8. Brady M, Kinn S, Ness V, O'Rourke K, Randhawa N, Stuart P. Preoperative fasting for preventing perioperative complications in children. *Cochrane Database Syst Rev* 2009; CD005285.

9. Maltby JR, Pytka S, Watson NC, Cowan RA, Fick GH. Drinking 300 mL of clear fluid two hours before surgery has no effect on gastric fluid volume and pH in fasting and non-fasting obese patients. *Can J Anaesth* 2004; **51**: 111–15.

10. Cook-Sather SD, Gallagher PR, Kruge LE, *et al*. Overweight/obesity and gastric fluid characteristics in pediatric day surgery: implications for fasting guidelines and pulmonary aspiration risk. *Anesth Analg* 2009; **109**: 727–36.

11. Meisner M, Ernhofer U, Schmidt J. Liberalisation of preoperative fasting guidelines: effects on patient comfort and clinical practicability during elective laparoscopic surgery of the lower abdomen. *Zentralbl Chir* 2008; **133**: 479–85.

12. Chung F, Yuan H, Yin L, Vairavanathan S, Wong DT. Elimination of preoperative testing in ambulatory surgery. *Anesth Analg* 2009; **108**: 467–75.

13. Nygren J, Soop M, Thorell A, Sree Nair K, Ljungqvist O. Preoperative oral carbohydrates and postoperative insulin resistance. *Clin Nutr* 1999; **18**: 117–20.

14. Ljungqvist O. Modulating postoperative insulin resistance by preoperative carbohydrate loading. *Best Pract Res Clin Anaesthesiol* 2009; **23**: 401–9.

15. Holte K, Klarskov B, Christensen DS, *et al*. Liberal versus restrictive fluid administration to improve recovery after laparoscopic cholecystectomy: a randomized, double-blind study. *Ann Surg* 2004; **240**: 892–9.

16. Dagher CF, Abboud B, Richa F, *et al*. Effect of intravenous crystalloid infusion on postoperative nausea and vomiting after thyroidectomy: a prospective, randomized, controlled study. *Eur J Anaesthesiol* 2009; **26**: 188–91.

17. Holte K, Jensen P, Kehlet H. Physiologic effects of intravenous fluid administration in healthy volunteers. *Anesth Analg* 2003; **96**: 1504–9.

18. Chaudhary S, Sethi AK, Motiani P, Adatia C. Pre-operative intravenous fluid therapy with crystalloids or colloids on postoperative nausea & vomiting. *Indian J Med Res* 2008; **127**: 577–81.

19. McCaul C, Moran C, O'Cronin D, *et al*. Intravenous fluid loading with or without supplementary dextrose does not prevent nausea, vomiting and pain after laparoscopy. *Can J Anaesth* 2003; **50**: 440–4.

20. Ead H. From Aldrete to PADSS: Reviewing discharge criteria after ambulatory surgery. *J Perianesth Nurs* 2006; **21**: 259–67.

21. Yogendran S, Asokumar B, Cheng DC, Chung F. A prospective randomized double-blinded study of the effect of intravenous fluid therapy on adverse outcomes on outpatient surgery. *Anesth Analg* 1995; **80**: 682–6.

22. Elhakim M, el-Sebiae S, Kaschef N, Essawi GH. Intravenous fluid and postoperative nausea and vomiting after day-case termination of pregnancy. *Acta Anaesthesiol Scand* 1998; **42**: 216–19.

23. Bennett J, McDonald T, Lieblich S, Piecuch J. Perioperative rehydration in ambulatory anesthesia for dentoalveolar surgery. *Oral Surg Oral Med Oral Pathol Oral Radiol Endod* 1999; **88**: 279–84.

24. Ali SZ, Taguchi A, Holtmann B, Kurz A. Effect of supplemental pre-operative fluid on postoperative nausea and vomiting. *Anaesthesia* 2003; **58**: 780–4.

25. Magner JJ, McCaul C, Carton E, Gardiner J, Buggy D. Effect of intraoperative intravenous crystalloid infusion on

postoperative nausea and vomiting after gynaecological laparoscopy: comparison of 30 and 10 ml/kg. *Br J Anaesth* 2004; **93**: 381–5.

26. Maharaj CH, Kallam SR, Malik A, *et al.* Preoperative intravenous fluid therapy decreases postoperative nausea and pain in high risk patients. *Anesth Analg* 2005; **100**: 675–82.

27. Chohedri AH, Matin M, Khosravi A. The impact of operative fluids on the prevention of postoperative anesthetic complications in ambulatory surgery – high dose vs low dose. *Middle East J Anesthesiol* 2006; **18**: 1147–56.

28. Goodarzi M, Matar MM, Shafa M, Townsend JE, Gonzalez I. A prospective randomized blinded study of the effect of intravenous fluid therapy on postoperative nausea and vomiting in children undergoing strabismus surgery. *Paediatr Anaesth* 2006; **16**: 49–53.

29. Lambert KG, Wakim JH, Lambert NE.Preoperative fluid bolus and reduction of postoperative nausea and vomiting in patients undergoing laparoscopic gynecologic surgery. *AANA J* 2009; **77**: 110–14.

Chapter 8

Pediatrics

Isabelle Murat

Perioperative fluid therapy is aimed at providing maintenance fluid requirements, at correcting fluid deficit and at providing the volume of fluid needed to maintain adequate tissue perfusion. Old concepts, e.g., age-related changes in body fluid composition as well as relatively new concerns such as the danger of hyponatremia, support modern management of perioperative fluid therapy in pediatrics. Neonates (0–28 days) and premature infants represent a subgroup with special requirements that differ considerably from common guidelines described for infants and children.

Children are not small adults

Throughout fetal life and during the first two years of life the distribution of body fluid undergoes a gradual but significant change [1]. Total body water represents as much as 80% of body weight in premature infants, 78% in full-term newborns and 65% in infants of 12 months of age compared with 60% in adults. These age-related changes of total body water mainly reflect changes in extracellular fluid with growth. Extracellular fluid volume represents 50% of body weight in premature infants, 45% in full-term newborns and 25% in infants of 12 months of age compared with 20% in adults.

Maturation of renal function is basically achieved by the end of the first month of life. After birth renal vascular resistances decrease abruptly, while systemic vascular resistances and arterial pressure increase. As a consequence, renal blood flow increases dramatically. This explains why glomerular filtration rate, still low during the first 24 h of life, rises very soon thereafter. Tubular function is less mature than glomerular function at birth. At birth, the newborn is unable to effectively concentrate urine. Clearance of free water is lower than that of adults, thus explaining the impaired ability of newborn infants to cope with excessive water loading or water deprivation.

Newborns and premature infants have limited cardiovascular reserves in response to increased preload or afterload. Cardiac output is high to compensate for the high oxygen affinity of fetal hemoglobin and to match the high oxygen consumption. Cardiac output is highly dependent on heart rate in the neonatal period.

Clinical Fluid Therapy in the Perioperative Setting, ed. Robert G. Hahn. Published by Cambridge University Press. © Cambridge University Press 2011.

Maintenance requirements

Calorie requirement

In 1957, Holliday and Segar estimated the metabolic requirements for children at bed rest, and this estimation is still used today [2]. The daily calorie expenditure is: 100 kcal/kg for infants weighing 3 to 10 kg; 1000 kcal + 50 kcal/kg for each kg over 10 kg for children ranging from 10 to 20 kg; and 1500 kcal + 20 kcal/kg for each kg over 20 kg for children 20 kg and up. Half of those calories are required for basic metabolic needs and the remainder is required for growth. General anesthesia essentially mimics calorie requirements at closer to basal metabolic rate [3].

Water requirement

Under normal conditions, 1 ml of water is required to metabolize 1 kcal. Therefore, in the awake child calorie and water consumption are considered equal. The corresponding rule for hourly water requirement is well known as the *4/2/1 rule*. Hourly water requirements are: 4 ml/kg/h for infants weighing 3 to 10 kg; 40 ml/h plus 2 ml/kg/h for each kg over 10 kg for children ranging from 10 to 20 kg; and 60 ml/h plus 1 ml/kg/h for each kg over 20 kg for children 20 kg and up. Insensible water loss increases with decreasing body weight in premature infants.

Electrolyte requirements

Holliday and Segar calculated maintenance electrolytes from the amount delivered by the same volume of human milk [2]. Daily sodium and potassium requirements are 3 mmol/kg and 2 mmol/kg, respectively, in children. Thus, the combination of maintenance fluid requirements and electrolyte requirements results in a hypotonic electrolyte solution. Since the publication of this paper, the usual intravenous maintenance fluid given to children by pediatricians for decades was one quarter- to one third-strength saline. This is inappropriate in many clinical situations (see below).

Preoperative assessment

The preoperative assessment of fluid volume and state of hydration varies from elective surgery patients, with no or slowly developing fluid deficit, to the severely traumatized patient who is undergoing a dynamic deficit in blood and interstitial volume, and in whom it is more difficult to evaluate fluid balance. Only some specific pediatric situations will be reviewed.

Fasting guidelines

There is now a large body of evidence that free intake of clear fluids up to 2 h preoperatively does not affect the pH or volume of gastric contents at induction of anesthesia in children or adults [4].

While there have been relatively few studies in infants, these suggest that they may be allowed clear fluids up to 2 h and breast milk 4 h preoperatively. There is also evidence that infants aged less than 3 months may safely be given infant formula up to 4 h preoperatively. By contrast, there is little evidence to support a reduction in the present 6 h fasting time for cow's milk or solid food in older infants and children.

Dehydration

Dehydration is observed in many common clinical situations such as vomiting, diarrhea and fever. Estimation of the degree of dehydration is based on classical clinical signs. In an acute clinical situation, the weight loss of the child is usually a very good indication of total water loss. Correction of one percent of dehydration requires about 10 ml/kg of fluids. Rate of fluid administration depends on seriousness and on rapidity of dehydration.

The ultimate goal of perioperative fluid therapy is to maintain a correct fluid and electrolyte balance and, as a consequence, normal cardiovascular stability. Indeed, dehydration and some medical conditions associated with third space sequestration of fluids (e.g., intestinal occlusion) will, in turn, affect vascular fluid volume. Replacement of intravascular volume loss should be performed by administration of normotonic and normo-osmolar solution. Crystalloid solutions, such as lactated Ringer's or normal saline, or even a colloid solution, can be used. The prognosis of some medical conditions such as septic shock depends on the quantity and the rapidity of vascular loading: the younger the child, the greater the quantity of fluid loading related to body weight [5,6].

Intraoperative fluid management

Quantity of intraoperative fluids

Intraoperative fluid therapy is aimed at providing basal metabolic requirements (maintenance fluids), at compensating for preoperative fasting deficit and at replacing losses from the surgical field.

When the new fasting guidelines are followed the preoperative fluid deficit is expected to be minimal. Fasting deficit is calculated by multiplying the hourly maintenance fluid requirement by the number of hours of restriction. In 1975, Furman *et al.* proposed to replace 50% of the fasting deficit in the first hour and 25% in the second and third hours [7].

In 1986, Berry suggested simplified guidelines for fluid administration, indicated in Table 8.1, according to the child's age and the severity of surgical trauma [8]. The amount of hydrating solutions required during the first hour of anesthesia was greater in infants and young children than in older children, taking into account the larger deficit due to larger losses of extracellular fluid volume. These guidelines are only guidelines and should be adapted to the clinical situation. Third-space losses may vary from 1 ml/(kg h) for a minor surgical procedure, to as much as 15–25 ml/(kg h) for major abdominal procedures. Blood losses are replaced with either a 1:1 ratio of blood or colloid, or 3:1 ratio for crystalloid.

Glucose: necessary or harmful?

The next question is whether or not administration of *dextrose* is necessary during surgery. In the past 20 years, there has been a complete re-evaluation of the place of glucose in routine intraoperative solutions.

Hypoglycemia is known to induce brain damage, especially in newborn infants [9]. However, the risk of preoperative hypoglycemia has been demonstrated to be low in normal healthy infants and children (1 to 2%), despite prolonged fasting periods [10]. Thus, it would appear that in the vast majority of patients there is no need to administer glucose in the perioperative period, nor is there a need to monitor blood glucose in these patients.

Conversely, the danger of hyperglycemia in the perioperative period is a real clinical issue that has been extensively reviewed [11,12]. Hyperglycemia can induce osmotic diuresis

Table 8.1. Guidelines for fluid administration of balanced salt solution in children according to the age and to the severity of tissue trauma.

First hour
25 ml/kg in children aged 3 years and under
15 ml/kg in children aged 4 years and over
All other hours
maintenance + mild trauma = 6 ml/(kg h)
maintenance + moderate trauma = 8 ml/(kg h)
maintenance + severe trauma = 10 ml/(kg h)
Berry, 1986 [8]

and consequently dehydration and electrolyte disturbances. Several animal studies have also demonstrated that hyperglycemia will increase the risk of hypoxic-ischemic brain or spinal cord damage. Thus, intraoperative hyperglycemia should be avoided.

The rationale for choosing isotonic hydrating solutions

Most of the fluids required during surgery are needed for replacing either fasting deficit or third-space losses. Both losses consist mainly of extracellular fluids as discussed previously. Thus hydrating solutions should contain a high concentration of sodium and chloride, and a low concentration of bicarbonate, calcium and potassium. As discussed below, polyionique B66 [13] presents only minor differences from standard lactated Ringer's solutions: its sodium concentration is slightly lower at 120 instead of 130 mmol/l. This difference allows maintenance of the osmolarity of the solution close to that of the plasma, despite the presence of 0.9% dextrose.

The history of manufacturing polyionique B66 comes from a series of clinical studies done in the early 1990s [14,15]. The main study [14] compared blood glucose and plasma sodium values after administration of three different hydrating solutions: a mixture in equal parts of lactated Ringer's (LR) and D5 (LR0.5D2.5), LR alone and LR with 1% dextrose (LRD1). As expected, blood glucose values were maintained within acceptable values with the two lactated Ringer's solutions. Plasma sodium values were also maintained within normal values with the two lactated Ringer's solutions, but a significant decrease in plasma sodium values was observed when LR0.5D2.5 was administered. This led us to promote the use of isotonic solutions during surgery in order to maintain normal plasma sodium values [16].

Clinical guidelines for intraoperative fluid therapy

Intraoperative administration of glucose-free isotonic hydrating solutions should be the routine practice for most procedures in children over 4 to 5 years of age. In infants and young children, 5% dextrose solutions should be avoided, but 1% or 2% dextrose in lactated Ringer's is appropriate [14,15]. Glucose infusion at a rate of 120 to 300 mg/(kg h) is sufficient to maintain an acceptable blood glucose level and to prevent lipid mobilization in infants and children [17,18]. Polyionique B66 contains 0.9% dextrose that is adequate to maintain normal blood glucose values in infants and young children during surgery.

Volume replacement during infancy: indications and choice of fluid

Crystalloids (normal saline or lactated Ringer's) are first administered to treat absolute or relative blood volume deficits frequently observed during surgery in children. This practice should also apply to premature and newborn infants. Indeed, recent studies performed in hypotensive premature infants or polycythemic newborns have demonstrated that normal saline is as effective as albumin to restore and maintain arterial pressure or to treat neonatal polycythemia [19,20]. The rate of fluid administration will be indicated by the cardiovascular condition. Normally, 15–20 ml/kg of lactated Ringer's solution over 15–20 min will re-establish cardiovascular stability. After administration of a total of 50 ml/kg of crystalloid solution, the administration of a colloid solution to maintain intravascular osmotic pressure is indicated.

Hydroxyethylstach (HES) preparations are becoming very popular for vascular loading in adults and children. However the main limiting factor for using HES in fluid loading is the quantity of fluid required to resuscitate young children, especially those in septic shock. Indeed three rapid administrations of 20 ml/kg are recommended at the initial stage of septic shock in children, i.e., 60 ml/kg, prior to introducing vasopressors [5].

In most countries, the permissible daily quantity of HES administration is limited by health authorities. Only third-generation HES (130/0.4 or 130/0.42) are now available in most countries, and only limited pediatric studies are available [21–24]. In these studies, children received only 10–15 ml/kg HES, and efficacy was similar to that of other colloids without undesirable side effects.

Only one study evidenced moderate effects on coagulation in infants and young children [23]. A recent study randomized 119 infants and young children (5–46 months) undergoing cardiac surgery to receive 50 ml/kg of either HES 130/0.4 or 4% albumin [24]. The authors found similar bleeding in both groups, but fluid balance favoured the HES group. Finally, a multicentric observational study reported the use of HES 130/0.42 in more than 300 children. Mean dose received was 11 ± 4.8 ml/kg. No side effects were reported but all patients included had normal preoperative renal function and coagulation. All these recent studies do not indicate any superiority of third-generation HES over other colloids, but side effects were minimal when standard low doses were used. The use of HES in neonates remains a subject of controversy owing to their immature renal function.

Gelatins have been used for many years in children and also in early infancy to treat intravascular fluid deficits. Haemaccel was demonstrated to be as effective as 4.5% albumin to maintain blood pressure during major surgery in neonates, but less effective to maintain plasma colloid osmotic pressure and plasma albumin concentration [25].

Although the use of albumin has been challenged, it remains the main colloid used for volume expansion in the neonatal period and early infancy [26,27]. In hypotensive premature infants, 4.5% albumin was demonstrated to be as effective as fresh frozen plasma to restore blood pressure, but more effective than 20% albumin [28]. This suggests that the volume of albumin administered is more important than its concentration to maintain or restore cardiovascular stability. Thus, 5% albumin is the preferred colloid in newborn infants as it is iso-oncotic to plasma and very effective to maintain blood pressure and plasma colloid perfusion pressure [25].

Postoperative fluid therapy: consensus and controversies

Consensus

Oral fluid intake is usually allowed within the first 3 postoperative hours in most pediatric patients. If oral intake should be delayed (e.g., after abdominal surgery), fluid therapy should be administered usually on a peripheral venous access if duration of intravenous infusion is not expected to exceed 5 days or on a central venous access when long-term parenteral nutrition is necessary.

Postoperative hyponatremia is the most frequent electrolyte disorder in the postoperative period. Severe hyponatremia (< 120–125 mmol/l) may result in transient or permanent brain damage [29]. Most postoperative hyponatremia observed in ASA 1 children is due to the administration of hypotonic fluids when capacities of free water elimination are impaired.

Acute symptomatic hyponatremia is a medical emergency that requires immediate therapy. Hypertonic NaCl should be administered to increase plasma sodium up to 125 mmol/l, as the risk of seizure decreases above this value. Postoperative hyponatremia should be prevented by avoiding hypotonic solutions during surgery and in the early postoperative period.

Controversies

Two opposite attitudes have emerged in the recent literature regarding both the volume and the composition of postoperative fluid therapy after the report of numerous cases of severe hyponatremia in children.

Some are defending the use of isotonic saline in 5% dextrose in hospitalized children except those with plasma sodium values above 140 mmol/l [30,31]. The maintenance rate should be reduced only in children with plasma sodium concentration less than 138 mmol/l and in those at risk for non-osmotic secretion of antidiuretic hormone (ADH).

Conversely, Holliday et al. have changed their recommendations for maintenance fluid therapy especially for surgical patients [32,33]. They recommend first correcting fluid deficit with 20–40 ml/kg normal saline, then to give half of the average maintenance fluid for the first 24 h and to monitor daily plasma sodium concentration.

Clinical guidelines

Basically, by combining the two approaches, these simple recommendations could be proposed.

- Hypovolemia should be treated rapidly.
- After major surgery in patients at risk of high ADH secretion, daily maintenance fluids are to be reduced by one third during the first postoperative day provided the child is normovolemic.
- Composition of fluids is a compromise between high sodium requirements, energy requirements and osmolarity of the solution. All extra losses (gastric tube, chest tubes, etc.) are to be replaced with lactated Ringer's solution.
- Plasma sodium and glucose concentrations should be monitored at least once daily in acute patients.
- Finally, one should keep in mind that recommendations are just a framework and that it is of critical importance to individualize fluid therapy in unstable children.

Conclusion

Old concepts such as age-related changes in body composition explain the necessity to provide larger volumes of fluid during infancy than later in life, but also to administer larger quantities of fluids to compensate for third space losses or to restore effective vascular volume in septic shock. Recent studies have re-evaluated the risk of hyponatremia, the most frequent postoperative electrolyte disorder, being likely to promote or to aggravate permanent or transient brain damage.

References

1. Friis-Hansen B. Body composition during growth. In vivo measurements and biochemical data correlated to differential anatomical growth. *Pediatrics* 1971; **47**: 264–74.

2. Holliday M, Segar W. The maintenance need for water in parenteral fluid therapy. *Pediatrics* 1957; **19**: 823–32.

3. Lindahl SG. Energy expenditure and fluid and electrolyte requirements in anesthetized infants and children. *Anesthesiology* 1988; **69**: 377–82.

4. Soreide E, Eriksson LI, Hirlekar G, *et al.* Pre-operative fasting guidelines: an update. *Acta Anaesthesiol.Scand.* 2005; **49**: 1041–7.

5. Brierley J, Carcillo JA, Choong K, *et al.* Clinical practice parameters for hemodynamic support of pediatric and neonatal septic shock: 2007 update from the American College of Critical Care Medicine. *Crit Care Med.* 2009; **37**: 666–88.

6. Carcillo JA, Tasker RC. Fluid resuscitation of hypovolemic shock: acute medicine's great triumph for children. *Intensive Care Med.* 2006; **32**: 958–61.

7. Furman E, Roman D, Lemmer L, Hairabet J, Jasinska M, Laver M. Specific therapy in water, electrolyte and blood-volume replacement during pediatric surgery. *Anesthesiology* 1975; **42**: 187–93.

8. Berry F. Practical aspects of fluid and electrolyte therapy. In Berry F, ed. *Anesthetic Management of Difficult and Routine Pediatric Patients.* New York: Churchill Livingstone, 1986, pp. 107–35.

9. Loepke AW, Spaeth JP. Glucose and heart surgery: neonates are not just small adults. *Anesthesiology* 2004; **100**: 1339–41.

10. Welborn LG, McGill WA, Hannallah RS, Nisselson CL, Ruttimann UE, Hicks JM. Perioperative blood glucose concentrations in pediatric outpatients. *Anesthesiology* 1986; **65**: 543–7.

11. Sieber FE, Smith DS, Traystman RJ, Wollman H. Glucose: a reevaluation of its intraoperative use. *Anesthesiology* 1987; **67**: 72–81.

12. Leelanukrom R, Cunliffe M. Intraoperative fluid and glucose management in children. *Paediatr Anaesth* 2000; **10**: 353–9.

13. Berleur MP, Dahan A, Murat I, Hazebroucq G. Perioperative infusions in paediatric patients: rationale for using Ringer-lactate solution with low dextrose concentration. *J Clin Pharm Ther* 2003; **28**: 31–40.

14. Dubois M, Gouyet L, Murat I. Lactated Ringer with 1% dextrose: an appropriate solution for perioperative fluid therapy in children. *Paediatr Anaesth* 1992; **2**: 99–104.

15. Hongnat J, Murat I, Saint-Maurice C. Evaluation of current paediatric guidelines for fluid therapy using two different dextrose hydrating solutions. *Paediatr Anaesth* 1991; **1**: 95–100.

16. Murat I, Dubois MC. Perioperative fluid therapy in pediatrics. *Paediatr Anaesth* 2008; **18**: 363–70.

17. Mikawa K, Maekawa N, Goto R, Tanaka O, Yaku H, Obara H. Effects of exogenous intravenous glucose on plasma glucose and lipid homeostasis in anesthetized children. *Anesthesiology* 1991; **74**: 1017–22.

18. Nishina K, Mikawa K, Maekawa N, Asano M, Obara H. Effects of exogenous intravenous glucose on plasma glucose and lipid homeostasis in anesthetized infants. *Anesthesiology* 1995; **83**: 258–63.

19. So KW, Fok TF, Ng PC, Wong WW, Cheung KL. Randomised controlled trial of colloid or crystalloid in hypotensive preterm infants. *Arch Dis.Child Fetal Neonatal Ed* 1997; **76**: F43-6.

20. Wong W, Fok TF, Lee C, Ng P, So KW, Ou Y, *et al.* Randomised controlled trial: comparison of colloid or crystalloid for partial exchange transfusion for treatment of neonatal polycythaemia. *Arch Dis Child Fetal Neonatal* 1997; **76**: F115-18.

21. Standl T, Lochbuehler H, Galli C, Reich A, Dietrich G, Hagemann H. HES 130/0.4 (Voluven) or human albumin in children younger than 2 yr undergoing non-cardiac surgery. A prospective, randomized, open label, multicentre trial. *Eur J Anaesthesiol.* 2008; **25**: 437–45.

22. Sumpelmann R, Kretz FJ, Gabler R, *et al.* Hydroxyethyl starch 130/0.42/6:1 for perioperative plasma volume replacement in children: preliminary results of a European Prospective Multicenter Observational Postauthorization Safety Study (PASS). *Paediatr Anaesth* 2008; **18**: 929–33.

23. Haas T, Preinreich A, Oswald E, *et al.* Effects of albumin 5% and artificial colloids on clot formation in small infants. *Anaesthesia* 2007; **62**: 1000–7.

24. Hanart C, Khalife M, De Ville A, Otte F, De Hert S, Van der Linden P. Perioperative volume replacement in children undergoing cardiac surgery: albumin versus hydroxyethyl starch 130/0.4. *Crit Care Med.* 2009; **37**: 696–701.

25. Stoddart PA, Rich P, Sury MR. A comparison of 4.5% human albumin solution and Haemaccel in neonates undergoing major surgery. *Paediatr Anaesth* 1996; **6**: 103–6.

26. Roberton NR. Use of albumin in neonatal resuscitation. *Eur J Pediatr* 1997; **156**: 428–31.

27. Greenough A. Use and misuse of albumin infusions in neonatal care. *Eur J Pediatr* 1998; **157**: 699–702.

28. Emery E, Greenough A, Gamsu H. Randomised controlled trial of colloid infusions in hypotensive preterm infants. *Arch Dis Child* 1992; **67**: 1185–90.

29. Arieff AI, Ayus J, Fraser C. Hyponatraemia and death or permanent brain damage in healthy children. *BMJ* 1992; **304**: 1218–22.

30. Moritz ML, Ayus JC. Hospital-acquired hyponatremia – why are hypotonic parenteral fluids still being used? *Nat Clin Pract Nephrol* 2007; **3**: 374–82.

31. Halberthal M, Halperin ML, Bohn D. Lesson of the week: Acute hyponatraemia in children admitted to hospital: retrospective analysis of factors contributing to its development and resolution. *BMJ* 2001; **322**: 780–2.

32. Holliday MA, Ray PE, Friedman AL. Fluid therapy for children: facts, fashions and questions. *Arch Dis Child* 2007; **92**: 546–50.

33. Holliday MA, Friedman AL, Segar WE, Chesney R, Finberg L. Acute hospital-induced hyponatremia in children: a physiologic approach. *J Pediatr* 2004; **145**: 584–7.

Chapter

9

Hypertonic fluids

Eileen M. Bulger

Hypertonic fluids have been under investigation for the resuscitation of injured patients for over 30 years. Several studies have suggested a potential benefit for the use of these fluids in the resuscitation of patients with hypovolemic shock and traumatic brain injury [1–3]. In addition, there have been a number of reports describing the use of hypertonic fluids in the perioperative setting including aortic surgery, cardiac surgery, transplant surgery and spinal surgery [4,5].

Hypertonic fluids include a wide spectrum of products with a varying range of hypertonic saline solutions from 1.6% to 23.4% sodium chloride. In addition, hypertonic saline is also available coupled with a variety of colloid solutions including dextran 70 and hetastarch.

This review seeks to describe the mechanisms of action of hypertonic fluids that may portend benefit to acute resuscitation and perioperative management of patients undergoing major surgery and to review the current clinical trial evidence in this regard.

Mechanism of action

Hypertonic fluids have several physiologic and immunologic effects that suggest potential benefit in management of severely injured patients. Because these agents have an osmotic effect, when administered intravenously they draw interstitial fluid into the intravascular space thus restoring tissue perfusion in the setting of hypovolemic shock. This allows improvement in blood pressure with a smaller volume of fluid than traditional isotonic crystalloid solutions. Furthermore, several in vitro and animal studies suggest that these fluids reduce endothelial cell edema and enhance microcirculatory flow following hemorrhagic shock.

In addition to these physiologic changes, a wide body of literature describes the significant impact of hypertonic solutions on the inflammatory response. Several animal studies have demonstrated that resuscitation with hypertonic solutions attenuates the activation of neutrophils after injury and reduces remote inflammatory lung injury. This effect appears to be due to downregulation of the adhesion molecule CD 11b and enhanced shedding of L-selectin.

These observations have also been made in humans receiving hypertonic saline early after severe injury [6,7]. Modulation of circulating monocyte function has also been described, which may downregulate the production of pro-inflammatory cytokines and enhance production of anti-inflammatory cytokines such as interleukin (IL)-10. This suppression of

Clinical Fluid Therapy in the Perioperative Setting, ed. Robert G. Hahn. Published by Cambridge University Press. © Cambridge University Press 2011.

the innate immune response appears to be transient and resolves once the serum osmolarity returns to normal. While the innate immune response appears to be inhibited, the cellular response, as manifested by changes in T-cell function, appears to be enhanced. Extensive work by Junger *et al.* has demonstrated that hypertonicity increases T-cell proliferation, enhances mitogen-stimulated IL-2 production and rescues T-cells from suppressive cytokines [8]. Taken together, these studies suggest a potential role for hypertonic fluids to modulate the immunosuppressive response observed after severe injury or insult.

Finally, a large body of research has focused on the mechanism of action of hypertonic fluids to reduce cerebral edema and improve cerebral perfusion after brain injury. In addition to the obvious physiologic effects, hypertonic fluids have been associated with improved cerebral vasoregulation resulting in reduced vasospasm, modulation of cerebral leukocytes and inhibition of the sodium glutamate exchanger leading to reduced extracellular glutamate accumulation which is neurotoxic [9]. These studies, coupled with animal models showing reduction of intracranial pressure in brain-injured animals, have led to a number of clinical studies of these fluids for the management of patients with severe traumatic brain injury.

In summary, there is compelling scientific evidence that hypertonic fluids have physiologic and anti-inflammatory effects that may prove beneficial for the management of a number of perioperative concerns including resuscitation of hypovolemic shock, management of traumatic brain injury and management of ischemia and reperfusion injury such as occurs following cardiopulmonary bypass or transplant surgery. This has led to numerous clinical reports.

Clinical trial experience

Clinical studies of hypertonic solutions have largely been focused on three areas: early resuscitation of hemorrhagic shock in the prehospital or emergency department setting, management of increased intracranial pressure largely in the intensive care unit setting, and operative reports in a variety of major surgical interventions. Each of these areas is addressed separately.

Hemorrhagic shock

There have been ten clinical trials of hypertonic fluids for the management of hemorrhagic shock following injury (Table 9.1). These studies were conducted in the prehospital or early hospital setting. It was hypothesized that the earlier the fluid is given after injury the more likely one would be to observe a significant effect. These studies used a 7.5% saline solution with or without the addition of 6% dextran 70. The early investigations were largely too small to demonstrate a definitive difference in outcome. However, meta-analysis of the studies conducted before 1997 suggested an overall survival benefit from hypertonic saline with dextran (HSD), with an odds ratio of 1.47 (95% confidence interval 1.04–2.08) [1].

These early studies led to the regulatory approval of HSD in several European countries, but did not afford approval by the US Food and Drug Administration. Two subsequent studies have been conducted. The first was a study by Bulger *et al.*, which focused the impact of HSD on the development of acute respiratory distress syndrome (ARDS) in a blunt trauma population with evidence of hypovolemic shock [10]. This study closed after enrollment of 209 patients because of futility, with no overall difference in the rate of 28-day ARDS-free survival between the treatment groups.

A pre-defined subgroup analysis did suggest a potential benefit in those patients at highest risk for ARDS as defined by the need for > 10 units of blood transfusion in the first 24 h. This led to a subsequent trial conducted by the Resuscitation Outcomes Consortium, a clinical trial network in the US and Canada. This trial sought to enroll injured patients with more severe shock based on a prehospital systolic blood pressure of < 70 mmHg or 70–90 mmHg with a heart rate > 108 beats/min. This study was also closed before reaching its full proposed sample size after enrolling 895 patients randomized to either 7.5% saline (HS), HSD or normal saline (NS). The results of this study show no difference in overall 28-day survival (HSD 74.5%, HS 73.0%, NS 74.4%, $p = 0.91$) [11].

In addition there was a concern raised by the Data Safety Monitoring Board regarding a higher mortality seen among the post-randomization subgroup of patients who did not receive any blood transfusions in the first 24 h. Subsequent analysis suggested a higher proportion of early deaths such that some patients in the hypertonic groups appeared to expire prior to the availability or administration of blood products. This difference was no longer evident 6 h after injury. Thus, despite a large number of clinical trials in this patient population, there remains no compelling evidence to support the routine use of hypertonic fluids in the early management of these patients in the civilian community.

Traumatic brain injury

There have been a number of studies examining the use of hypertonic fluids ranging in concentration from 1.6% to 23.4%, given as both bolus and continuous infusions for the management of patients with intracranial hypertension. Most of these studies are case series or descriptive studies, which describe improved intracranial pressure (ICP) with the use of hypertonic fluids in patients who have been refractory to conventional therapy. There have been few randomized controlled trials.

The first trial, by Shackford et al., randomized patients to hypertonic saline (HTS) vs. lactated Ringer's along with conventional therapies for increased ICP [12]. They were unable to demonstrate any major differences between the treatment groups but were hampered by the randomization of more severely injured patients into the HTS group.

Francony et al. compared equimolar doses of 20% mannitol and 7.45% hypertonic saline for management of patients with sustained elevations in ICP and found them to be equally effective [13]. Despite the lack of definitive data in this area, many neurosurgeons are now using hypertonic saline routinely for management of elevated ICP.

Three randomized controlled trials have specifically focused on the *prehospital administration* of hypertonic saline to patients with suspected traumatic brain injury. All of these studies utilized the Glasgow Outcome Score (GOS) as a measure of the long-term neurologic outcome for these patients.

The first of these studies, by Cooper et al., enrolled injured patients with a prehospital Glasgow Coma Scale (GCS) value < 8 and systolic blood pressure < 100 mmHg [14]. This trial, which compared 7.5% saline with normal saline, was closed for futility ($n = 229$) with no difference in extended GOS between the treatment groups six months after injury. Because this study included patients who had both severe traumatic brain injury and shock they were limited by a 50% mortality in the study cohort.

A second trial recently completed in Toronto, Canada was also closed with limitations in obtaining long-term outcome data [15].

The largest trial in this patient population was recently completed by the Resuscitation Outcomes Consortium. The study was closed early for futility after enrolling 1331 patients

Table 9.1. Human trials of hypertonic saline as a resuscitation fluid for hemorrhagic shock.

Reference	Population	Design	n	Hypertonic fluid	Outcome
Holcroft *et al.*, 1987 [30]	prehospital trauma patients	prospective, randomized	49	7.5% NaCl/ 6% dextran 70	improved SBP and overall survival
Holcroft *et al.*,1989 [31]	hypotensive trauma pts in ED (SBP < 80)	prospective, randomized	32	7.5% NaCl/ 6% dextran 70	no difference in survival
Vassar *et al.*, 1991 [32]	prehospital trauma patients (SBP < 100)	prospective, randomized	166	7.5% NaCl/ 6% dextran 70	improved SBP & improved survival for pts with traumatic brain injury
Mattox *et al.*, 1991 [33]	prehospital trauma patients (SBP < 90) 72% penetrating	prospective, randomized	359	7.5% NaCl/ 6% dextran 70	improved SBP, Trend toward improved survival
Younes *et al.*, 1992 [34]	hypovolemic shock in ED (SBP < 80)	prospective, randomized	105	7.5% NaCl and 7.5% NaCl/ 6% dextran 70	improved SBP, no difference in survival
Vassar *et al.*, 1993 [35]	prehospital trauma patients (SBP < 90)	prospective, randomized	258	7.5% NaCl and 7.5% NaCl/ 6% dextran 70	improved survival vs. predicted historical controls

Study	Population	Design	N	Fluid	Outcome
Vassar et al., 1993 [36]	prehospital trauma patients (SBP < 90)	prospective, randomized	194	7.5% NaCl and 7.5% NaCl/ 6% dextran 70	improved survival vs. historical controls and for patients with traumatic brain injury
Younes et al., 1997 [37]	hypovolemic shock in ED	prospective, randomized	212	7.5% NaCl/ 6% dextran70	improved survival for pts with SBP < 70
Bulger et al., 2008 [10]	prehospital blunt trauma patients (SBP < 90)	prospective, randomized	209	7.5%NaCl/ 6% dextran 70	no difference in ARDS free survival
Bulger et al., 2011 [11]	prehospital trauma patients (SBP <70 or SBP 70–90, HR > 108)	prospective, randomized	895	7.5% NaCl and 7.5% NaCl/ 6% dextran 70	no difference in 28 day mortality

ARDS, acute respiratory distress syndrome; ED, emergency department; HR, heart rate; pts, patients; SBP, systolic blood pressure with no difference in the GOS at 6 months after injury [16]. Importantly, this trial enrolled patients with a GCS value < 8 but no prehospital hypotension. Thus like the hypovolemic shock studies, despite a large body of preclinical evidence supporting these resuscitation strategies, clinical trials have been unable to show convincing evidence of improved outcome.

Intraoperative studies

A number of small studies have been reported regarding the use of hypertonic solutions in *operative cases*. Most of these have been conducted during either cardiac or aortic surgery. For patients undergoing cardiopulmonary bypass surgery, the most consistent finding has been a significant decrease in the positive fluid balance with the use of hypertonic fluids [4]. This finding was also noted in a recent Cochrane review of this literature [5].

Many of these studies have also demonstrated improvement in *cardiac index* (CI) with hypertonic fluids, but the duration of this effect has been variable. Two studies noted improved CI up to 48 h after surgery [17,18], while others suggested a transient effect as short as 1–3 h [19,20]. This variability may be due to variations in the dose of hypertonic fluids used and additional fluid given. These studies have been too small to identify any significant improvement in outcome.

Nine studies have examined the use of hypertonic solutions during *aortic surgery*. Like the studies in cardiac surgery, these studies also supported a lower overall fluid requirement in patients receiving hypertonic fluids. Auler *et al.* reported a small case series ($n = 10$) describing the administration of hypertonic saline vs. isotonic saline at the time of removal of the aortic clamp [21]. These authors report improved physiologic endpoints and lower overall volumes of fluid required in the patients given HTS.

In another study, Shackford *et al.* randomized 58 patients undergoing elective aortic reconstruction to lactated Ringer's vs. a hypertonic saline (250 mEq sodium/l) solution during operative repair [22]. The hypertonic group required on average half the amount of intraoperative fluid as the lactated Ringer's group but there was no difference in clinical outcomes.

The most recent study by Bruegger *et al.* ($n = 28$) compared HTS with hydroxyethyl starch in normal saline for administration during the period of aortic clamping and found no difference between the groups [23]. Several other studies have also shown improved hemodynamic parameters (for review, see Azoubel *et al.* [4]), but none were large enough to demonstrate improved outcome.

Other operative scenarios explored have included transplantation, elective hysterectomy and spinal surgery. One case series has been reported describing the use of 7.5% saline for patients with fulminant hepatic failure and Grade IV encephalopathy while undergoing orthotopic liver transplant [24]. These authors compare these patients with historical controls, and suggest that patients receiving HTS had more favorable hemodynamics and improved intracranial pressure. Another study examined the immune effect of hypertonic saline administration for patients undergoing elective hysterectomy and did not find any significant changes [25].

Finally a retrospective, case-controlled study compared outcomes for patients undergoing major spinal surgery who received intraoperative hypertonic saline with those that did not, and suggested an association with lower postoperative infections rates [26]. A few studies have also examined the role of preloading patients undergoing spinal anesthesia with hypertonic fluids [27–29]. These studies have had mixed results with some demonstrating improved hemodynamic parameters, while others did not. All of these studies are limited by very small sample size.

Conclusion

In conclusion, despite a wide body of supportive preclinical data suggesting that hypertonic fluids are associated with improved hemodynamic response, reduction in cerebral edema, reduced fluid requirements and modulation of the inflammatory response, clinical trials have been disappointing in the lack of definitive improvement in overall patient outcome with this resuscitation strategy. In particular, studies of the intraoperative use of these fluids are very limited. Future studies need to focus carefully on the patient selection and ensure a randomized, placebo-controlled design, and adequate sample size to observe a meaningful difference in clinical outcome.

References

1. Wade C, Grady J, Kramer G. Efficacy of hypertonic saline dextran (HSD) in patients with traumatic hypotension: meta-analysis of individual patient data. *Acta Anaesthesiol Scand* Suppl. 1997; **110**: 77–9.

2. Wade CE, Grady JJ, Kramer GC, Younes RN, Gehlsen K, Holcroft JW. Individual patient cohort analysis of the efficacy of hypertonic saline/dextran in patients with traumatic brain injury and hypotension. *J Trauma* 1997; **42**: S61–5.

3. Wade CE, Kramer GC, Grady JJ, Fabian TC, Younes RN. Efficacy of hypertonic 7.5% saline and 6% dextran-70 in treating trauma: a meta-analysis of controlled clinical studies. *Surgery* 1997; **122**: 609–16.

4. Azoubel G, Nascimento B, Ferri M, Rizoli S. Operating room use of hypertonic solutions: a clinical review. Clinics (Sao Paulo) 2008; **63**: 833–40.

5. McAlister V, Burns KE, Znajda T, Church B. Hypertonic saline for perioperative fluid management. *Cochrane Database Syst Rev.* (1):CD005576.

6. Bulger EM, Cuschieri J, Warner K, Maier RV. Hypertonic resuscitation modulates the inflammatory response in patients with traumatic hemorrhagic shock. *Ann Surg* 2007; **245**: 635–41.

7. Rizoli SB, Rhind SG, Shek PN, *et al.* The immunomodulatory effects of hypertonic saline resuscitation in patients sustaining traumatic hemorrhagic shock: a randomized, controlled, double-blinded trial. *Ann Surg* 2006; **243**: 47–57.

8. Junger WG, Coimbra R, Liu FC, *et al.* Hypertonic saline resuscitation: a tool to modulate immune function in trauma patients? *Shock* 1997; **8**: 235–41.

9. Doyle JA, Davis DP, Hoyt DB. The use of hypertonic saline in the treatment of traumatic brain injury. *J Trauma* 2001; **50**: 367–83.

10. Bulger EM, Jurkovich GJ, Nathens AB, *et al.* Hypertonic resuscitation of hypovolemic shock after blunt trauma: a randomized controlled trial. *Arch Surg* 2008; **143**: 139–48.

11. Bulger EM, May S, Kerby J, *et al.* Out of hospital hypertonic resuscitation following traumatic hypovolemic shock: a randomized, placebo controlled trial. *Ann Surg* 2011; **253**: 431–41.

12. Shackford SR, Bourguignon PR, Wald SL, Rogers FB, Osler TM, Clark DE. Hypertonic saline resuscitation of patients with head injury: a prospective, randomized clinical trial. *J Trauma* 1998; **44**: 50–58.

13. Francony G, Fauvage B, Falcon D, *et al.* Equimolar doses of mannitol and hypertonic saline in the treatment of increased intracranial pressure. *Crit Care Med* 2008; **36**: 795–800.

14. Cooper DJ, Myles PS, McDermott FT, *et al.* Prehospital hypertonic saline resuscitation of patients with hypotension and severe traumatic brain injury: a randomized controlled trial. *JAMA* 2004; **291**: 1350–7.

15. Morrison LJ, Rizoli SB, Schwartz B, et al. The Toronto prehospital hypertonic resuscitation-head injury and multi organ dysfunction trial (TOPHR HIT) – methods and data collection tools. Trials 2009; 10: 105.

16. Bulger EM, May S, Brasel KJ, et al. Out-of-hospital hypertonic resuscitation following severe traumatic brain injury: a randomized, placebo controlled trial. JAMA 2010; 304: 1455–64.

17. Bueno R, Resende AC, Melo R, Neto VA, Stolf NA. Effects of hypertonic saline-dextran solution in cardiac valve surgery with cardiopulmonary bypass. Ann Thorac Surg 2004; 77: 604–611; discussion 611.

18. Boldt J, Zickmann B, Ballesteros M, et al. Cardiorespiratory responses to hypertonic saline solution in cardiac operations. Ann Thorac Surg 1991; 51: 610–15.

19. Sirieix D, Hongnat JM, Delayance S, et al. Comparison of the acute hemodynamic effects of hypertonic or colloid infusions immediately after mitral valve repair. Crit Care Med 1999; 27: 2159–65.

20. Jarvela K, Kaukinen S. Hypertonic saline (7.5%) after coronary artery bypass grafting. Eur J Anaesthesiol 2001; 18: 100–7.

21. Auler JO, Jr, Pereira MH, Gomide-Amaral RV, et al. Hemodynamic effects of hypertonic sodium chloride during surgical treatment of aortic aneurysms. Surgery 1987; 101: 594–601.

22. Shackford SR, Sise MJ, Fridlund PH, et al. Hypertonic sodium lactate versus lactated ringer's solution for intravenous fluid therapy in operations on the abdominal aorta. Surgery 1983; 94: 41–51.

23. Bruegger D, Bauer A, Rehm M, et al. Effect of hypertonic saline dextran on acid-base balance in patients undergoing surgery of abdominal aortic aneurysm. Crit Care Med 2005; 33: 556–63.

24. Filho JA, Machado MA, Nani RS, et al. Hypertonic saline solution increases cerebral perfusion pressure during clinical orthotopic liver transplantation for fulminant hepatic failure: preliminary results. Clinics 2006; 61: 2318.

25. Kolsen-Petersen JA, Nielsen JO, Tonnesen EM. Effect of hypertonic saline infusion on postoperative cellular immune function: a randomized controlled clinical trial. Anesthesiology 2004; 100: 1108–18.

26. Charalambous MP, Swoboda SM, Lipsett PA. Perioperative hypertonic saline may reduce postoperative infections and lower mortality rates. Surg Infect 2008; 9: 67–74.

27. Jarvela K, Honkonen SE, Jarvela T, Koobi T, Kaukinen S. The comparison of hypertonic saline (7.5%) and normal saline (0.9%) for initial fluid administration before spinal anesthesia. Anesth Analg 2000; 91: 1461–65.

28. Jarvela K, Koobi T, Kauppinen P, Kaukinen S. Effects of hypertonic 75 mg/ml (7.5%) saline on extracellular water volume when used for preloading before spinal anaesthesia. Acta Anaesthesiol Scand 2001; 45: 776–81.

29. Durasnel P, Cresci L, Madougou M, et al. [Practice of spinal anesthesia in a developing country: usefulness of vascular preloading with a 7.5% hypertonic saline solution]. Ann Fr Anesth Reanim 1999; 18: 631–5.

30. Holcroft JW, Vassar MJ, Turner JE, Derlet RW, Kramer GC. 3% NaCl and 7.5% NaCl/dextran 70 in the resuscitation of severely injured patients. Ann Surg 1987; 206: 279–88.

31. Holcroft JW, Vassar MJ, Perry CA, Gannaway WL, Kramer GC. Use of a 7.5% NaCl/6% Dextran 70 solution in the resuscitation of injured patients in the emergency room. Prog Clin Biol Res 1989; 299: 331–8.

32. Vassar MJ, Perry CA, Gannaway WL, Holcroft JW. 7.5% sodium chloride/dextran for resuscitation of trauma patients undergoing helicopter transport. Arch Surg 1991; 126:1065–72.

33. Mattox KL, Maningas PA, Moore EE, et al. Prehospital hypertonic saline/dextran infusion for post-traumatic hypotension. The U.S.A. Multicenter Trial. Ann Surg 1991; 213: 482–91.

34. Younes RN, Aun F, Accioly CQ, et al. Hypertonic solutions in the treatment of hypovolemic shock: a prospective, randomized study in patients admitted

to the emergency room. *Surgery* 1992; **111**: 380–5.

35. Vassar MJ, Perry CA, Holcroft JW. Prehospital resuscitation of hypotensive trauma patients with 7.5% NaCl versus 7.5% NaCl with added dextran: a controlled trial. *J Trauma* 1993; **34**: 622–32.

36. Vassar MJ, Fischer RP, O'Brien PE, *et al.* A multicenter trial for resuscitation of injured patients with 7.5% sodium chloride. The effect of added dextran 70. The Multicenter Group for the Study of Hypertonic Saline in Trauma Patients. *Arch Surg* 1993; **128**: 1003–11.

37. Younes RN, Aun F, Ching CT, *et al.* Prognostic factors to predict outcome following the administration of hypertonic/ hyperoncotic solution in hypovolemic patients. *Shock* 1997; **7**: 79–83.

Chapter 1

Invasive hemodynamic monitoring

Philip E. Greilich and William E. Johnston

The clinical assessment of a patient's volume status using physical examination and vital signs is often misleading. Bedside patient examination is only 30–50% accurate and clinical tests for assessing hypovolemia suffer from excessive observer bias and variability as well as poor reproducibility, interobserver agreement and sensitivity.

Consequently, invasive hemodynamic monitoring has evolved to allow a more accurate assessment of intravascular fluid status and cardiac output (CO).

Pulmonary artery catheterization

Since its introduction into clinical medicine in the 1970s, the pulmonary artery catheter (PAC) has provided bedside assessment of filling pressures and CO. A recent meta-analysis of all randomized controlled trials with PACs indicates that their use has increased inotropic and vasodilator drug therapy without altering patient mortality or duration of hospitalization [1].

The PAC should be regarded as a diagnostic and not a therapeutic tool, and will only be beneficial if the derived data drive treatment protocols of proven benefit. Recently, the use of PACs has steadily declined by nearly 65% in medical and surgical patients, particularly in patients with myocardial infarction [2]. Standard PACs provide hemodynamic data relating to filling pressure (pulmonary artery wedge pressure, or PAWP) and thermodilution CO.

Pulmonary artery wedge pressure

In order for PAWP to accurately reflect left ventricular end-diastolic volume (LVEDV) requires several assumptions. The relationship between end-diastolic volume and pressure reflects myocardial compliance, which is curvilinear and shifts unpredictably depending on illness and treatment with positive end-expiratory pressure and vasoactive drugs [3]. Accordingly, any accurate assessment of LVEDV using pressure measurement is frequently unreliable.

Another basic requirement for PAWP to accurately reflect left ventricular end-diastolic pressure is a continuous column of blood between the catheter tip and left ventricle; any interruption of this fluid column can cause overestimation of left heart pressures. Such interruption may occur with the use of positive end-expiratory pressure if alveolar pressure exceeds pulmonary venous pressure (zone 2 lung condition). A low pressure reading may reflect reduced LV preload, but normal or high values do not necessary imply that the heart is maximally filled.

Clinical Fluid Therapy in the Perioperative Setting, ed. Robert G. Hahn. Published by Cambridge University Press. © Cambridge University Press 2011.

Because of these influences, an accurate reflection of LV filling volume by PAWP remains problematic. No significant relationship was found between PAWP and LV end-diastolic area assessed by transesophageal echocardiography in cardiac surgery patients ($r = 0.35$; not statistically significant) or in critically ill patients ($r = 0.21$; not significant) [4]. In healthy volunteers, both right- and left-sided filling pressures as well as changes in filling pressure after a 3 l fluid infusion failed to correlate with ventricular volumetric measures [5]. These findings underscore problems using PAC-derived filling pressures alone for patient management.

Thermodilution cardiac output

Thermodilution CO uses the Stewart–Hamilton equation where a known quantity of thermal indicator is injected above the right atrium and detected by a thermistor located 4 cm from the PAC tip. The ensuing change in thermistor temperature allows calculation of the area under the thermodilution curve by:

$$CO = (V_1 (T_B - T_1) K_1 K_2) \div {}_0\int \infty \Delta T_B (t) dt$$

where V_1 = injectate volume; T_B = blood temperature; T_1 = injectate temperature; K_1 = density factor defined as the product of the specific heat and specific gravity of the injectate divided by the product of the specific heat and gravity of blood; K_2 is a computation constant reflecting catheter dead space, heat exchange during transit and injection rate. The denominator of this equation reflects the change in blood temperature as a function of time, which represents the area under the thermodilution curve.

Any error that causes less cold solution to be injected, such as injecting less than the prescribed fluid volume, will falsely reduce the area under the curve causing overestimation of CO. In contrast, any factor which increases the amount of negative thermal energy injected, such as a simultaneous fluid infusion with the injectate solution, will falsely increase the area under the curve causing underestimation of CO [3].

Due to the effect of thoracic pressure on right ventricular filling, an average of three CO measurements should be made randomly throughout the ventilatory cycle to reduce the inherent error to 12–14% [6].

Another factor introducing variability in CO measurements is tricuspid valvular regurgitation. Tricuspid regurgitation can prevent complete and uniform passage of the negative thermal bolus from the right ventricle, causing progressive underestimation (0.5–1.0 L/min) of the actual CO values as the amount of tricuspid regurgitation becomes severe.

Underestimation of thermodilution CO can occur with a rapid change in baseline body temperature following rewarming and termination of hypothermic cardiopulmonary bypass. During the initial 10–20 min after bypass, temperature equilibration lowers baseline pulmonary artery temperature, so that false lower values of CO of 10–15% are obtained [7]. With the development of other techniques for CO measurement, the placement of PACs solely for the measurement of CO may be no longer justified.

Continuous cardiac output

Embedding a thermal filament in the PAC allows continuous CO to be determined by releasing small, intermittent thermal pulses every 30–60 s and detecting changes in blood temperature using a rapid-response thermistor on the distal catheter tip [8]. CO is calculated using the area under the thermodilution curve and trended to reflect average pulmonary blood flow over the previous 3–6 min sampling period. The effects from other thermal noise such as respiration, drug or fluid infusions, or gradual body temperature changes are minimized.

Clinical studies over a wide range of heart rate and CO values show close correlation with the traditional thermodilution technique. Intrinsic errors may be introduced immediately after termination of hypothermic cardiopulmonary bypass due to a shift of cold blood from the gastrointestinal tract.

Transpulmonary thermodilution cardiac output

The transpulmonary artery technique to measure left-side CO involves injecting an indicator through a peripheral (lithium) or central (thermal) vein with sampling from a specialized arterial catheter [9]. Excellent correlation has been established comparing PAC thermodilution CO with that measured by a femoral artery thermistor. Advantages of transpulmonary indicator dilution include less respiratory-induced changes in CO during mechanical ventilation, as well as the derivation of volumetric data including global end-diastolic volume, extravascular lung water and intrathoracic blood volume. Extravascular lung water exceeding 10 ml/kg may indicate patients at risk for developing respiratory failure.

Fluid management guided by extravascular lung water can reduce the need for mechanical ventilation in critically ill patients and length of stay in the intensive care unit. Volumetric measurements more accurately reflect preload and blood volume status than filling pressures, although both are static measurements with limited ability to accurately predict the need for volume loading [5]. Potential errors using the transpulmonary CO technique occur in patients with large thoracic aortic aneurysms, intracardiac shunts, pulmonary embolism or recent pulmonary resection.

Arterial waveform pulse contour cardiac output

Less invasive techniques to measure CO have been recently introduced that use pressure waveform analysis from an arterial catheter. Pulse contour analysis is based on the concept that stroke volume is proportionate to the arterial waveform contour and can be calculated from the area under the systolic portion of the pressure wave [10]. Accurately converting a pressure tracing to a volume calculation requires independent calibration due to the non-linear relationship between measured pressure and arterial compliance [11].

Calibrated techniques require initial CO determination using transpulmonary dilution either by peripheral lithium indicator injection (LiDCO plus system; LiDCO, Cambridge, UK) or central thermal indicator injection (PiCCO plus system; Pulsion, Munich, Germany). An uncalibrated system (FloTrac; Edwards Lifesciences, Irvine, CA, USA) does not require manual calibration but uses a proprietary algorithm based on patient demographic data.

Contraindications to pulse contour CO include arrhythmia, intra-aortic balloon counterpulsation and severe aortic valve disease. Each technique has advantages and disadvantages and the clinician needs to understand inherent limitations to consistently obtain reliable data.

Calibrated pulse contour analysis by lithium dilution

The LiDCO system calculates stroke volume from pulse power analysis of the arterial waveform after initial calibration with lithium indicator [12]. Continuous CO can then be determined using beat-to-beat pulse contour analysis. This technique requires an initial single calibration with 0.3 mmol lithium chloride solution injected by peripheral or central vein with sampling from a special femoral or radial arterial catheter. Averaging three lithium dilution curves allows changes in cardiac output exceeding 14% to be reliably detected [13]. Recalibration is recommended every 8 h or during hemodynamic instability.

Limitations include a maximum daily dose of 3 mmol lithium, and inability to use in patients receiving chronic lithium medication or neuromuscular blockers due to sensor interactions.

Calibrated pulse contour analysis by thermodilution

The PiCCO system analyzes the systolic portion of the arterial waveform using Fourier transformation after manual calibration by transpulmonary thermodilution. Central venous and major (femoral) artery catheters are necessary but volumetric data such as extravascular lung water can also be calculated (see above). Recalibration is recommended every 8 h or more frequently with hemodynamic instability [13]. Experimental studies indicate that recalibration is also needed with hemorrhage and during vasopressor support. A recent study shows the coefficient of variation for CO using this technique is similar to the LiDCO apparatus [14].

Non-calibrated pulse contour analysis

The FloTrac system requires no manual calibration but has automatic internal calibration using a proprietary software program based on the patient's height, weight, gender and age. Recalibration is automatic and updated every 60 s. A peripheral arterial catheter can be used and the system is easy to set up and use.

Software versions 1.07 and greater have, in general, shown good agreement with other techniques to measure CO, including PAC thermodilution [15], although there continues to be some concern regarding acceptability for general clinical use [9] and reliability and accuracy in hemodynamically unstable patients [16]. The coefficient of variation with the FloTrac system is nearly double that of other pulse contour modes [14].

Dynamic indices from arterial pressure waveform analysis

In addition to CO, continuous pulse contour systems also provide dynamic indices that assess the adequacy of left-ventricular preload and in particular the predictive response to subsequent volume infusion.

These dynamic indices have replaced the use of static indices of measuring filling pressures or end-diastolic ventricular dimensions for predicting fluid responsiveness. The current focus of patient management is no longer trying to assess ventricular preload but to predict the subsequent hemodynamic improvement from fluid (usually colloid) administration [17].

It is known that positive pressure ventilation causes cyclical changes in arterial blood pressure due to acute alterations in right- and left-ventricular preload and afterload. Patients operating on the steep portion of the Frank–Starling curve typically show larger swings in arterial blood pressure during mechanical ventilation. These biphasic differences in systolic blood pressure with positive pressure ventilation represent dynamic indices and are more sensitive than heart rate, mean blood pressure, urine output or filling pressures to identify reduced preload.

Dynamic indices reflect intravascular volume status as well as lung and chest wall compliances, tidal volume, method of ventilation (spontaneous or mechanical), abdominal pressure, arrhythmias, and underlying myocardial function. If all of these factors are maintained relatively constant in a patient, an acute change will inversely reflect fluid status and the response to volume challenge. This technique is applicable only to subjects receiving total mechanical ventilation and patients must maintain sinus rhythm.

Systolic pressure variation

The biphasic difference in systolic arterial pressure is termed systolic pressure variation and represents the difference between maximal and minimal values of systolic blood pressure during a single positive pressure breath. A proposed threshold value > 8.5 mmHg predicts a positive response to subsequent colloid infusion with an improvement in stroke volume exceeding 15%. A study in elective cardiac surgical patients found this value had a sensitivity of 82% and specificity of 86% [18].

Respiratory systolic variation test

The respiratory systolic variation test examines the line of best fit drawn between minimal systolic blood pressures obtained at four successive pressure-controlled breaths of increasing magnitude (5, 10, 15 and 20 cm H_2O).

This test alleviates the need for an apneic period and is not influenced by tidal volume or the early inspiratory increase in systolic pressure. The downslope ($mmHg/cmH_2O$) is calculated as the decrease in systolic blood pressure at each increment in airway pressure, and a threshold value > 0.5 $mmHg/cmH_2O$ predicts a positive response to subsequent volume loading with 93% sensitivity and 89% specificity [18].

Pulse pressure variation

Pulse pressure variation measures the difference in maximal and minimal arterial pulse pressures over one respiratory cycle relative to the mean pulse pressure where pulse pressure is the difference between systolic and diastolic arterial pressures in the same cardiac cycle.

Pulse pressure variation exceeding 12% can accurately predict a positive benefit from subsequent volume expansion in patients with a sensitivity of 94% and specificity of 96% [18]. Pulse pressure variation can predict with greater accuracy the hemodynamic response to subsequent fluid administration than systolic pressure variation.

Stroke volume variation

Using an arterial pulse contour monitoring system, the variations in beat-to-beat stroke volume throughout a respiratory cycle can be calculated and automatically displayed.

Stroke volume variation is calculated continuously as the difference between maximal and minimal values of left ventricular stroke volume relative to the mean stroke volume.

The PiCCO system determines stroke volume variation over a 7.5 s period and displays the floating mean of a 30 s window. Values exceeding 11.5% predict a positive response to subsequent fluid administration with 81% sensitivity and 82% specificity [18].

Cardiovascular ultrasound

Transesophageal echocardiography and esophageal Doppler monitoring use ultrasound technology to provide dynamic measurements of preload-recruitable cardiac performance. Echocardiographic measurements do not rely on "pressure" measurements to make

(a)

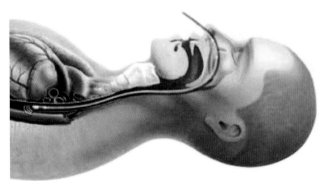

Figure 11.3a. Esophageal Doppler: (a) Schematic representation of esophageal Doppler probe in a patient, demonstrating the close relation between esophagus and descending thoracic aorta.

(b)

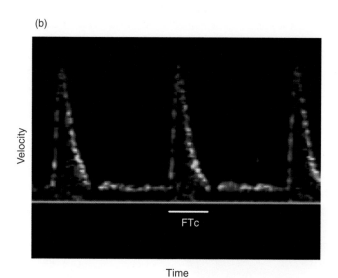

Figure 11.3b. Esophageal Doppler: (b) Characteristic velocity waveform obtained in the descending aorta.

volumetric determinations, and as such they are not subject to the confounding influence of differences in ventricular compliance associated with PAC interpretation.

Transesophageal echocardiography (TEE)

Ninety percent (90%) of stroke volume is derived from shortening of the ventricular short axis [19]. Left ventricle (LV) end-diastolic *area* (using a single mid-transgastric short-axis view) can provide an acceptable estimate of LV end-diastolic *volume* [20].

Although regional wall motion abnormalities and markedly depressed LV function can influence this relationship, *serial* measurements of LV end-diastolic area can be used to minimize this effect [21]. In practice, most clinicians use qualitative assessments of LV end-diastolic area since significant changes are usually readily apparent.

The emergence of the multiplane probe makes determination of TEE-derived CO feasible in more than 95% of patients [22,23]. Cardiac output is determined by calculating the cross-sectional area (using midesophageal long axis [LAX] view) and stroke distance (using deep transgastric long axis or transgastric LAX). A continuous-wave Doppler beam aligned parallel with the left ventricular outflow tract (LVOT) is used to generate a spectral velocity profile for each cardiac systole; the area under this curve represents the maximal velocity–time integral (VTI) or stroke distance. The CO is then calculated using the VTI, cross-sectional area of the LVOT and heart rate as follows:

CO (ml/min) = (velocity–time integral [cm]) (cross-sectional area [cm^2]) (heart rate [beats/min])

Several authors have shown that CO can be accurately measured using TEE (r = 0.90–0.98) [22, 23]. The time required to make *repeat* CO measurements is usually less than 1 min for individuals having intermediate TEE skills. Since the average adult LVOT has a radius of 1 cm, stroke volume can be rapidly *estimated* by multiplying the VTI or stroke distance by three (since $\prod r^2$ or cross-sectional area = 3.14 when the radius or r = 1).

Transesophageal echocardiography is superior to the pulmonary artery catheter in diagnosing the etiology of hemodynamic instability in surgical patients [24,25]. The ability to directly visualize the relative size of cardiac chambers is particularly useful in patients having valvular abnormalities, poor left ventricular function or right heart failure. The use of TEE is considered a Class I indication for patients with hemodynamic instability [26].

Assessment of LV end-diastolic area by TEE can be used to optimize preload recruitable cardiac performance [27,28]. The responsiveness of LV end-diastolic area to interventions that alter preload (blood loss, volume expansion) is universally superior to PAWP measurement [27]. Once optimal LV filling is established, the associated central venous pressure (CVP) can be communicated to those caring for the patient after the probe has been removed.

The fixed cost and training required for this technology represents its chief limitations. The emergence of less expensive TEE solutions, advanced software (image optimization, automated border detection, etc.) and inclusion of basic TEE training during core residency training (in anesthesiology) will likely overcome some of these limitations. Although contraindications for TEE use do exist (esophageal malformations, recent surgery, etc.), the incidence of major adverse events is very low (< 0.05%).

Esophageal Doppler monitoring (EDM)

EDM assesses blood flow in the descending thoracic aorta during each cardiac cycle using Doppler ultrasound. A small, disposable probe is placed into the esophagus (via a nasal approach) and adjusted so that its echo beam is aligned with the aorta. The corrected flow time (FTc) derived from the flow velocity profile is used to assess preload [29]. The flow time represents the time needed for the LV to eject each stroke volume with the presumption that the larger the LV end-diastolic volume or preload, the longer the flow time. Since flow time is also dependent on the cycle time or heart rate, a corrected flow time (flow time/square root of the cycle time) is calculated to adjust for this factor. The EDM FTc has a modest correlation with preload when PAWP is low, yet this relationship is lost when PAWP is normal or elevated especially in patients with poor LV function [29].

Esophageal Doppler monitoring can also be used to calculate the CO. The VTI or stroke distance can be determined using the continuous spectral display in a manner analogous to that used for TEE CO. Esophageal Doppler-derived CO measurements compare favorably with those made using a pulmonary artery catheter [30] and electromagnetic flow probes (placed on the ascending aorta) [31].

EDM-driven protocols have been used in a variety of surgical populations to guide fluid management in both the anesthetized and awake patient [32]. These treatment algorithms use the corrected flow time and CO measurements to detect hypovolemia and guide fluid administration [33,34]. These algorithms have consistently observed reductions in major complications and hospital length of stay [32–35].

The chief limitation of EDM is the need for frequent probe manipulation to insure alignment of the Doppler beam with the aorta. There have been no reported major adverse events directly associated with probe placement.

Conclusion

This chapter summarizes the relative strengths and weaknesses of currently available technologies for monitoring intravascular volume status and preload-recruitable cardiac performance. More dynamic, less invasive modalities are emerging which may overcome the confounding influence of significant variations in LV diastolic pressure–volume relationship between individuals.

The ability of a given monitoring system to effectively drive treatment protocols and improve clinical outcome must be demonstrated before widespread adoption of any technology. Anesthesiologists need to play an active role in performing these studies if evidence-based guidelines are to be established for this fundamental aspect of perioperative care.

References

1. Shah MR, V. Hasselblad V, Stevenson LW, *et al.* Impact of the pulmonary artery catheter in critically ill patients: Meta-analysis of randomized clinical trials. *JAMA* 2005; **294**: 1664–70.

2. Weiner RS, Welch HG. Trends in the use of the pulmonary artery catheter in the United States, 1993–2004. *JAMA* 2007; **298**: 423–9.

3. Greilich PG, W.E. Johnston WE. Invasive hemodynamic monitoring. In: Hahn RG, Prough DS, Svensen CH, eds. *Perioperative Fluid Therapy*. New York: Informa Healthcare, 2007, pp. 29–47.

4. Tousignant CP, Walsh F, Mazer CD. The use of transesophageal echocardiography for preload assessment in critically ill patients. *Anesth Analg* 2000; **90**: 351–5.

5. Kumar A, Anel R, Bunnell E, *et al.* Pulmonary artery occlusion pressure and central venous pressure fail to predict ventricular filling volume, cardiac performance, or the response to volume infusion in normal subjects. *Crit Care Med* 2004; **32**: 691–9.

6. Stetz CW, Miller RG, Kelly GE, *et al.* Reliability of the thermodilution method in the determination of cardiac output in clinical practice. *Am Rev Resp Dis* 1982; **126**: 1001–4.

7. Bazaral MG, Petre J, Novoa R. Errors in thermodilution cardiac output measurements caused by rapid pulmonary artery temperature decreases after cardiopulmonary bypass. *Anesthesiology* 1992: **77**; 31–7.

8. de Waal EC, Wappler F, Buhre WF. Cardiac output monitoring. *Curr Opin Anaesthesiol* 2009; **22**: 71–7.

9. Benington S, Ferris P, Nirmalan M. Emerging trends in minimally invasive haemodynamic monitoring and optimization of fluid therapy. *Eur J Anaesthesiol* 2009; **26**: 893–905.

10. Van Lieshout JJ, Wesseling KH. Continuous cardiac output by pulse contour analysis? *Br J Anaesth* 2001; **86**: 467–9.

11. Morgan P, Al-Subaie N, Rhodes A. Minimally invasive cardiac output monitoring. *Curr Opin Crit Care* 2008; **14**: 322–6.

12. Cecconi M, Dawson D, Grounds RM, *et al.* Lithium dilution cardiac output measurement in the critically ill patient: Determination of precision of the technique. *Intensive Care Med* 2009; **35**: 498–504.

13. Mayer J, Suttner S. Cardiac output derived from arterial pressure. *Curr Opin Anaesthesiol* 2009; **22**: 804–8.

14. Cecconi M, Dawson D, Casaretti R, *et al.* A prospective study of the accuracy and precision of continuous cardiac output monitoring devices as compared to intermittent thermodilution. *Minerva Anaesthesiol* 2010; **76**: 1–8.

15. Mayer J, Boldt J, Poland R, *et al.* Continuous arterial pressure waveform-based cardiac output using the FloTrac/Vigileo: A review and meta-analysis. *J Cardiothorac Vasc Anesth* 2009; **23**: 401–6.

16. Singh S, Taylor MA. Con: The FloTrac device should not be used to follow cardiac output in cardiac surgical patients. *J Cardiothorac Vasc Anesth* 2010; **24**: 709–11.

17. Marik PE, Cavallazzi R, Vasu T, *et al.* Dynamic changes in arterial waveform derived variables and fluid responsiveness in mechanically ventilated patients: A systematic review of the literature. *Crit Care Med* 2009; **37**: 2642–7.

18. Preisman S, Kogan S, Berkenstadt H, *et al.* Predicting fluid responsiveness in patients undergoing cardiac surgery: Functional haemodynamic parameters including the Respiratory Systolic Variation Test and static preload indicators. *Br J Anaesth* 2005; **95**: 746–55.

19. Rankin JS, McHale PA, Arentzen CE. Three-dimensional dynamic geometry of the left ventricle in the conscious dog. *Circulation Research* 1976; **39**: 304–13.

20. Ryan T, Burwash I, Lu J, *et al.* The agreement between ventricular volumes and ejection fraction by transesophageal echocardiography or a combined radionuclear and thermodilution technique in patients after coronary artery surgery. *J Cardiothorac Vasc Anesth* 1996; **10**: 323–8.

21. Cheung AT, Savino JS, Weiss SJ, Aukburg SJ, Berlin JA. Echocardiographic and hemodynamic indexes of left ventricular preload in patients with normal and abnormal ventricular function. *Anesthesiology* 1994; **81**: 376–87.

22. Perrino AC, Harris SN, Luther MA. Intraoperative determination of cardiac output using multiplane transesophageal echocardiography. *Anesthesiology* 1998; **89**: 350–7.

23. Darmon PL, Hillel Z, Mogtader A, Mindich B, Thys D. Cardiac output by transesophageal echocardiography using continuous-wave Doppler across the aortic valve. *Anesthesiology* 1994; **80**: 796–805.

24. Glower DD, Spratt JA, Snow ND, *et al.* Linearity of the Frank–Starling relationship in the intact heart: the concept of preload-recruitable stroke work. *Circulation* 1985; **71**: 994–1009.

25. Tousignant CP, Walsh F, Mazer CD. The use of transesophageal echocardiography for preload assessment in critically ill patients. *Anesth Analg* 2000; **90**: 351–5.

26. Practice guidelines for perioperative transesophageal echocardiography: an updated report by the American Society of Anesthesiologists and the Society of Cardiovascular Anesthesiologists Task Force on Transesophageal Echocardiography. *Anesthesiology* 2010; **112**: 1–13.

27. Reich DL, Konstadt SN, Nejat M, Abrams HP, Bucek J. Intraoperative transesophageal echocardiography for the detection of cardiac preload changes induced by transfusion and phlebotomy in pediatric patients. *Anesthesiology* 1993; **79**: 10–15.

28. Swenson JD, Harkin C, Pace NL, Astle K, Bailey P. Transesophageal echocardiography: an objective tool in defining maximum ventricular response to intravenous fluid therapy. *Anesth Analg* 1996; **83**: 1149–53.

29. Singer M, Allen MJ, Webb AR, Bennett ED. Effects of alterations in left ventricular filling, contractility and systemic vascular resistance on the ascending aortic blood velocity waveform of normal subjects. *Crit Care Med* 1991; **19**: 1138–45.

30. Singer M. Esophageal Doppler monitoring of aortic blood flow: Beat-by-beat cardiac output monitoring. *Int Anesth Clin* 1993; **31**: 99–125.

31. DiCorte CJ, Latham P, Greilich PE, *et al.* Esophageal Doppler monitor determinations of cardiac output and preload during cardiac operations. *Ann Thorac Surg* 2000; **69**: 1782–6.

32. Laupland KB, Bands CJ. Utility of esophageal Doppler as a minimally invasive hemodynamic monitor: a review. *Can J Anesth* 2002; **49**: 393–401.

33. Conway DH, Mayall R, Abdul-Latif MS, Gilligan S, Tackaberry C. Randomised controlled trial investigating the influence of intravenous fluid titration using oesophageal Doppler monitoring during bowel surgery. *Anaesthesia* 2002; **57**: 845–9.

34. Gan TJ, Soppitt A, Maroof M, *et al.* Goal-directed intraoperative fluid administration reduces length of hospital stay after major surgery. *Anesthesiology* 2002; **97**: 820–6.

35. Venn R, Steele A, Richardson P, *et al.* Randomized controlled trial to investigate influence of the fluid challenge on duration of hospital stay and perioperative morbidity in patients with hip fractures. *Br J Anaesth* 2002; **88**: 65–71.

Goal-directed fluid therapy

Timothy E. Miller and Tong J. Gan

High-risk surgery is associated with significant morbidity and mortality. From a database of over 4 million patients it has recently been shown that 80% of deaths occur in only 12.5% of surgical procedures [1]. In these high-risk patients the expected mortality was 5%, either due to the type of surgery, the patient comorbidities or both. Optimization of the high-risk surgical patient during the perioperative period aims to improve outcomes in this patient population.

Goal-directed therapy (GDT) is a term that has been used for nearly 30 years to describe methods of optimizing fluid and hemodynamic status. Unfortunately the term GDT has not been standardized, and therefore can mean different things to people causing a significant amount of confusion.

The term was first used to describe early oxygen-targeted GDT in the 1980s and 1990s which used the pulmonary artery catheter (PAC) to augment oxygen delivery to supranormal levels in high-risk surgical patients. More recently, goal-directed fluid therapy aims to maximize stroke volume (SV) and therefore cardiac output using a minimally invasive cardiac output monitor.

This review will concentrate on the increasing evidence for the benefits of goal-directed fluid therapy during major surgery.

Early goal-directed therapy: supranormal oxygen delivery

The first major GDT study was conducted by Shoemaker and colleagues in 1988 [2]. This landmark paper looked at patients undergoing high-risk surgery, and compared standard of care with supramaximal oxygen delivery. The hypothesis was proposed that increased cardiac index (CI) and oxygen delivery (DO_2) are necessary circulatory compensations needed to cope with high postoperative metabolism. To do this in the protocol group a PAC was used to obtain targets of CI > 4.5 l/(min m²), oxygen delivery index (DO_2I) > 600 ml/(min m²) and oxygen consumption index (VO_2I) > 170 ml/(min m²). This was achieved through a combination of fluids, inotropes (principally dobutamine) and vasopressors. Targets were based on physiological values that they had observed in survivors after high-risk surgery [3], and the results showed a significant reduction in mortality.

This led to further studies of supranormal oxygen delivery in high-risk surgery, using the same oxygen delivery target of 600 ml/(min m²). Boyd *et al.*, in 1993, showed a reduction in mortality of 75% with GDT [4]. Mortality benefits were also seen with preoperative optimization [5], as well as in cardiac [6] and general surgery patients [7].

Clinical Fluid Therapy in the Perioperative Setting, ed. Robert G. Hahn. Published by Cambridge University Press. © Cambridge University Press 2011.

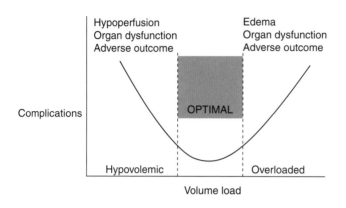

Hypoperfusion
Organ dysfunction
Adverse outcome

Edema
Organ dysfunction
Adverse outcome

Figure 11.1. Fluid load vs. complications (modified from Bellamy) [9].

Complications

OPTIMAL

Hypovolemic

Overloaded

Volume load

The underlying mechanisms for the success of GDT are thought to relate to avoidance of episodes of hypovolemia, hypoxia or decreased blood flow that may cause mitochondrial damage and subsequent organ dysfunction. Therefore, adequate tissue oxygen supply throughout the perioperative period is the key to successful outcomes.

Despite these promising results, the technique was not widely adopted. The reasons for this are almost certainly multi-factorial. Early GDT required significant resources, was very labor intensive and most importantly was reliant on information from the PAC. Catheterization of the right heart began falling out of favor in intensive care units in the 1990s after the publication of several observational studies showing increased mortality [8]. As early GDT was linked so closely with the use of PAC it became embroiled in this controversy.

Thus, despite the fact that numerous trials have shown that mortality, morbidity and length of hospital stay can be reduced with early GDT, widespread use remained a pipedream for enthusiasts.

Modern goal-directed therapy – individualized volume optimization

The past 20 years has seen the arrival of a number of minimally invasive cardiac output monitors that can enable clinicians to guide perioperative volume therapy and cardiocirculatory support. Goal-directed fluid therapy uses these monitors to trend and optimize stroke volume and therefore cardiac output.

Perioperative morbidity has been linked to the amount of fluid administered, with both insufficient and excess fluid leading to increased morbidity, resulting in a characteristic U-shaped curve [9] (see Figure 11.1). Episodes of hypovolemia during surgery can lead to organ hypoperfusion, ischemia and adverse outcomes. Conversely, a number of studies have shown that perioperative fluid excess, particularly crystalloid, can result in tissue edema and increased complications [10].

The challenge for us as clinicians is to keep our patients in the optimal range at all times during the perioperative period. Episodes of hypovolemia or edema, if severe, can cause major morbidity. However, more commonly these changes can be subtle, with bowel mucosa ischemia or edema causing gastrointestinal tract dysfunction and prolonged postoperative ileus, with resultant inability to tolerate a normal diet and increased length of hospital stay [11].

Traditional monitoring techniques are not useful to accurately detect and optimize the volume status of patients. Healthy volunteers can lose 25% of their blood volume without

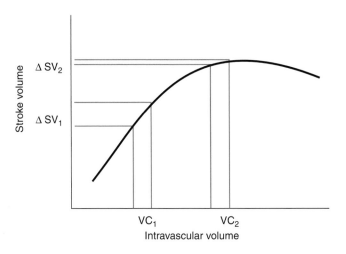

Figure 11.2. Frank–Starling-based stroke volume optimization.

any discernible change in heart rate or blood pressure, whilst at the same time advanced monitors show a significant reduction in stroke volume and gastric intramucosal pH, inferring a degree of ischemia [12]. Central venous pressure (CVP) monitoring has also been shown to be a poor predictor of volume responsiveness [13]. A recent systematic review showed that CVP is not able to identify which patients need more fluid, and concluded that CVP should no longer be routinely measured in the intensive care unit, operating room or emergency department [14].

Advanced monitors in goal-directed fluid therapy can be used to non-invasively measure cardiac output (CO) and SV, and thereby use fluid challenges to achieve SV optimization (see Figure 11.2).

When a patient is hypovolemic and on the steep part of the Starling curve, an intravenous fluid challenge (VC_1 in Figure 11.2) will lead to a greater than 10% increase in SV. This patient has "recruitable" SV, and is in a fluid-responsive state. Fluid loading, typically with 250 ml boluses of intravenous colloid should continue until the increase in SV is less than 10% when the patient has reached the flat part of the Starling curve. This "Frank Starling fluid challenge" provides a sophisticated method of titrating intravenous fluids to complex patients.

A crucial difference from the earlier Shoemaker concept for optimization is that the present approach is individualized to optimize flow-related parameters, such as stroke volume, within the individual's cardiac capacity, as opposed to using predetermined supraphysiologic goals.

Esophageal Doppler

There are a number of technologies that can be used for goal-directed fluid therapy. The most widely studied is undoubtedly the esophageal Doppler monitor (EDM; Deltex Medical, Chichester, UK). The Doppler probe is placed in the esophagus and focused at the descending thoracic aorta, where it uses the Doppler principle to measure blood flow, and produce a waveform (see Figure 11.3). This is then converted to SV using a nomogram of height, weight and age to estimate the cross-sectional area of the descending aorta. EDM-derived SV measurements have been well validated in different environments and clinical scenarios [15–20].

(a)

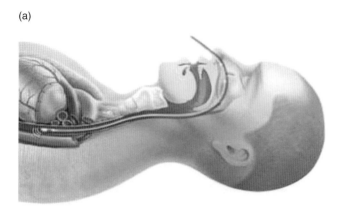

Figure 11.3. Esophageal Doppler: (a) Schematic represen-tation of esophageal Doppler probe in a patient, demonstrat-ing the close relation between esophagus and descending thoracic aorta. (b) Characteristic velocity waveform obtained in the descending aorta. (See also colour figure section.)

(b)

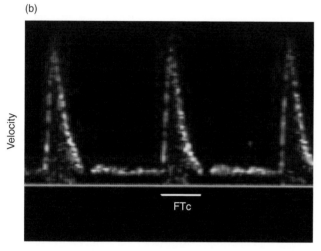

Time

Another useful measurement is the corrected flow time (FTc), which is the width of the waveform, or length of systole in ms, corrected to a HR of 60. An FTc < 350 ms is an add-itional indicator of recruitable stroke volume.

There are a number of studies that show improved outcomes with EDM-guided fluid optimization, as demonstrated by a faster return in gastrointestinal function, a reduction in postoperative complications and reduced length of stay.

These studies are summarized in Table 11.1. Five studies were in a major general/colorec-tal study population [21–25], two in cardiac surgery [26,27] and two in patients scheduled for repair of fractured neck of femur [28,29]. All of these studies used a 10% algorithm to opti-mize SV, often combined with assessment of FTc, to predict fluid responsiveness. Although there are small differences between the studies, a typical algorithm is shown in Figure 11.4.

Mythen and Webb demonstrated a reduction in the incidence of gastrointestinal muco-sal hypoperfusion and major complications in cardiac surgery patients who received plasma volume optimization [26]. The GDT-group also had shorter intensive care unit and hospital length of stay.

Gan *et al.* [22] randomized 100 major elective noncardiac surgical patients with an expected blood loss > 500 ml to either routine care or EDM-guided GDT. As with other

Table 11.1 Summary of the perioperative esophageal Doppler monitor-guided GDT studies.

Reference	Surgical group	Patients (n)	Outcome
Mythen and Webb (1995) [26]	cardiac	60	⇓ gastric acidosis in GDT ⇓ complications in GDT ⇓ LOS (3.5 days) in GDT
Sinclair et al. (1997) [28]	neck of femur fracture	40	⇓ time FFD (5 days) in GDT ⇓ LOS (8 days) in GDT
Conway et al. (2002) [21]	major bowel	57	⇑ ICU admissions in control no difference in LOS
Gan et al. (2002) [22]	major general	100	⇑ PONV in control ⇓ time to tolerating oral intake in GDT ⇓ LOS (2 days) in GDT
Venn et al. (2002) [29]	neck of femur fracture	90	⇓ time FFD (6.2 days) in GDT (vs. control) ⇓ time FFD (3.9 days) in CVP (vs. control)
McKendry et al. (2004) [27]	cardiac surgery	174	⇓ LOS (2.5 days) in GDT no difference in complications
Wakeling et al. (2005) [23]	colorectal	128	⇓ morbidity (GI and overall) in GDT ⇓ time to full diet (1 day) in GDT ⇓ LOS (1.5 days) in GDT
Noblett et al. (2006) [24]	colorectal	108	⇓ morbidity in GDT ⇓ time to tolerating diet (2 days) in GDT ⇓ time FFD (3 days) in GDT ⇓ LOS (2 days) in GDT
Senagore et al. (2009) [25]	laparoscopic colorectal	64	no difference in LOS no difference in complications

CVP, central venous pressure ; FFD, medical/surgical fitness for discharge; GDT, goal directed therapy; GI, gastrointestinal; ICU, intensive care unit; LOS, length of stay; PONV, postoperative nausea and vomiting

studies they observed significant improvement in SV and CO in the GDT group. Patients in the GDT group had significantly shorter median length of stay (5 vs. 7 days) and an earlier ability to tolerate solid food (3 vs. 5 days, $p < 0.05$).

The studies by Wakeling et al. [23] and Noblett et al. [24] showed a similar reduction in the length of hospital stay in colorectal surgical patients, as well as a shorter time to full oral diet, suggesting improved gastrointestinal perfusion. Interestingly, the Noblett study patients also had, in the GDT-group, low levels of interleukin-6, indicating an attenuated inflammatory response to surgery [24]. Conversely, Conway et al. [21] showed no difference in the length of hospital stay in major bowel surgery patients; however, they did observe less requirement for intensive care in the GDT group.

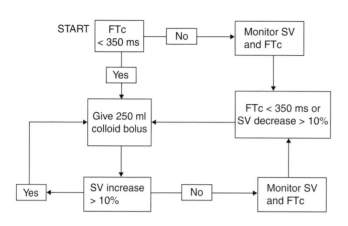

Figure 11.4. A typical combined FTc and SV optimization algorithm.

Venn *et al.* [29] created a 3-group, 90-patient study in patients undergoing repair of fractured neck of femur under general anesthesia, comparing conventional fluid management, dynamic CVP-based volume expansion and EDM-guided GDT. When compared with the CVP group, EDM-guided patients had less intraoperative hypotension and were considered medically fit for discharge sooner. Sinclair *et al.* [28] also looked at this patient population and showed the GDT group had significantly increased SV and CO, as well as a shorter hospital length of stay.

The McKendry *et al.* study [27] was a little different in that the protocol group received EDM-volume optimization as well as inotropes and vasodilators in the first 4 h after admission to the intensive care unit post-cardiac surgery. The investigators showed fewer complications and a 2-day reduction in median hospital length of stay in the protocol group.

The major limitation of the esophageal Doppler is the occasional need for frequent repositioning of the probe to optimize the signal, which can be time consuming. There is a learning curve for positioning the probe, and as such it is somewhat user dependent. The use of electrocautery can also interfere with the signal.

Nevertheless the evidence base behind its use is relatively strong, and its incorporation into Enhanced Recovery After Surgery (ERAS) programs is currently a major driving force for increased interest [30]. Recently the Center for Medicare Services in the USA have reviewed the literature and supported a professional fee being paid to clinicians using EDM-guided perioperative volume optimization [31]. The Centre for Evidence-Based Purchasing division of the NHS Purchasing and Supply Agency in the UK has also recommended the EDM [32].

Crystalloids and colloids

A common theme between the studies is the use of background crystalloid infusions with colloid boluses in the GDT groups to optimize stroke volume. Patients in the GDT groups generally received greater colloid and less crystalloid. Noblett *et al.* is the only study where no differences were found in intraoperative crystalloids and colloids between the study and control groups [24]. However, the timing of fluid administration was different, with greater volumes administered in the GDT group early in the surgical procedures. The hypothesis is that timing of fluid administration is as important as the total volume.

The crystalloid/colloid debate is a long-running and largely erroneous discussion. Crystalloids and colloids are different fluids with different indications and side effects. We eat balanced diets, give balanced analgesic and antiemetic regimens, and it follows that we should be using a balanced fluid regimen.

Recent literature suggests that the amount of crystalloid that is needed perioperatively has been greatly exaggerated in the past. This has largely been due to the theory proposed by Shires in the 1960s that there is an all-consuming third space where fluid is sequestered and therefore needs to be replaced. We now know that a classic third space does not exist [33].

Crystalloids when given intravenously will quickly leave the vascular space to be distributed across the entire extracellular compartment, primarily in the interstitium. Further crystalloid infusions will increase this effect so that the amount of crystalloid given is directly related to perioperative weight gain [33]. The primary indication for crystalloids intraoperatively is to replace preoperative fasting deficits, insensible perspiration and urine output. This can easily be achieved with a background crystalloid infusion.

Colloids, by comparison, contain much larger molecules and are designed to primarily remain in the plasma. Goal-directed fluid therapy uses colloid boluses to replace blood loss and protein losses from the circulation; thereby optimizing intravascular volume, CO and oxygen delivery. Animal models have shown that GDT with colloid significantly increases microcirculatory blood flow and tissue oxygen tension in healthy and injured colon compared with goal-directed or restricted crystalloid fluid therapy [34]. In most patients this is best achieved with a third-generation lower-molecular weight starch with fewer concerns regarding coagulation dysfunction [35].

Arterial pressure waveform analysis

The other major monitoring technique used in goal-directed fluid therapy is arterial pressure waveform analysis. There are several monitors available that are able to analyze the arterial waveform to calculate stroke volume and cardiac output, and therefore use the "10% algorithm" in response to a fluid challenge.

Arterial waveform analysis is also able to derive dynamic parameters of fluid responsiveness, based on cardiopulmonary interactions such as stroke volume variation (SVV) and pulse pressure variation (PPV). These dynamic variables are superior to traditional static indices such as central venous pressure in predicting volume responsiveness in mechanically ventilated patients [36].

The physiology behind SVV and PPV is relatively simple. Positive pressure ventilation induces cyclical changes in the loading conditions of the right ventricle, with a reduction in preload during mechanical insufflation. This will lead to cyclical changes in stroke volume. If the ventricle is operating on the steep part of the Starling curve, the magnitude of the change in SV and blood pressure will be greater, and will manifest itself as a characteristic "swing" in the arterial line pressure with respiration (see Figure 11.5).

Pulse pressure variation and SVV represent "virtual" preload challenges occuring during each respiratory cycle in ventilated patients. There is no need to administer fluid to predict responders, with an SVV or PPV > 10% accurately predicting a positive response to a fluid challenge [37]. As these metrics predict responders with more accuracy than CVP or pulmonary artery occlusion pressure (PAOP) there is less need for invasive central lines.

Although the physiology is robust and well validated, there are to date limited outcome studies with the arterial waveform devices. Targeting a PPV < 10% has been shown to improve postoperative outcomes, and reduce length of intensive care and hospital stay in high-risk surgical patients [38]. However this study was small, with several limitations and the results of larger ongoing studies are awaited.

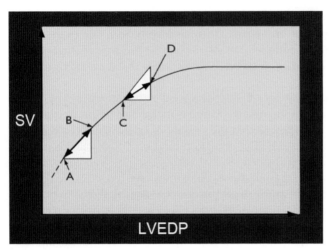

Figure 11.5. A Starling Curve of left ventricular SV against LVEDP demonstrating the change in stroke volume that occurs with positive pressure ventilation. The starting position on the curve determines the magnitude of the change in SV, and hence the stroke volume variation. If the patient is hypovolemic, the LVEDP will cycle between A and B with respiration causing a cyclical change in SV, and a swing in the arterial line. If the patient is euvolemic LVEDP will cycle between C and D causing a much smaller change in SV. FTc, corrected flow time; LVEDP, left ventricular end-diastolic pressure; SV, stroke volume.

Benes *et al.* recently performed a larger study in 120 high-risk patients undergoing elective intra-abdominal surgery [39]. The authors used the Flotrac/Vigileo (Edwards, Irving, USA) to maintain SVV < 10%, and optimize CI. The primary intervention consisted of colloid boluses of 3ml/kg, with dobutamine reserved for patients with a CI < 2.5ml/min/m². Patients in the study group received more colloid, and a lower number of hypotensive episodes were observed. Lactate levels at all time points were consistently lower in the study group, and fewer patients developed postoperative complications (30% vs. 58%, p = 0.0033). However hospital length of stay was not significantly different between the two groups.

Pearse and colleagues used the LiDCOplus system (LiDCO Ltd, Cambridge, UK) to optimize high-risk surgical patients postoperatively, using colloid and inotropes to obtain Shoemaker's original DO_2I target of 600 ml/(min m²) [40]. There were fewer complications (44% vs. 68%) and a shorter length of stay in the GDT group.

The PiCCO system (Pulsion Medical Systems, Munich, Germany) is an alternative device that has been shown to be reliable at assessing fluid responsiveness [41]. Recently another technology, the respiratory variations in pulse oximeters waveform, has been shown to be strongly related to PPV, and may prove useful in assessing fluid status [42].

There are several limitations to the use of SVV and PPV. Firstly, the patient needs to be in sinus rhythm. Secondly, cyclical changes in stroke volume or pulse pressure rely on significant variations in intrathoracic pressure. If the patient has small tidal volumes, is breathing spontaneously, or has an open chest the changes in intrathoracic pressure are usually too small to induce significant changes in venous return. Conversely, high intrathoracic or intra-abdominal pressure may exaggerate SVV and PPV. These limitations apply to the measurement of SVV/PPV, and not analysis of the waveform to calculate SV and CO.

In the perioperative environment where most high-risk patients are mechanically ventilated with "normal" airway pressures, these limitations do not commonly apply, and dynamic monitoring appears to be the ideal method to titrate fluid resuscitation. However further outcome studies are needed before these waveform-based devices will be universally recommended.

Other technologies

There are an increasing number of new technologies that have recently been marketed which have the ability to monitor CO noninvasively and, in some cases, assess fluid responsiveness.

The NICOM (Cheetah Medical, Israel) is a continuous noninvasive cardiac output monitor based on chest bioreactance that is totally noninvasive and accurate when compared with the PAC [43].

The BioZ (Cardiodynamics Intl., San Diego, CA, USA) uses thoracic bioimpedance and was not as robust [44].

The Aesculon (Osypka Medical, LA Jolla, CA, USA) uses electrical velocimetry to interpret the maximal change in thoracic bioimpedance to calculate CO, and also has been shown to correlate poorly with the PAC [45]. The challenge for manufacturers is to produce not only a well-validated, reliable monitor, but also to show an outcome benefit in this increasingly competitive field.

Conclusion

As the population ages, the number of patients requiring high-risk non-cardiac surgery is only going to increase. The concept of individualized GDT for these patients seems to improve outcomes by ensuring adequate tissue perfusion at all times perioperatively.

The underlying mechanism behind the success of GDT is related to the optimization of oxygen delivery to the tissues. This avoids an oxygen debt, which can cause mitochondrial damage and organ dysfunction.

Many authors have described how the use of GDT can reduce morbidity and the length of hospital stay in high-risk surgical patients, although most of the studies have been performed on small sample sizes from single centers. Two recent meta-analyses focusing on renal function [46] and gastrointestinal function [47] have also shown that surgical patients receiving perioperative GDT are at decreased risk of renal and gastrointestinal impairment, which account for a significant proportion of postoperative morbidity.

Perioperative GDT has not become standard care for a variety of reasons. It remains a challenge to implement GDT because of the significant commitment and resources needed. However, with an increasing number of studies being published on the clinical utility of noninvasive hemodynamic monitoring, the use of GDT should continue to gain popularity.

References

1. Pearse RM, Harrison DA, James P, et al. Identification and characterisation of the high-risk surgical population in the United Kingdom. *Crit Care* 2006; **10**: R81.

2. Shoemaker WC, Appel PL, Kram HB, Waxman K, Lee TS. Prospective trial of supranormal values of survivors as therapeutic goals in high-risk surgical patients. *Chest* 1988; **94**: 1176–86.

3. Shoemaker WC, Montgomery ES, Kaplan E, Elwyn DH. Physiologic patterns in surviving and nonsurviving shock patients. Use of sequential cardiorespiratory variables in defining criteria for therapeutic goals and early warning of death. *Arch Surg* 1973; **106**: 630–6.

4. Boyd O, Grounds RM, Bennett ED. A randomized clinical trial of the effect of deliberate perioperative increase of oxygen delivery on mortality in high-risk surgical

patients. *JAMA* 1993; **270**: 2699–707.

5. Wilson J, Woods I, Fawcett J, *et al.* Reducing the risk of major elective surgery: randomised controlled trial of preoperative optimisation of oxygen delivery. *BMJ* 1999; **318**: 1099–103.

6. Polonen P, Ruokonen E, Hippelainen M, Poyhonen M, Takala J. A prospective, randomized study of goal-oriented hemodynamic therapy in cardiac surgical patients. *Anesth Analg* 2000; **90**: 1052–9.

7. Lobo SM, Salgado PF, Castillo VG, *et al.* Effects of maximizing oxygen delivery on morbidity and mortality in high-risk surgical patients. *Crit Care Med* 2000; **28**: 3396–404.

8. Connors AF, Jr., Speroff T, Dawson NV, *et al.* The effectiveness of right heart catheterization in the initial care of critically ill patients. SUPPORT Investigators. *JAMA* 1996; **276**: 889–97.

9. Bellamy MC. Wet, dry or something else? *Br J Anaesth* 2006; **97**: 755–7.

10. Brandstrup B, Tonnesen H, Beier-Holgersen R, *et al.* Effects of intravenous fluid restriction on postoperative complications: comparison of two perioperative fluid regimens: a randomized assessor-blinded multicenter trial. *Ann Surg* 2003; **238**: 641–8.

11. Bennett-Guerrero E, Welsby I, Dunn TJ, *et al.* The use of a postoperative morbidity survey to evaluate patients with prolonged hospitalization after routine, moderate-risk, elective surgery. *Anesth Analg* 1999; **89**: 514–19.

12. Hamilton-Davies C, Mythen MG, Salmon JB, Jacobsen D, Shukla A, Webb AR. Comparison of commonly used clinical indicators of hypovolaemia with gastrointestinal tonometry. *Intensive Care Med* 1997; **23**: 276–81.

13. Osman D, Ridel C, Ray P, *et al.* Cardiac filling pressures are not appropriate to predict hemodynamic response to volume challenge. *Crit Care Med* 2007; **35**: 64–8.

14. Marik PE, Baram M, Vahid B. Does central venous pressure predict fluid responsiveness? A systematic review of the literature and the tale of seven mares. *Chest* 2008; **134**: 172–8.

15. Davies JN, Allen DR, Chant AD. Non-invasive Doppler-derived cardiac output: a validation study comparing this technique with thermodilution and Fick methods. *Eur J Vasc Surg* 1991; **5**: 497–500.

16. Okrainec A, Bergman S, Demyttenaere S, *et al.* Validation of esophageal Doppler for noninvasive hemodynamic monitoring under pneumoperitoneum. *Surg Endosc* 2007; **21**: 1349–53.

17. Lafanechere A, Albaladejo P, Raux M, *et al.* Cardiac output measurement during infrarenal aortic surgery: echo-esophageal Doppler vs. thermodilution catheter. *J Cardiothorac Vasc Anesth* 2006; **20**: 26–30.

18. Chytra I, Pradl R, Bosman R, Pelnar P, Kasal E, Zidkova A. Esophageal Doppler-guided fluid management decreases blood lactate levels in multiple-trauma patients: a randomized controlled trial. *Crit Care* 2007; **11**: R24.

19. Rodriguez RM, Lum-Lung M, Dixon K, Nothmann A. A prospective study on esophageal Doppler hemodynamic assessment in the ED. *Am J Emerg Med* 2006; **24**: 658–63.

20. Dark PM, Singer M. The validity of trans-esophageal Doppler ultrasonography as a measure of cardiac output in critically ill adults. *Intensive Care Med* 2004; **30**: 2060–6.

21. Conway DH, Mayall R, Abdul-Latif MS, Gilligan S, Tackaberry C. Randomised controlled trial investigating the influence of intravenous fluid titration using oesophageal Doppler monitoring during bowel surgery. *Anaesthesia* 2002; **57**: 845–9.

22. Gan TJ, Soppitt A, Maroof M, *et al.* Goal-directed intraoperative fluid administration reduces length of hospital stay after major surgery. *Anesthesiology* 2002; **97**: 820–6.

23. Wakeling HG, McFall MR, Jenkins CS, *et al.* Intraoperative oesophageal Doppler guided fluid management shortens postoperative

hospital stay after major bowel surgery. *Br J Anaesth* 2005; **95**: 634–42.

24. Noblett SE, Snowden CP, Shenton BK, Horgan AF. Randomized clinical trial assessing the effect of Doppler-optimized fluid management on outcome after elective colorectal resection. *Br J Surg* 2006; **93**: 1069–76.

25. Senagore AJ, Emery T, Luchtefeld M, Kim D, Dujovny N, Hoedema R. Fluid management for laparoscopic colectomy: a prospective, randomized assessment of goal-directed administration of balanced salt solution or hetastarch coupled with an enhanced recovery program. *Dis Colon Rectum* 2009; **52**: 1935–40.

26. Mythen MG and Webb AR. Perioperative plasma volume expansion reduces the incidence of gut mucosal hypoperfusion during cardiac surgery. *Arch Surg* 1995; **130**: 423–9.

27. McKendry M, McGloin H, Sabery D, Caudwell L, Brady AR, Singer M. Randomised controlled trial assessing the impact of a nurse delivered, flow monitored protocol for optimisation of circulatory status after cardiac surgery. *BMJ* 2004; **329**: 258.

28. Sinclair S, James S, Singer M. Intraoperative intravascular volume optimisation and length of hospital stay after repair of proximal femoral fracture: randomised controlled trial. *BMJ* 1997; **315**: 909–12.

29. Venn R, Steele A, Richardson P, *et al.* Randomized controlled trial to investigate influence of the fluid challenge on duration of hospital stay and perioperative morbidity in patients with hip fractures. *Br J Anaesth* 2002; **88**: 65–71.

30. Lassen K, Soop M, Nygren J, *et al.* Consensus review of optimal perioperative care in colorectal surgery: Enhanced Recovery After Surgery (ERAS) Group recommendations. *Arch Surg* 2009; **144**: 961–9

31. US Department of Health and Human Services. Esophageal Doppler ultrasound-based cardiac output monitoring for real-time therapeutic management of

hospitalized patients. Rockville: Agency for Healthcare Research and Quality, Department of Health & Human Services, 2007.

32. Mowatt G, Houston G, Hernandex R. Evidence review: oesophageal Doppler monitoring in patients undergoing high-risk surgery and in critically ill patients. London: NHS Purchasing and Supply Agency – Centre for Evidence-Based Purchasing, 2008.

33. Chappell D, Jacob M, Hofmann-Kiefer K, Conzen P, Rehm M. A rational approach to perioperative fluid management. *Anesthesiology* 2008; **109**: 723–40.

34. Kimberger O, Arnberger M, Brandt S, *et al.* Goal-directed colloid administration improves the microcirculation of healthy and perianastomotic colon. *Anesthesiology* 2009; **110**: 496–504.

35. Westphal M, James MF, Kozek-Langenecker S, *et al.* Hydroxyethyl starches: different products – different effects. *Anesthesiology* 2009; **111**: 187–202.

36. Marik PE, Cavallazzi R, Vasu T, Hirani A. Dynamic changes in arterial waveform derived variables and fluid responsiveness in mechanically ventilated patients: a systematic review of the literature. *Crit Care Med* 2009; **37**: 2642–7.

37. Berkenstadt H, Margalit N, Hadani M, *et al.* Stroke volume variation as a predictor of fluid responsiveness in patients undergoing brain surgery. *Anesth Analg* 2001; **92**: 984–9.

38. Lopes MR, Oliveira MA, Pereira VO, *et al.* Goal-directed fluid management based on pulse pressure variation monitoring during high-risk surgery: a pilot randomized controlled trial. *Crit Care* 2007; **11**: R100.

39. Benes J, Chytra I, Altmann P, *et al.* Intraoperative fluid optimization using stroke volume variation in high risk surgical patients: results of prospective randomized study. *Crit Care* 2010; **14**(3): R118.

40. Pearse R, Dawson D, Fawcett J, *et al.* Early goal-directed therapy after major surgery reduces complications and duration of

hospital stay. A randomised, controlled trial. *Crit Care* 2005; **9**: R687–93.

41. Wiesenack C, Prasser C, Keyl C, Rodig G. Assessment of intrathoracic blood volume as an indicator of cardiac preload: single transpulmonary thermodilution technique vs. assessment of pressure preload parameters derived from a pulmonary artery catheter. *J Cardiothorac Vasc Anesth* 2001; **15**: 584–8.

42. Cannesson M, Besnard C, Durand PG, Bohe J, Jacques D. Relation between respiratory variations in pulse oximetry plethysmographic waveform amplitude and arterial pulse pressure in ventilated patients. *Crit Care* 2005; **9**: R562–8.

43. Squara P, Denjean D, Estagnasie P, *et al*. Noninvasive cardiac output monitoring (NICOM): a clinical validation. *Intensive Care Med* 2007; **33**: 1191–4.

44. Spiess BD, Patel MA, Soltow LO, Wright IH. Comparison of bioimpedance vs. thermodilution cardiac output during cardiac surgery: evaluation of a second-generation bioimpedance device. *J Cardiothorac Vasc Anesth* 2001; **15**: 567–73.

45. Petter H, Erik A, Björn E *et al*. Measurement of cardiac output with non-invasive Aesculon impedance versus thermodilution. *Clin Physiol Funct Imaging* 2011; **31**(1): 39–47.

46. Brienza N, Giglio MT, Marucci M, Fiore T. Does perioperative hemodynamic optimization protect renal function in surgical patients? A meta-analytic study. *Crit Care Med* 2009; **37**: 2079–90.

47. Giglio MT, Marucci M, Testini M, Brienza N. Goal-directed haemodynamic therapy and gastrointestinal complications in major surgery: a meta-analysis of randomized controlled trials. *Br J Anaesth* 2009; **103**: 637–46.

Chapter 2

Non-invasive guidance of fluid therapy

Maxime Cannesson

It is estimated that about 240 million anesthesia procedures are performed each year around the world [1]. Among them, 24 million (~10%) are conducted in high-risk patients. If this is a small percentage of the whole population, one has to remember that this sample accounts for more than 80% of the overall mortality related to surgery [2].

Moderate-risk surgery represents approximately 40% of the whole population (i.e., 96 million patients a year). Thankfully, most of these patients present with uncomplicated post-operative course. However, it is estimated that approximately 30% of them (i.e., ~29 million patients a year) present with "minor" postoperative complications mainly related to gut injury inducing delayed enteral feeding, abdominal distension, nausea, vomiting or wound complications such as wound dehiscence or pus from the operation wound [3]. Even if these complications are said to be "minor" they induce an increased postoperative medication, increased length of stay in hospital and finally an increase in the cost of the medicosurgical management. In most of these patients, postoperative complications are related to tissue hypoperfusion and inadequate perioperative resuscitation [3,4].

The function of the circulation system is to service the needs of the body tissues, to transport nutrients to the body tissues, to transport waste products away, to conduct hormones from one part of the body to another and, in general, to maintain an appropriate environment in all the tissue fluids of the body for optimal survival and function of the cells.

To be achieved, this goal requires two physiological objectives: adequate perfusion pressure in order to force blood into the capillaries of all organs and adequate cardiac output to deliver oxygen and substrates, and to remove carbon dioxide and other metabolic products [5,6]. This is so true that several studies have demonstrated that cardiac output maximization during high-risk surgery has the ability to improve postoperative patients' outcome and to decrease the cost of surgery [7–10].

It is obvious that optimization of oxygen delivery to the tissues during surgery cannot be conducted by monitoring arterial pressure alone. Because arterial pressure and cardiac output are both dependent on systemic vascular resistances, a normal or even supra-normal arterial pressure does not guarantee that cardiac output is not low. However, flow measurement is technologically not as straightforward as pressure measurements.

Therefore, apart from cardiac output monitoring, new parameters (called *functional hemodynamic parameters*) have recently been developed. These parameters rely on cardiopulmonary interactions in patients under general anesthesia and mechanical ventilation and can be obtained invasively from the arterial pressure waveform (pulse pressure variation

Clinical Fluid Therapy in the Perioperative Setting, ed. Robert G. Hahn. Published by Cambridge University Press. © Cambridge University Press 2011.

[11] or PPV [12]) or non-invasively from the plethysmographic waveform (ΔPOP [13] or PVI for pleth variability index [14]) [15,16].

In this chapter we describe the rationale and the potential applications of these non-invasive hemodynamic monitoring parameters during surgery and how they can improve patients' outcome by optimizing cardiac output and oxygen delivery during surgery.

Preload dependence

Hypovolemia induces hypotension, oliguria and tachycardia. That's a fact. But one has to be very careful: these signs are not related to hypovolemia, but they are related to severe hypovolemia [17]. Moreover, they are not specific and can be present even in the absence of hypovolemia. Consequently, they are neither sensitive nor specific and cannot be used for assessing a patient's fluid status with accuracy.

Central venous pressure (CVP) or pulmonary capillary wedge pressure (PCWP) have been used for years for monitoring patients' volemia. However, this assumption has been made because CVP and PCWP were supposed to reflect ventricular preload or preload dependence, which is actually wrong. And almost all the studies focusing on the ability of CVP and PCWP to predict fluid responsiveness have failed to demonstrate any accuracy of these parameters for predicting the effects of volume expansion on cardiac output [18].

The main question anesthesiologists and/or intensivists have to answer before they perform volume expansion is: "will my patient increase cardiac output in response to volume expansion?" What he or she wants to know is: "is my patient preload dependent or not?"

Preload dependence is defined as the ability of the heart to increase stroke volume in response to an increase in preload. To understand this concept, one has to be reminded of the Frank–Starling relationship. This relationship links preload to stroke volume and presents two distinct parts: a steep portion and a plateau (Figure 12.1). If the patient is on the steep portion of the Frank–Starling relationship, then an increase in preload (induced by volume expansion) is going to induce an important increase in stroke volume. If the patient is on the plateau of this relationship, then increasing preload will have no effect on stroke volume.

The Frank–Starling relationship does not only depend on preload and stroke volume, but it also depends on cardiac function. When cardiac function is impaired the Frank–Starling relationship is flattened and for the same level of preload the effects of volume expansion on stroke volume are going to be less important, explaining why preload parameters such as CVP or PCWP are not accurate predictors of fluid responsiveness (Figure 12.1). Instead of monitoring a given parameter, functional hemodynamic monitoring assesses the effects of a stress on this given parameter [19].

Functional hemodynamic parameters

For the assessment of preload dependence, the stress is a "fluid challenge" and the parameter is stroke volume or one of its surrogates (pulse pressure or plethysmographic waveform amplitude for instance). In mechanically ventilated patients under general anesthesia, the effects of positive-pressure ventilation on preload and stroke volume are used to detect fluid responsiveness. If mechanical ventilation induces important respiratory variations in stroke volume (SVV) or in PPV it is more likely that the patient is preload dependent [15] (Figure 12.2).

These dynamic parameters (SVV, PPV, passive leg raising [PLR]) have consistently been shown to be superior to static parameters (CVP, PCWP) for the prediction of fluid responsiveness. Today CVP and PCWP, as well as oliguria, hypotension and tachycardia, should not be used anymore for predicting the effects of volume expansion on cardiac output [18,20].

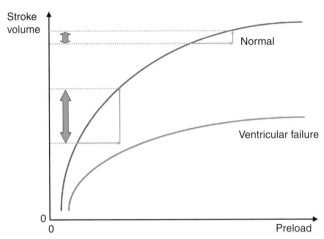

Figure 12.1. Frank–Starling relationship between ventricular preload and ventricular stroke volume. The first portion of this relationship is called the *steep portion* and the second portion is called the *plateau*. If the heart is working on the steep portion (low preload), then an increase in preload (induced by volume expansion) will induce a significant increase in stroke volume (here the heart is said to be preload dependent). If the heart is working on the plateau (elevated preload), then an increase in preload (induced by volume expansion) will not induce any significant increase in stroke volume (here the heart is said to be preload independent). The Frank–Starling relationship does not depend only on preload and stroke volume but it also depends on ventricular function, and the Frank–Starling curve is flattened when ventricular function is impaired. Consequently, for a given preload value, it is not possible to predict the effects of an increase in preload on stroke volume.

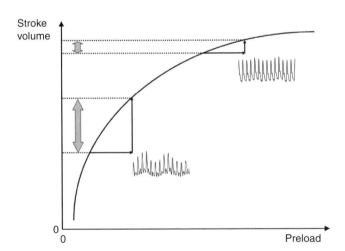

Figure 12.2. Frank–Starling relationship with associated respiratory variations in the arterial pressure waveform signal. Considering that respiratory variations in arterial pulse pressure are studied in adequate conditions, high respiratory variations reflect that the heart is working on the steep portion of the relationship (indicating a preload dependence), while low respiratory variations reflect that the heart is working on the plateau of the relationship (indicating a preload independence).

Theoretically, the main interest of these dynamic parameters is that they can be used as a surrogate for cardiac output monitoring. As a matter of fact, if one considers that knowing whether the patient is preload dependent (i.e., whether cardiac output can be improved using volume expansion) is more important than knowing the absolute cardiac output value, then monitoring these parameters could replace cardiac output monitoring itself (Figure 12.2).

However, dynamic parameters of fluid responsiveness based on cardiopulmonary inter-actions have several limitations that need to be clearly stated before they can be adequately used in the clinical setting.

First, these parameters have to be used in mechanically ventilated patients have under general anesthesia. Up to now, studies conducted in spontaneously breathing patients failed to demonstrate that PPV can predict fluid responsiveness in this setting [21]. Moreover, tidal volume has an impact on the predictive value of PPV and a tidal volume of 8 ml/kg of body weight is required [22]. Patients have to be in sinus rhythm, the chest must be closed (open chest as well as open pericardium strongly modify cardiopulmonary interactions) and the intra-abdominal pressure has to be within the normal ranges [24].

These dynamic indicators need to be further explored in children and in the setting of left ventricular failure and acute respiratory distress syndrome.

To summarize, the conditions of application of PPV for the purpose of fluid responsive-ness are:

- patient under general anesthesia and mechanical ventilation;
- tidal volume > 8 ml/kg of ideal body weight;
- sinus rhythm;
- no right ventricular failure;
- closed chest;
- normal intra-abdominal pressure.

Finally, PPV monitoring requires an arterial line and is more likely to be applied in high-risk surgery patients. In moderate-risk surgery patients, the pulse oximeter waveform can be used to assess preload dependence as described below.

Using the pulse oximeter to optimize fluid status

The pulse oximeter waveform is based on a signal proportional to light absorption between an emitter and a receptor, which are usually placed on the fingertip, on the forehead or on the earlobe. Light absorption increases with the amount of hemoglobin present in the stud-ied tissue.

The amplitude of the pulse oximeter plethysmographic waveform depends particularly on the vessel volume (venous, arterial and microcirculation volume) and on the transmural pressure applied on the probe [24]. This waveform presents two components: the first com-ponent is said to be constant (DC as direct current) and is due to light absorption by bone, tissue, pigments, non-pulsatile blood (venous) and skin. The second component is said to be pulsatile absorption (AC as alternating current) and is mainly related to arterial pulse.

Venous blood is responsible for a slight pulsatile absorption on the plethysmographic waveform recorded at the forehead when the pulse oximetry sensor is not pressed by an elastic tensioning headband [25,26] (i.e., when the transmural pressure is low). In this case, venous saturation can induce false low-saturation readings. At the finger, the pulsatile com-ponent is due primarily to arterialized blood and the venous pulse is less frequently seen. Low-frequency oscillations due to changes in capillary density (sympathetic tone) have also been reported [27] and can alter the waveform quality.

Shamir et al. were the first to describe the respiratory variations in the plethysmographic waveform (SPVpleth) and in its Δdownpleth component (by analogy with the arterial Δdown) in patients presenting with various degrees of hypovolemia [28]. Then, in 2005 our team showed the relationship between the respiratory variations in the ΔPOP and in the PPV in mechanically ventilated patients under general anesthesia in the intensive care unit [29]. In this study, we showed that both indices were strongly related and that ΔPOP was easily measurable at the bedside. Using the PPV formula rather than the variations in the peak of the waveform for quantifying the respiratory variations in the plethysmographic waveform allowed us to get rid of the fact that this waveform has no unit. By dividing the difference in amplitude by the mean of these amplitudes we observe a mathematical simplification for the unit and then ΔPOP is expressed as a percentage.

Pulse oximeter waveform amplitude was then tested in clinical settings and was shown to be sensitive to venous return in mechanically ventilated patients [30] and to be an accurate predictor of fluid responsiveness in various settings [13], including in the intensive care unit [31] and in the postoperative period following cardiac surgery [32]. In the operating room, a ΔPOP greater than 13% before volume expansion allowed discrimination between responders and nonresponders with 80% sensitivity and 90% specificity [30].

In the intensive care unit, in a septic hypotensive cohort, Feissel *et al.* showed that a ΔPOP value of 14% before volume expansion allowed discrimination between responders and nonresponders with 94% and 80% specificity, respectively [31]. It is interesting to underline that patients were all under vasoactive drugs in this last study and that it did not seem to impact the ability of this index to predict fluid responsiveness.

We now have numerous evidences showing that ΔPOP has the ability to predict fluid responsiveness in mechanically ventilated patients under general anesthesia despite some limitations related to vasomotor tone [27]. The most recently published study comes from Pizov *et al.* and shows that respiratory variations in the plethysmographic waveform are early detectors of hypovolemia and that this parameter increases before arterial pressure decreases and heart rate increases in patients in whom occult bleeding occurs [33].

Pleth variability index

Most pulse oximeter waveforms displayed by conventional monitor screens are smoothed and filtered because it is impossible to accurately eyeball the respiratory variations in this waveform and to draw any reliable informations regarding patients' fluid status from these screens [34].

Recently, a new parameter extracted from this waveform allows clinicians to continuously and automatically monitor these respiratory variations. The PVI is continusoulsy displayed as a percentage on Radical 7 Masimo Monitors (Masimo Corp., Irvine, CA, USA). Pleth variability index is an automatic measure of the dynamic change in perfusion index (PI) that occurs during a complete respiratory cycle.

For the measurement of SpO_2 via pulse oximetry, red and infrared lights are used. A constant amount of light (DC) from the pulse oximeter is absorbed by skin, other tissues and non pulsatile blood, while a variable amount of blood (AC) is absorbed by the pulsatile arterial inflow. For PI calculation, the infrared pulsatile signal is indexed against the non-pulsatile infrared signal and expressed as a percentage (PI = [AC/DC] x 100) reflecting the amplitude of the pulse oximeter waveform. Then PVI calculation is accomplished by measuring changes in PI over a time interval sufficient to include one or more complete respiratory cycles as $PVI = [(PI_{max} - PI_{min})/PI_{max}] \times 100$.

Several studies have now validated the ability of PVI to predict fluid responsiveness in mechanically ventilated patients undergoing general anesthesia [14,35,36]. A PVI higher than 10–15% is suggestive of preload dependence and indicates that volume expansion is more likely to increase cardiac output.

Functional hemodynamic monitoring and clinical outcome

In 2007, the literature regarding the influence of goal-directed therapy based on cardiac output maximization on postoperative outcome was reviewed [37]. The authors concluded that individualized goal-directed therapy in the perioperative period improves gut function and reduces postoperative nausea and vomiting, morbidity and hospital length of stay.

More recently, a 15-year follow-up study of high-risk surgical patients even found that short-term goal-directed therapy based on cardiac output monitoring in the perioperative period may improve long-term outcomes, in part due to the ability of such therapy to reduce the number of perioperative complications [38].

Growing evidence indicates that goal-directed therapy using appropriate fluid monitoring methods, such as PPV and PVI, is effective in optimizing patient outcomes [15]. For example, in a randomized controlled trial published in 2007, monitoring and minimizing PPV by volume loading during high-risk surgery improved postoperative outcome and decreased hospital length of stay [39]. The median duration of postoperative hospital stay was lower in the intervention group than the control group (7 vs. 17 days, $p < 0.01$), as were the number of postoperative complications per patient (1.4 ± 2.1 vs. 3.9 ± 2.8, $p < 0.05$) and the median duration of mechanical ventilation (1 vs. 5 days, $p < 0.05$) and stay in the intensive care unit (3 vs. 9 days, $p < 0.01$).

Similarly, in a randomized controlled trial in 60 high-risk patients undergoing major abdominal surgery, a goal-directed hemodynamic optimization protocol using the FloTrac/ Vigileo device was associated with a shorter median length of stay: 15 days for the goal-directed group vs. 19 days for the control group receiving a standard management protocol ($p = 0.006$) [10]. The goal-directed group also had a reduced incidence of perioperative complications (20%) relative to the control group (50%) ($p = 0.03$). In another study, high-risk patients undergoing major abdominal surgery whose fluid management was guided by SVV had fewer complications than those receiving routine intraoperative care ($p = 0.0066$) [40].

PVI may also play a role in optimizing hemodynamic status in patients undergoing major abdominal surgery [41]. In a recently published randomized controlled trial, patients scheduled for major abdominal surgery ($n = 82$) were randomized into two groups; a PVI group monitored for PVI and a control group receiving standard care. In the PVI group, authors aimed at maintaining PVI under 13% by iterative volume expansion. The primary outcome measure, the perioperative serum lactate level, was significantly lower in the PVI group, and peri- and postoperative volume infused were lower in the PVI group. It was concluded that PVI improved perioperative fluid management in abdominal surgery. Other studies focusing on the ability of non-invasive technologies to be used in goal-directed therapy protocols are now ongoing and should be published in a near future.

Conclusion

"From flying blind to flying right?" [42]

Hemodynamic optimization is of major importance during surgery. This concept requires arterial pressure monitoring and optimization and also cardiac output monitoring and optimization. High-risk surgery has been shown to benefit from cardiac output maximization

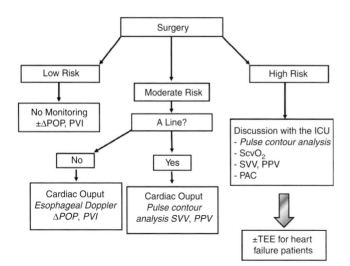

Figure 12.3. Proposed algorithm for hemodynamic monitoring during anesthesia depending on the type of surgery. ICU, intensive care unit; PAC, pulmonary artery catheter; ΔPOP, respiratory variations in pulse oximeter waveform amplitude; PPV, pulse pressure variation; PVI, pleth variability index; ScvO$_2$, mixed venous oxygen saturation; SVV, stroke volume variation; TEE, transesophageal echocardiography.

using semi-invasive technologies. Moderate-risk surgery patients may also benefit from this approach using non-invasive technologies. It is more likely that in the future, goal-directed therapy using more sophisticated and less invasive monitoring will help clinicians to optimize their patients' hemodynamic status during surgery (Figure 12.3).

References

1. Weiser TG, Regenbogen SE, Thompson KD, et al. An estimation of the global volume of surgery: a modelling strategy based on available data. *Lancet* 2008; **372**: 139–44.

2. Pearse RM, Harrison DA, James P, et al. Identification and characterisation of the high-risk surgical population in the United Kingdom. *Crit Care* 2006; **10**: R81.

3. Bennett-Guerrero E, Welsby I, Dunn TJ, et al. The use of a postoperative morbidity survey to evaluate patients with prolonged hospitalization after routine, moderate-risk, elective surgery. *Anesth Analg* 1999; **89**: 514–19.

4. Gan TJ, Mythen MG. Does perioperative gut-mucosa hypoperfusion cause postoperative nausea and vomiting? *Lancet* 1995; **345**: 1123–4.

5. Guyton AH, Hall JE. Heart muscle; The heart as a pump and function of the heart valves. In: Elsevier S, ed. *Textbook of Medical Physiology*, 11th edn. Philadelphia: Elsevier, Inc., 2006, pp.103–15.

6. Guyton AH, Hall JE. Overview of the circulation: medical physics of pressure, flow, and resistance. In: Elsevier S, ed. *Textbook of Medical Physiology*, 11th edn. Philadelphia: Elsevier, Inc., 2006, pp. 161–70.

7. Gan TJ, Soppitt A, Maroof M, et al. Goal-directed intraoperative fluid administration reduces length of hospital stay after major surgery. *Anesthesiology* 2002; **97**: 820–6.

8. Pearse R, Dawson D, Fawcett J, et al. Early goal-directed therapy after major surgery reduces complications and duration of hospital stay. A randomised, controlled trial. *Crit Care* 2005; **9**: R687–93.

9. Wakeling HG, McFall MR, Jenkins CS, et al. Intraoperative oesophageal Doppler guided fluid management shortens postoperative hospital stay after major bowel surgery. *Br J Anaesth* 2005; **95**: 634–42.

10. Mayer J, Boldt J, Mengistu AM, Rohm KD, Suttner S. Goal-directed intraoperative therapy based on autocalibrated arterial pressure waveform analysis reduces

hospital stay in high-risk surgical patients: a randomized, controlled trial. *Crit Care* 2010; **14**: R18.

11. Michard F, Boussat S, Chemla D, *et al.* Relation between respiratory changes in arterial pulse pressure and fluid responsiveness in septic patients with acute circulatory failure. *Am J Respir Crit Care Med* 2000; **162**: 134–8.

12. Cannesson M, Slieker J, Desebbe O, *et al.* The ability of a novel algorithm for automatic estimation of the respiratory variations in arterial pulse pressure to monitor fluid responsiveness in the operating room. *Anesth Analg* 2008; **106**: 1195–2000.

13. Cannesson M, Attof Y, Rosamel P, *et al.* Respiratory variations in pulse oximetry plethysmographic waveform amplitude to predict fluid responsiveness in the operating room. *Anesthesiology* 2007; **106**: 1105–11.

14. Cannesson M, Desebbe O, Rosamel P, *et al.* Pleth variability index to monitor the respiratory variations in the pulse oximeter plethysmographic waveform amplitude and predict fluid responsiveness in the operating theatre. *Br J Anaesth* 2008; **101**: 200–6.

15. Cannesson M. Arterial pressure variation and goal-directed fluid therapy. *J Cardiothorac Vasc Anesth* 2010; **24**: 487–97.

16. Michard F. Changes in arterial pressure during mechanical ventilation. *Anesthesiology* 2005; **103**: 419–28.

17. Perel A, Pizov R, Cotev S. Systolic blood pressure variation is a sensitive indicator of hypovolemia in ventilated dogs subjected to graded hemorrhage. *Anesthesiology* 1987; **67**: 498–502.

18. Marik PE, Baram M, Vahid B. Does central venous pressure predict fluid responsiveness?: a systematic review of the literature and the tale of seven mares. *Chest* 2008; **134**: 172–8.

19. Pinsky MR, Payen D. Functional hemodynamic monitoring. *Crit Care* 2005; **9**: 566–72.

20. Marik PE, Cavallazzi R, Vasu T, Hirani A. Dynamic changes in arterial waveform derived variables and fluid responsiveness in mechanically ventilated patients: a systematic review of the literature. *Crit Care Med* 2009; **37**: 2642–7.

21. De Backer D, Pinsky MR. Can one predict fluid responsiveness in spontaneously breathing patients? *Intensive Care Med* 2007; **33**: 1111–13.

22. De Backer D, Heenen S, Piagnerelli M, Koch M, Vincent JL. Pulse pressure variations to predict fluid responsiveness: influence of tidal volume. *Intensive Care Med* 2005; **31**: 517–23.

23. Duperret S, Lhuillier F, Piriou V, *et al.* Increased intra-abdominal pressure affects respiratory variations in arterial pressure in normovolaemic and hypovolaemic mechanically ventilated pigs. *Intensive Care Med* 2007; **33**: 163–71.

24. Reisner A, Shaltis PA, McCombie D, Asada HH. Utility of the photoplethysmogram in circulatory monitoring. *Anesthesiology* 2008; **108**: 950–8.

25. Shelley KH, Dickstein M, Shulman SM. The detection of peripheral venous pulsation using the pulse oximeter as a plethysmograph. *J Clin Monit* 1993; **9**: 283–7.

26. Agashe GS, Coakley J, Mannheimer PD. Forehead pulse oximetry: Headband use helps alleviate false low readings likely related to venous pulsation artifact. *Anesthesiology* 2006; **105**: 1111–16.

27. Landsverk SA, Hoiseth LO, Kvandal P, *et al.* Poor agreement between respiratory variations in pulse oximetry photoplethysmographic waveform amplitude and pulse pressure in intensive care unit patients. *Anesthesiology* 2008; **109**: 849–55.

28. Shamir M, Eidelman LA, Floman Y, Kaplan L, Pizov R. Pulse oximetry plethysmographic waveform during changes in blood volume. *Br J Anaesth* 1999; **82**: 178–81.

29. Cannesson M, Besnard C, Durand PG, Bohe J, Jacques D. Relation between respiratory variations in pulse oximetry plethysmographic waveform amplitude and arterial pulse pressure in ventilated patients. *Crit Care* 2005; **9**: R562–8.

30. Cannesson M, Desebbe O, Hachemi M, *et al*. Respiratory variations in pulse oximeter waveform amplitude are influenced by venous return in mechanically ventilated patients under general anaesthesia. *Eur J Anaesthesiol* 2007; **24**: 245–51.

31. Feissel M, Teboul JL, Merlani P, *et al*. Plethysmographic dynamic indices predict fluid responsiveness in septic ventilated patients. *Intensive Care Med* 2007; **33**: 993–9.

32. Wyffels PA, Durnez PJ, Helderweirt J, Stockman WM, De Kegel D. Ventilation-induced plethysmographic variations predict fluid responsiveness in ventilated postoperative cardiac surgery patients. *Anesth Analg* 2007; **105**: 448–52.

33. Pizov R, Eden A, Bystritski D, *et al*. Arterial and plethysmographic waveform analysis in anesthetized patients with hypovolemia. *Anesthesiology* 2010; **113**: 83–91.

34. Feldman JM. Can clinical monitors be used as scientific instruments? *Anesth Analg* 2006; **103**: 1071–2.

35. Cannesson M, Delannoy B, Morand A, *et al*. Does the pleth variability index indicate the respiratory induced variation in the plethysmogram and arterial pressure waveforms? *Anesth Analg* 2008; **106**: 1189–94.

36. Zimmermann M, Feibicke T, Keyl C, *et al*. Accuracy of stroke volume variation compared with pleth variability index to predict fluid responsiveness in mechanically ventilated patients undergoing major surgery. *Eur J Anaesthesiol* 2009; **27**: 555–61.

37. Bundgaard-Nielsen M, Holte K, Secher NH, Kehlet H. Monitoring of peri-operative fluid administration by individualized goal-directed therapy. *Acta Anaesthesiol Scand* 2007; **51**: 331–40.

38. Rhodes A, Cecconi M, Hamilton M, *et al*. Goal-directed therapy in high-risk surgical patients: a 15-year follow-up study. *Intensive Care Medicine* 2010: **36**: 1327–32.

39. Lopes MR, Oliveira MA, Pereira VO, *et al*. Goal-directed fluid management based on pulse pressure variation monitoring during high-risk surgery: a pilot randomized controlled trial. *Crit Care* 2007; **11**: R100.

40. Benes J, Chytra I, Altmann P, *et al*. Intraoperative fluid optimization using stroke volume variation in high risk surgical patients: results of prospective randomized study. *Crit Care* 2010; **14**: R118.

41. Forget P, Lois F, de Kock M. Goal-directed fluid management based on the pulse oximeter-derived pleth variability index reduces lactate levels and improves fluid management. *Anesth Analg* 2010; **111**: 910–14.

42. Cannesson M, Vallet B, Michard F. Pulse pressure variation and stroke volume variation: from flying blind to flying right? *Br J Anaesth* 2009; **103**: 896–7; author reply 7–9.

Hemodilution

Chapter 13

Philippe van der Linden

Acute normovolemic hemodilution (ANH) was introduced into clinical practice in the 1970s to reduce requirements for allogeneic blood products [1]. Acute normovolemic hemodilution entails the removal of blood either immediately before or shortly after the induction of anesthesia and its simultaneous replacement by an appropriate volume of crystalloids and/or colloids to maintain "isovolemic" conditions [2]. As a result, blood subsequently lost during surgery will contain proportionally less red blood cells (RBCs), thus reducing the loss of autologous erythrocytes.

Acute normovolemic hemodilution therefore presents all the advantages associated with a reduction in allogeneic blood exposure, including a reduction of transfusion reactions from exposure to donor's blood antigens and a decreased exposure to bloodborne pathogens, but also offers several advantages in comparison with other blood conservation techniques. It is quite inexpensive and easily available, it improves tissue oxygenation through its microcirculatory effects and it provides fresh autologous blood units for later transfusion after the achievement of surgical hemostasis. However, the real efficacy of ANH in reducing allogeneic blood transfusion remains to be discussed. The aim of this article is to describe the physiology, limits and efficacy of ANH.

Physiological compensatory mechanisms

The acute reduction in RBC concentration induced by hemodilution elicits intrinsic compensatory mechanisms, allowing the maintenance of adequate tissue oxygenation [3,4]. The development of these mechanisms is closely related to the improvement of whole blood fluidity achieved by the hemodilution process, providing the maintenance of "isovolemic" conditions. Basic determinants of blood fluidity are the red cell concentration, the plasma viscosity, the cell-to-cell interactions and the prevailing shear rate (i.e., the mean linear flow velocity). The lower the shear rate, the more pronounced the improvement in blood fluidity based on changes in hematocrit [5]. The sympathetic nervous system also plays an important role in the maintenance of optimal oxygen delivery during ANH [6]. Elicited compensatory mechanisms mainly involve an increase in cardiac output and an increase in tissue oxygen extraction.

Increase in cardiac output

At the systemic level, improvement in blood fluidity results in an increase of venous return and a reduction of left ventricular afterload. Enhancement of shear rate with subsequent

Clinical Fluid Therapy in the Perioperative Setting, ed. Robert G. Hahn. Published by Cambridge University Press. © Cambridge University Press 2011.

release of nitric oxide may also contribute to systemic vasodilation, while hemodilution-induced stimulation of aortic chemoreceptors increases the sympathetic activity of the heart, resulting in improved myocardial performance [7]. These entire phenomena are responsible for the increase in cardiac output, mainly through a rise in stroke volume, but also to some extent through an increase in heart rate.

Increase in tissue oxygen extraction

The second compensatory mechanism aims at a better matching of oxygen delivery to oxygen demand at the tissue level. This mechanism entails physiologic alterations at both the systemic and the microcirculatory level. At the systemic level, a redistribution of blood flow to areas of high metabolic demand from areas of low demand has been repeatedly demonstrated during isovolemic ANH [8]. This regional redistribution of blood flow is partly due to α-adrenergic stimulation, but seems unaltered in the presence of β-adrenergic blockade.

At the microcirculatory level, several physiologic alterations develop to provide a more efficient utilization of the remaining blood oxygen content. Increased RBC velocity appears the most important, resulting from increased arteriolar pressure, which, alone, stimulates arterial vasomotion [9]. Both phenomena provide a better spatial and temporal distribution of RBCs within the capillary network, and result in improved tissue oxygen extraction capacity [10]. Lastly, a right shift of the oxygen dissociation curve may reduce the affinity of hemoglobin for oxygen and therefore improve oxygen availability. This shift, related to a rise in RBC 2,3-diphosphoglycerate level, takes some hours to occur and has been demonstrated only in chronic anemia [11].

Effects of anesthesia

Anesthesia can alter the physiologic adjustments to isovolemic hemodilution at several levels (Table 13.1). The most striking effect of anesthesia appears to be a decreased cardiac output response, mainly related to a complete blunting of the increase in heart rate [12,13] (Figure 13.1). This reduced cardiac output response resulted in a decreased oxygen delivery, but oxygen consumption remained unchanged as the oxygen extraction ratio increased (Figure 13.2).

Interestingly, ANH appears to be associated with increased oxygen consumption in awake patients, which could be related at least in part to an increase in myocardial oxygen demand. In the study of Ickx *et al.*, when the patients undergoing ANH while awake were anesthetized, all the measured parameters returned to values similar to those obtained in patients undergoing hemodilution while anesthetized [13]. Therefore, performing ANH before or after induction of anesthesia did not result in a significant different physiologic response at the time of surgery.

Limits of hemodilution

As described above, maintenance of tissue oxygenation during ANH results from an increase in cardiac output and oxygen extraction. Several experimental and clinical studies have demonstrated the involvement of both mechanisms even in the early stage of ANH [14]. The relative contribution of these mechanisms will depend on the ability of the organism to recruit them. They allow the maintenance of adequate tissue oxygenation until the hemoglobin concentration falls to about 3–4 g/dl (hematocrit 10–12%). Below this "critical" value, oxygen delivery can no longer match tissue oxygen demand and cellular hypoxia will

Table 13.1. Effects of anesthesia on the physiologic response to hemodilution.

1. Effects on **cardiac output response**:
   a. alteration in cardiac preload and afterload conditions;
   b. negative inotropic effect;
   c. depressed autonomic nervous system activity.
2. Effects on **O_2 extraction response**:
   a. vasodilation;
   b. depressed sympathetic nervous system activity.
3. Effects on **gas exchange**:
   a. decreased functional residual capacity.
4. Effects on **tissue oxygen demand**:
   a. relief of pain, stress, anxiety;
   b. decreased muscular activity;
   c. decreased myocardial O_2 demand (negative chronotropic and inotropic effect).

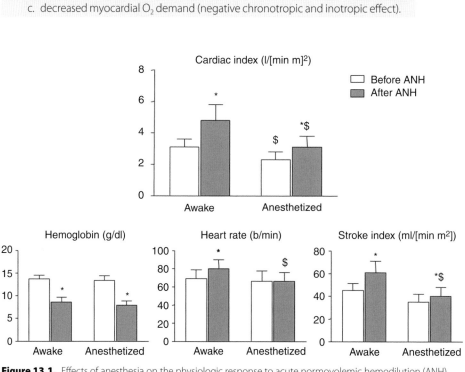

Figure 13.1. Effects of anesthesia on the physiologic response to acute normovolemic hemodilution (ANH). * $p < 0.05$ after ANH vs. before ANH; $ $p < 0.05$ anesthetized vs. awake. Adapted from Ickx et al., 2000 [13].

develop as demonstrated in several experimental studies [15–17]. Van Woerkens et al. studied a Jehovah's Witness patient who died from extreme hemodilution, and reported a critical hemoglobin concentration of 4 g/dl [18].

The efficacy of the mechanisms maintaining tissue oxygen delivery when the oxygen-carrying capacity of the blood is reduced depends primarily on the maintenance of an adequate circulating blood volume. Indeed, hypovolemia blunts the effects of decreased

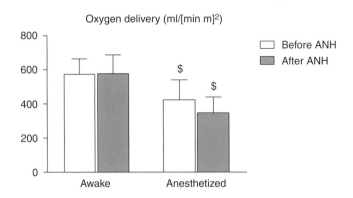

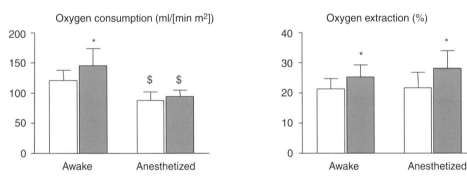

Figure 13.2. Effects of anesthesia on the oxygen delivery/oxygen consumption balance during acute normovolemic hemodilution (ANH). * $p < 0.05$ after ANH vs. before ANH; $ $p < 0.05$ anesthetized vs. awake. Adapted from Ickx et al., 2000 [13].

blood viscosity on venous return [19]. Although "normovolemic" conditions are difficult to define, replacement of the blood and fluid losses with at least a volume of substitute having the same expanding effect on the intravascular volume is required. Only a few studies have compared the effects of different plasma substitutes on the hemodynamic response to ANH: colloids appeared superior to crystalloids [20,21].

Tolerance to acute isovolemic hemodilution depends, not only on the integrity of the compensatory mechanisms described above, but also on the level of tissue oxygen demand. For a given cardiac output and oxygen extraction response, any increase in tissue oxygen demand will require a higher hemoglobin concentration.

Acute normovolemic hemodilution and the cardiac patient

Maintenance of myocardial oxygen delivery during ANH depends essentially on the increase in the coronary blood flow as oxygen extraction is already nearly maximal at the level of the heart under resting conditions [8]. This is achieved by a reduction in coronary vascular resistance related to decreased blood viscosity and to specific coronary vasodilation. Heart rate and possibly myocardial contractility have been shown to increase during hemodilution [22], which results in an augmentation of myocardial oxygen demand. When the hematocrit is reduced to about 10%, myocardial oxygen consumption more than doubles, and coronary vasodilation is nearly maximal. Below such a hematocrit, coronary blood flow can no longer match myocardial oxygen demand and ischemia develops, ultimately resulting in cardiac failure.

The dependency of myocardial oxygen supply on coronary blood flow highlights the vulnerability of the heart during ANH, especially in patients with coronary artery disease (CAD) in whom coronary blood flow could not increase. The lowest tolerable hemoglobin concentration in CAD patients remains unknown and probably depends on several factors, including the severity of the disease [23]. There is, however, increased evidence that tolerance of CAD patients to isovolemic anemia closely depends on the level of myocardial oxygen demand.

In anesthetized patients scheduled for coronary surgery, several studies demonstrated that moderate ANH (target hematocrit value 27–33%) is well tolerated, and may be even cardioprotective if associated with a decreased myocardial oxygen demand [24]. Myocardial oxygen balance is profoundly influenced by the level of heart rate, and recent clinical data confirm that tolerance of CAD patients to moderate anemia is closely related to the level of heart rate [25]. The anesthetic technique may also play a role [26]. The early postoperative period is certainly critical in hemodiluted CAD patients, because they have to face an increased tissue metabolic demand [27].

Acute normovolemic hemodilution and hemostasis

Hemodilution could affect hemostasis in different ways. First, it will dilute not only plasmatic factors, but also cellular coagulation factors, like platelets and, of course, RBCs. Red blood cells have been shown to interfere with hemostasis through a mechanical effect and also through biological effects related to the release of intracellular adenosine diphosphate and to the generation of thrombin [28]. The clinical consequences (i.e., importance of perioperative bleeding) of these interactions between RBCs and hemostasis remain to be determined.

Hemodilution could also affect hemostasis through the direct effects of plasma substitution fluids on the platelets and the coagulation mechanisms [29]. These effects are more marked with colloids than with crystalloids. Among colloids, they are more marked with dextrans than with gelatins and albumin. For hydroxyethyl starches, these effects appear closely related to the intrinsic properties of the different solutions, such as a high in vitro molecular weight and a high degree of hydroxyethyl substitution [30]. Several in vitro studies have confirmed these effects in the context of ANH [31,32]. In addition, patients with type O blood may demonstrate more coagulation compromise than those with non-O blood when undergoing hemodilution with low-molecular weight hydroxyethyl starch [33].

Despite the evidence that ANH may directly interfere with normal hemostasis, there is no evidence from the literature that ANH is associated with increased perioperative bleeding [34,35].

Efficacy
Theoretical aspects

The basic concept behind ANH is that patients undergoing such a procedure will lose fewer erythrocytes per milliliter of lost blood during surgery and after transfusion of the collected autologous blood in the immediate postoperative period [5].

Several equations have been developed to calculate the efficacy of ANH as a function of surgical blood loss, initial hematocrit, target post-ANH hematocrit and hematocrit used as the transfusion trigger. Presuming a "usual" surgical patient without preoperative anemia, and a transfusion decision based exclusively on a trigger hemoglobin concentration of 6–7 g/dl, Weiskopf calculated that 55–77% of patient's total blood volume must be lost during surgery in order to achieve savings of about 180 ml of RBCs, which represents one standard blood unit [36]. However, the usefulness of the different published equations in clinical practice remains limited, as several factors have not been always taken into account in the proposed formulas [2].

Results from the literature

Efficacy of ANH as a blood conservation technique remains highly debated [34,35,37]. Most of the studies reviewed were performed in the setting of cardiac or orthopedic surgery. Adequate evaluation of the published results was hampered by the relatively poor quality of the studies and the marked heterogeneity observed between trials, partly explained by study factors (patient populations, target hematocrit values, transfusion triggers, ANH techniques, etc.). Efficacy of ANH was found to be relatively modest in terms of likelihood of exposure to allogeneic blood and units transfused. It closely depends on the use or not of protocols to guide transfusion practice. There was no obvious increase in adverse events with ANH, but the incidence of complications was poorly reported.

Studies having demonstrated a clear efficacy of ANH in reducing the likelihood of patient's exposure to allogeneic blood in the perioperative period have been performed in major liver resection [38,39] or major abdominal surgery [40]. In all of them, a large volume of blood was collected. Surgery was associated with significant blood loss and a low hemoglobin concentration (7–8 g/dl) was used as the transfusion trigger. All these observations indicate that efficient ANH requires quite significant expertise in the field from the care giving team.

Conclusions

Acute normovolemic hemodilution entails the removal of blood from a patient shortly after the beginning of the surgical procedure, and its replacement with crystalloids or colloids to maintain the circulating blood volume. It is a relatively simple, cheap and effective tool to avoid or reduce allogeneic blood transfusion. Factors that influence the efficacy of the technique have been clearly identified. This reduces the field of application of ANH to patients undergoing high bleeding-risk surgery in whom a large volume of blood can be collected.

Knowledge of the physiologic compensatory mechanisms that occur during normovolemic hemodilution and their limits are essential for the safe use of the technique. In addition, the anesthesiologist must be familiar with its practical aspects. Although ANH has a place in different types of surgery, it must be regarded as an integral part of a blood conservation strategy tailored to the individual patient's needs and adapted to specific surgical procedures.

References

1. Klövekorn WP, Laks H, Pilon RN, *et al.* Effects of acute hemodilution in man. *Eur Surg Res* 1973; **5**: 27–8.

2. Jamnicki M, Kocian R, van der Linden P, Zaugg M, Spahn DR. Acute normovolemic hemodilution: physiology, limitations, and clinical use. *J Cardiothorac Vasc Anesth* 2003; **17**: 747–54.

3. Van der Linden P.: The physiology of acute isovolaemic anaemia. *Acta Anaesthesiol Belg* 2002; **53**: 97–103.

4. Hébert PC, Van der Linden P, Biro GP, Qun Hu L: Physiologic aspects of anemia. *Crit Care Clin* 2004; **20**: 187–212.

5. Kreimeier U, Messmer K. Perioperative hemodilution. *Transfusion and Apheresis Science* 2002; **27**: 59–72.

6. Tsui AK, Dattani ND, Marsden PA, *et al.* Reassessing the risk of hemodilutional anemia: Some new pieces to an old puzzle. *Can J Anaesth* 2010; **57**: 779–91.

7. Chapler CK, Cain CM. The physiologic reserve in oxygen carrying capacity: studies in experimental hemodilution. *Can J Physiol Pharmacol* 1986; **64**: 7–12.

8. Fan FC, Chen RYZ, Schuessler GB, Chien S. Effects of hematocrit variations on regional hemodynamics and and oxygen transport in the dog. *Am J Physiol* 1980; **238**: H545–52.

9. Messmer K, Gutierrez G, Vincent JL. Blood rheology factors and capillary blood flow, *Tissue Oxygen Utilization*. Berlin, Heidelberg, New-York: Springer-Verlag, 1991, pp. 103–13.

10. Van der Linden P, Gilbart E, Paques P, Simon C, Vincent JL. Influence of hematocrit on tissue O2 extraction capabilities during acute hemorrhage. *Am J Physiol* 1993; **264**: H1942–7.

11. Rodman T, Close HP, Purcell MK. The oxyhemoglobin dissociation curve in anemia. *Ann Intern Med* 1960; **52**: 295–301.

12. Kungys G, Rose DD, Fleming NW. Stroke volume variation during acute normovolemic hemodilution. *Anesth Analg* 2009; **109**: 1823–30.

13. Ickx B, Rigolet M, Van der Linden P. Cardiovascular and metabolic response to acute normovolemic anemia: effects of anesthesia. *Anesthesiology* 2000; **93**: 1011–16.

14. Spahn DR, Leone BJ, Reves JG, Pasch T. Cardiovascular and coronary physiology of acute isovolemic hemodilution: a review of nonoxygen-carrying and oxygen-carrying solutions. *Anesth Analg* 1994; **78**: 1000–21.

15. Räsänen J. Supply-dependent oxygen consumption and mixed venous oxyhemoglobin saturation during isovolemic hemodilution in pigs. *Chest* 1992; **101**: 1121–4.

16. Van der Linden P, De Groote F, Mathieu N, *et al.* Critical haemoglobin concentration in anaesthetized dogs: comparison of two plasma substitutes. *Br J Anaesth* 1998; **81**: 556–62.

17. Van der Linden P, De Hert S, Mathieu N, *et al.* Tolerance to acute isovolemic hemodilution: effect of anesthetic depth. *Anesthesiology* 2003; **99**: 97–104.

18. van Woerkens ECSM, Trouwborst A, van Lanschot JJB. Profound hemodilution: what is the critical level of hemodilution at which oxygen delivery-dependent oxygen consumption starts in an anesthetized human? *Anesth Analg* 1992; **75**: 818–21.

19. Richardson TQ, Guyton AC. Effects of polycythemia and anemia on cardiac output and other circulatory factors. *Am J Physiol* 1959; **197**: 1167–70.

20. Otsuki DA, Fantoni DT, Margarido CB, *et al.* Hydroxyethyl starch is superior to lactated Ringer as a replacement fluid in a pig model of acute normovolaemic haemodilution. *Br J Anaesth* 2007; **98**: 29–37.

21. Arya VK, Nagdeve NG, Kumar A, Thingnam SK, Dhaliwal RS. Comparison of hemodynamic changes after acute normovolemic hemodilution using Ringer's lactate versus 5% albumin in patients on beta-blockers undergoing coronary artery bypass surgery. *J Cardiothorac Vasc Anesth* 2006; **20**: 812–18.

22. Weiskopf RB, Feiner J, Hopf H, *et al.* Heart rate increases linearly in response to acute isovolemic anemia. *Transfusion* 2003; **43**: 235–40.

23. Tircoveanu R, Van der Linden P. Hemodilution and anemia in patients with cardiac disease: what is the safe limit? *Curr Opin Anaesthesiol* 2008; **21**: 66–70.

24. Licker M, Ellenberger C, Sierra J, Kalangos A, Diaper J, Morel D. Cardioprotective effects of acute normovolemic hemodilution in patients undergoing coronary artery bypass surgery. *Chest* 2005; **128**: 838–47.

25. Cromheecke S, Lorsomradee S, Van der Linden PJ, De Hert SG. Moderate acute isovolemic hemodilution alters myocardial

function in patients with coronary artery disease. *Anesth Analg* 2008; **107**: 1145–52.

26. De Hert SG, Cromheecke S, Lorsomradee S, Van der Linden PJ. Effects of moderate acute isovolaemic haemodilution on myocardial function in patients undergoing coronary surgery under volatile inhalational anaesthesia. *Anaesthesia* 2009; **64**: 239–45.

27. Hogue CW, Goodnough LT, Monk T. Perioperative myocardial ischemic episodes are related to hematocrit level in patients undergoing radical prostatectomy. *Transfusion* 1998, pp. **38**: 1070–7.

28. Ouakine-Orlando B, Samama CM, Samama CM, *et al.* Hématocrite et hémostase, *Hémorragies et thromboses périopératoires: approche pratique.* Paris: Masson, 2000, pp. 113–119.

29. Van der Linden P, Ickx BE. The effects of colloid solutions on hemostasis. *Can J Anaesth* 2006, pp. **53**: S30–9.

30. Westphal M, James MF, Kozek-Langenecker S, Stocker R, Guidet B, Van Aken H: Hydroxyethyl starches: different products – different effects. *Anesthesiology* 2009; **111**: 187–202.

31. Jones SB, Whitten CW, Despotis GJ, Monk TG: The influence of crystalloid and colloid replacement solutions in acute normovolemic hemodilution: a preliminary survey of hemostatic markers. *Anesth Analg* 2003; **96**: 363–8.

32. Thyes C, Madjdpour C, Frascarolo P, *et al.* Effect of high- and low-molecular-weight low-substituted hydroxyethyl starch on blood coagulation during acute normovolemic hemodilution in pigs. *Anesthesiology* 2006; **105**: 1228–37.

33. Kang JG, Ahn HJ, Kim GS, *et al.* The hemostatic profiles of patients with Type O and non-O blood after acute normovolemic hemodilution with 6% hydroxyethyl starch (130/0.4). *Anesth Analg* 2006; **103**: 1543–8.

34. Bryson GL, Laupacis A, Wells GA. Does acute normovolemic hemodilution reduce perioperative allogeneic transfusion? A meta-analysis. *Anesth Analg* 1998; **86**: 9–15.

35. Segal JB, Blasco-Colmenares E, Norris EJ, Guallar E. Preoperative acute normovolemic hemodilution: a meta-analysis. *Transfusion* 2004; **44**: 632–44.

36. Weiskopf RB: Efficacy of acute normovolemic hemodilution assessed as a function of fraction of blood volume lost. Anesthesiology 2001; **94**: 439–46.

37. Carless P, Moxey A, O'Connell D, Henry D. Autologous transfusion techniques: a systematic review of their efficacy. *Transfusion Medicine* 2004; **14**: 123–44.

38. Matot I, Scheinin O, Jurim O, Eid A. Effectiveness of acute normovolemic hemodilution to minimize allogeneic blood transfusion in major liver resections. *Anesthesiology* 2002; **97**: 794–800.

39. Wuest D, Kundu K, Blumgart LH, Fischer M. A prospective randomized trial of acute normovolemic hemodilution compared to standard intraoperative management in patients undergoing major hepatic resection. *Ann Surg* 2008; **248**: 360–9.

40. Spahn DR, Waschke KF, Standl T, *et al.* Use of perflubron emulsion to decrease allogeneic blood transfusion in high-blood-loss non-cardiac surgery: results of a European phase 3 study. *Anesthesiology* 2002; **97**: 1338–49.

Microvascular fluid exchange

Per-Olof Gründe and Johan Persson

Fluid and protein exchange from the intravascular space to the extravascular space is a continuous process with a net fluid flow across the capillary membranes and the venules, the rate of which is called the *transcapillary escape rate* (TER) [1].

Under normal circumstances, accumulation of fluid and proteins in the interstitium is prevented by recirculation back to the intravascular space via the *lymphatic system*. The entire plasma volume passes the vascular membranes to the extravascular space and back to the circulation at least once a day, and even several times a day under pathophysiological conditions such as after trauma and during sepsis/systemic inflammatory response syndrome (SIRS).

This means that accumulation of plasma in the interstitium that results in hypovolemia and tissue edema is not only a question of microvascular permeability to fluid and proteins, but also a question of the capacity of the lymphatic system. As discussed below, other factors may also be involved, such as hydrostatic capillary pressure, types of plasma volume expanders and the infusion strategy.

The present chapter is an attempt to explain the mechanisms controlling microvascular fluid exchange under physiological and pathophysiological conditions and the relationship between the volumes of the intravascular and the extravascular spaces. This knowledge is of importance not only for an adequate treatment of hypovolemia, but also to reduce side effects of the fluid treatment.

Transvascular fluid exchange outside the brain

Fluid exchange across the capillary membrane has been described by the classical Starling fluid equation for transcapillary fluid exchange:

$$Jv = LpS(\Delta P - \sigma\Delta\pi)$$

where Lp represents hydraulic permeability (fluid conductivity), S is the surface area available for fluid exchange, reflecting the number of perfused capillaries, ΔP is the net transcapillary hydrostatic force for filtration, σ is the reflection coefficient for macromolecules (plasma proteins) and $\Delta\pi$ is the transcapillary oncotic absorbing pressure force.

The reflection coefficient for plasma proteins describes the effective part of the transcapillary oncotic pressure counteracting fluid filtration and represents the difficulty with which proteins pass the exchange vessels relative to water. The reflection coefficient is 1.0 when the

Clinical Fluid Therapy in the Perioperative Setting, ed. Robert G. Hahn. Published by Cambridge University Press. © Cambridge University Press 2011.

membrane is impermeable to molecules and 0 when molecules pass through the membrane without any hindrance.

The reflection coefficient for proteins is below 1.0 in all organs of the body except the brain. For albumin it is 0.90–0.95 in skeletal muscle, 0.50–0.65 in the lung and 0.80 in the intestine and in the subcutis. A reflection coefficient below 1.0 means a continuous leakage of proteins to the interstitium. A system with recirculation of proteins between blood vessels and tissue and back to the intravascular space is essential to allow access of antibodies, protein-bound hormones, cytokines and other macromolecules to the interstitial space. The reflection coefficient can be reduced significantly under a state of inflammation, leading to increased loss of albumin and other macromolecules to the interstitium. Tissue edema is formed when the leakage of plasma fluid is greater than the recirculating capacity of the lymphatic system and hypovolemia develops in parallel.

The Starling formula, however, gives no information about the mechanisms responsible for protein leakage. There has been a general belief for decades that active (energy-consuming) trancytosis (vesicle transport) across the endothelial membrane of capillaries is responsible for a large part of protein loss to the interstitium [2].

However, it is unlikely that the relatively small capacity of an active vesicle transporting mechanism would be responsible for transport of *all* the plasma proteins in one day – and under inflammatory states, several times a day. The capacity of an energy-consuming process is also normally reduced by inflammation. Furthermore, blockade of transcytosis by cooling or pharmacological inhibition in the rat was not found to reduce TER [3,4]. Most likely, transport of proteins across the capillary membrane is therefore mainly a *passive process* independent of energy-consuming activities.

The 2-pore theory

By the 2-pore theory for transcapillary fluid and protein exchange [5], the large loss of proteins from intravascular to the extravascular space can be explained by *passive mechanisms*. According to this theory, fluid and small solutes pass the capillary membrane through all the pores along the entire capillary bed and in venules, whereas proteins pass the membrane mainly through the 10–30×10^3 times less common large pores on the venous side of the capillary network, and in the venules (Figure 14.1).

While the small pores, with their radius of 40–45 Å, are freely permeable to electrolytes and other small molecules and much less permeable to proteins, the large pores with their radius of about 250 Å are also freely permeable to proteins. This means that the oncotic pressure gradient across the large pore is low. The protein loss to the interstitium can partly be explained by diffusion, but the main mechanism is *convection* when the proteins follow the large-pore fluid stream with the transcapillary/transvenular hydrostatic pressure as the major driving force. This means that protein loss depends on both the number and size of large pores (large pore permeability) and the transcapillary/transvenular hydrostatic pressure.

The lymphatic system

The capacity of the lymphatic system is of great importance for maintenance of a balance between the intravascular and the extravascular space. A normal TER of 5–8% of plasma volume per hour, corresponding to 150–200 ml plasma per hour for an adult, is in the range of the capacity of the lymphatic system under normal circumstances [1]. The capacity of the

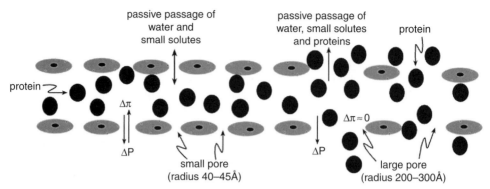

Figure 14.1. A schematic illustration of the principles used in control of transvascular exchange of fluid and macromolecules. Absence of an oncotic absorbing force across the large pore means that the hydrostatic transcapillary force (ΔP) is the main force creating a "jet" stream of protein-rich fluid through each large pore, mainly via convection from the intravascular space to the extravascular space. An increase in the number and the area of large pores and an increase in the hydrostatic transcapillary pressure will increase the loss of proteins.

lymphatic drainage increases with increase in skeletal muscle activity and it can be reduced by inactivity, such as in immobile patients.

If TER is increased, such as after trauma and during sepsis/SIRS, the capacity of the lymphatic system may be too low to transfer all the leaking plasma fluid back to the circulation, and *tissue edema* in combination with *hypovolemia* develops. The situation will be aggravated in immobile patients by the reduced recirculating capacity of the lymphatic system.

Physiotherapy might improve this capacity and help to counteract tissue edema, hypovolemia and the need for plasma volume expanders in critically ill patients.

Transvascular fluid exchange in the brain

The volume regulation of the *brain* is more effective than that of other organs of the body. This is important, as there is no room for expansion in volume of the brain as it is tightly enclosed in the cranium. The brain also lacks a lymphatic drainage system [6]. The sophisticated regulation of brain volume can be ascribed to the low permeability of cerebral capillaries, which creates the so-called *blood–brain barrier* (BBB).

The intact BBB means that the cerebral capillaries are impermeable to passive transport of all molecules except water. Thus, neither macromolecules such as proteins nor small solutes such as sodium or chloride ions can pass the cerebral capillary passively. This means that a disturbed balance between the hydrostatic and the oncotic pressures will result in transfer of *only water* across the cerebral capillaries, and the subsequent dilution/concentration of the crystalloid osmotic pressure of brain interstitium will result in immediate stoppage of further fluid exchange [6].

In the injured brain with a disrupted BBB – in the sense that it has been passively permeable for small solutes – there will be much less dilution during filtration. The filtration continues for a longer period of time, creating a vasogenic brain edema, and it will finally be balanced by the increase in intracranial pressure [7].

Crystalloids and colloids as plasma volume expanders

While the healthy patient is normovolemic and needs no extra plasma volume expanders, most critically ill patients develop hypovolemia due to increased leakage of plasma fluid that exceeds the capacity of the lymphatic system. However, there is still debate regarding which plasma volume expander should be used to maintain or achieve normovolemia. In this chapter we attempt to describe the advantages and drawbacks of using crystalloids and various colloids as plasma volume expanders.

Due to the small radius of electrolytes (< 2–3 Å) relative to the radius of the small pores (40–45 Å), the reflection coefficient of electrolytes is very small. A *crystalloid solution* is therefore distributed relatively quickly over the whole extracellular space after infusion, and more or less independently of the prevailing microvascular permeability, also resulting in reduction in plasma and interstitial oncotic pressure. Only 20–25% of the infused solution can be used for plasma volume expansion and the rest will result in tissue edema. A simultaneous increase in urine production must be compensated by further infusions to maintain normovolemia.

Tissue edema not only has cosmetic consequences, but it can be a real drawback in terms of pulmonary edema, acute respiratory distress syndrome and increased intercapillary distances. It may also compromise perfusion from an increase in tissue pressure, and there is a risk of development of a compartment syndrome. Lowering of the plasma oncotic pressure may also result in further filtration according to the Starling formula.

Such a distribution to the interstitium will not occur in the normal brain due to the intact BBB, but it may occur to some extent in the injured brain if the cerebral capillaries become permeable to small solutes, aggravating a vasogenic brain edema [7,8].

Albumin is the predominant protein in plasma and the only natural colloid solution recommended for plasma volume expansion today, as transfusion with plasma is justified only to compensate for coagulation disturbances. The albumin molecule has a molecular weight of 69 kDa and solutions are available in various concentrations (3.5%, 4%, 5%, 20% and 25% solutions). The albumin molecule is negatively charged, which may moderate its distribution to the interstitium. It is transported back to the intravascular compartment via the lymphatic system. In contrast to synthetic colloids it is degraded very slowly, which can be of advantage by acting as a plasma volume expander for a longer time; but this can also be a disadvantage when it accumulates in the interstitium. The effectiveness of albumin as a plasma volume expander has been questioned, however, as some studies could not demonstrate a better outcome with albumin than with saline [9]. The effectiveness of albumin as a plasma volume expander can be improved and side effects reduced by adhering to specific rules in its administration, as will be described below. Allergic reactions are rare.

The *synthetic colloids* available today are dextran, hydroxyethyl starch (HES) and gelatin – and they are all cheaper than albumin. In contrast to albumin, they are all polydisperse with molecular weights ranging from low to higher values, and with the majority of molecules concentrated in the range of the average molecular weight. They are degraded in plasma and in the interstitium. Their recirculation back to the intravascular space via the lymphatic system is less effective than for albumin. When degraded to molecules with weights below their renal threshold, they are also lost via the kidneys.

Dextran solutions are produced by hydroxylation of polysaccharides. The predominant dextran solution is dextran 70, with an average molecular weight of 70 kDa. It is slowly degraded to CO_2 and water or lost via the kidneys. It improves the microcirculation and has the most effective and long-lasting plasma volume expanding effect of all synthetic colloids available for clinical use today [10,11]. The risk of anaphylaxis is significantly reduced on pretreatment with 1 kDa dextran molecules (hapten competitor dextran 1). By its influence on platelet function, dextran can exacerbate an underlying coagulopathy, which limits its use in larger volumes during surgery or other situations with bleeding. It is of great value preferentially in intensive care for its good and long-lasting plasma volume expanding effect, for improving microcirculation and through its prophylactic effect against thrombosis.

Due to side effects with *HES* solutions of higher molecular weights, the third generation of HES solutions – with a lower mean molecular weight of 130 kDa and molar substitution of approximately 0.4 – now predominate. HES molecules are degraded relatively rapidly by amylase to smaller molecules below the renal threshold and cleared from the circulation via the kidney. The half-life of the plasma concentration of HES130 after a bolus infusion is 1.5–2.0 h, and it is almost totally eliminated after 4 h [12]. This has made the third generation of HES solutions less effective as plasma volume expanders which, however, can be compensated for by repeating the infusion. Allergic reactions to modern HES solutions are less common. The coagulopathic effect appears to be smaller with HES than with dextran. Whether or not modern HES solutions have adverse renal effects is currently debated.

Gelatin solutions are derived from bovine collagen. The mean molecular weight of molecules in gelatin solutions is only 35 kDa. This fact in combination with the relatively fast degradation of gelatin molecules and loss via the kidneys explains their relatively poor and short-lasting plasma volume expanding effect. Gelatin has no or only moderate effects on coagulation, but anaphylactic reactions are more common with gelatin than with other synthetic colloids.

How can we reduce the need for colloids?

Maintenance of normovolemia by infusion of plasma volume expanders in critically ill patients is always associated with interstitial accumulation of fluid due to the increased TER, the reduced capacity of lymphatic recirculation in these patients and the fluid distribution to the extracellular space. The accumulation is associated with side effects in terms of tissue edema, compromised perfusion and respiratory insufficiency.

Increased amounts of macromolecules in the interstitium reduce the transcapillary oncotic pressure, resulting in further tissue edema. Besides maintenance of normovolemia by giving plasma volume expanders, an optimal strategy in the treatment of these patients must therefore be to simultaneously minimize the accumulation of fluid and proteins in the interstitial space.

There are no evidence-based measures to reduce the amount of fluid accumulated in the interstitium, and thereby reduce the need for colloids to maintain normovolemia. However, based on the 2-pore theory and other well-established physiological principles of hemodynamic vascular control, a few quite simple measures may help to maintain normovolemia with a relatively small amount of colloids infused. For example, high concentrations of albumin may be more effective as plasma volume expanders than low concentrations, as a result of their higher oncotic absorbing pressure and the smaller amount of fluid given for the same plasma-expanding effect.

As shown both experimentally in the rat and clinically in patients [13,14], the plasma volume is better preserved at a *normal arterial pressure* than at a high one. Increase in blood pressure by vasopressors may therefore increase the plasma volume loss, and avoidance of high arterial pressures by avoidance of vasopressors or the use of antihypertensive treatment can be an alternative to reduce the need for plasma volume expanders.

Due to the transient increase in arterial pressure by bolus infusions and the fact that a bolus infusion may result in an atrial natriuretic peptide-induced increase in microvascular permeability and increase in urine production [15] a more effective long-term plasma expansion may be obtained by giving the colloid *slowly* rather than using a faster infusion rate.

Stimulation of the lymphatic system with *physiotherapy* may also reduce the interstitial fluid accumulation by improving the recirculating capacity of leaking plasma fluid.

There is controversy regarding the lowest acceptable blood hemoglobin concentration [16], but arguments can be put forward in favor of the view that maintenance of a relatively normal hemoglobin concentration is beneficial. Red blood cells do not pass the capillary membrane and remain intravascular for a long time, thus contributing to preservation of blood volume. Due to the relatively smaller volume of plasma at a normal compared with a low hemoglobin concentration, the leakage and the need of intravascular volume to substitute may be smaller – a hypothesis supported from an experimental study in dogs [17] and one in rats [18].

Side effects of blood transfusions can be reduced by using leukocyte-depleted and recently stored blood. Blood cell transfusion has also been shown to be associated with improved outcome after subarachnoid hemorrhage, and also increases local cerebral oxygenation [19,20].

This chapter describes physiological hemodynamic principles of fluid exchange that form the basis of normovolemia, hypovolemia, edema formation and are fundamental for fluid therapy and for optimization of microcirculation and oxygenation. In view of the lack of appropriate evidence-based clinical studies in this field, such principles may be used as a guide in the use of colloids, crystalloids and erythrocytes in intensive care.

References

1. Haskell A, Nadel ER, Stachenfeld NS, Nagashima K, Mack GW. Transcapillary escape rate of albumin in humans during exercise-induced hypervolemia. *J Appl Physiol* 1997; **83**: 407–13.

2. Predescue D, Vogel SM, Malik AB. Functional and morphological studies of protein transcytosis in continuous endothelia. *Am J Physiol Cell Mol Physiol* 2004; **287**: L895-901.

3. Rippe B, Kamiya A, Folkow B. Is capillary micropinocytosis of any significance for the transcapillary transfer of plasma proteins? *Acta Physiol Scand* 1977; **100**: 258–60.

4. Rosengren BI, Al Rayyes O, Rippe B. Transendothelial transport of low-density lipoprotein and albumin across the rat peritoneum in vivo: effects of the transcytosis inhibitors NEM and filipin. *J Vasc Res* 2002; **39**: 230–7.

5. Rippe B, Haraldsson B. Transport of macromolecules across microvascular walls: the two-pore theory. *Physiol Rev* 1994; **74**: 163–219.

6. Fenstermacher JD. Volume regulation of the central nervous system. In: Staub NC, Taylor AE (eds). Edema, NC: Raven Press, 1984, pp. 383–404.

7. Gründe PO. The Lund concept for treatment of a severe brain trauma – a physiological approach. *Intensive Care Med* 2006: **32**: 1475–84.

8. Jungner M. Gründe PO, Mattiasson G, Bentzer P. Effects on brain edema of crystalloid and albumin fluid resuscitation after brain trauma and hemorrhage in the rat. *Anaesthesiology* 2010; **112**: 1194–203.

9. The SAFE study investigators. Saline or albumin för fluid resuscitation in patients with traumatic brain injury. *New Engl J Med* 2007; **357**: 874–84.

10. Lamke LO, Liljedahl SO. Plasma volume changes after infusion of various plasma expanders. *Resuscitation* 1976; **5**: 93–102.

11. Persson J, Gründe PO. Plasma volume expansion and transcapillary fluid exchange in skeletal muscle of albumin, dextran, gelatin, hydroxyethyl starch, and saline after trauma in the cat. *Crit Care Med* 2006; **34**: 2456–62.

12. Waitzinger J, Bepperling F, Pabst G, *et al.* Pharmacokinetics and tolerability of a new hydroxyethyl starch (HES) specification [HES (130/0.4)] after single-dose infusion of 6% or 10% solutions in healthy volunteers. *Clin Drug Investig* 1998; **16**: 151–60.

13. Dubniks M, Persson J, Grände PO. Effect of blood pressure on plasma volume loss in the rat under increased permeability. *Intensive Care Med* 2007; **33**: 2192–8.

14. Nygren A, Redfors B, Thoren A, Ricksten SE. Norepinephrine causes a pressure-dependent plasma volume decrease in clinical vasodilatory shock. *Acta Anaetshesiol Scand* 2010; **54**: 814–20.

15. Curry FR, Rygh CB, Karlsen T, *et al.* Atrial natriuretic peptide modulation of albumin clearance and contrast agent permeability in mouse skeletal muscle and skin: role in regulation of plasma volume. *J Physiol* 2010; **588**: 325–39.

16. Hébert P, Wells G, Blajchman A, *et al.* A multicenter, randomized, controlled clinical trial of transfusion requirements in critical care. *New Eng J Med* 1999; **340**: 409–18.

17. Valeri CR, Donahue K, Feingold HM, Cassidy GP, Altschule MD. Increase in plasma volume after the transfusion of washed erythrocytes. *Surg Gynecol Obstet* 1986; **162**: 30–6.

18. Persson J, Grände PO. Volume expansion of albumin, gelatin, HES, saline and erythrocytes after haemorrhage in the rat. *Intensive Care Med* 2005; **31**: 296–301.

19. Naidech A, Jovanovic B, Wartenberg K, *et al.* Higher hemoglobin is associated with improved outcome after subarachnoid hemorrhage. *Crit Care Med* 2007; **35**: 2383–9.

20. Smith M, Stiefel M, Magge S, *et al.* Packed red blood cell transfusion increases local cerebral oxygenation. *Crit Care Med* 2005; **33**: 1104–8.

Chapter

15

Body volumes and fluid kinetics

Robert G. Hahn

Infusion fluids exert their therapeutic effects primarily by expanding one of the three body fluid compartments (spaces), namely the *plasma volume* and the *interstitial* and *intracellular* fluid (ICF) volumes. The sum of the plasma and interstitial fluid volumes is called the *extracellular fluid* (ECF) volume.

The sizes of these body fluid volumes have been measured under steady state conditions by the use of *tracer methods*. In an adult weighing 70 kg, they average 3 l for the plasma, 11 l for the interstitial fluid and 28 l for the ICF volume. Hence, the sum of the plasma and interstitial fluid volumes (the ECF volume) amounts to 14 l or 20% of the body weight.

Tracers

Substances known to distribute solely within one body fluid compartment can be injected and the size of the compartment can be calculated by means of *dilution* of the substance.

The substance is then used as a *tracer*. The basic equation for such calculations is:

$$\text{Size of compartment} = \frac{\text{Injected dose of tracer}}{\text{Plasma concentration of tracer}}$$

Examples of such tracers include bromide and iohexol for measurements of the ECF volume and radioiodated albumin for measurement of the plasma volume.

Bromide has a very slow turnover, which means that the measurement might be problematic to repeat several times. *Iohexol* has a shorter half-life, only 100 min, but this also implies that an estimation of the ECF volume has to be based on several plasma samples to account for the elimination during the period of mixing. Sampling cannot start within 30–40 min because the kinetics shows a clear distribution phase [1].

The *total body water* (sum of ECF and ICF) can be measured with water isotopes, which include *tritium* (radioactive) and *deuterium* (not radioactive). One problem is that even distribution of these molecules in the body requires about 3 h to be completed.

An alternative approach is to use *ethanol*, but the relatively short half-life requires frequent sampling in blood or in the expired air [2].

The *plasma volume* has frequently been measured by radioactive *iodated albumin*. After 10 min of distribution of the injected substance, 3–4 samples are taken every 10 min to account for the exponential elimination. The radioiodated albumin method slightly

Clinical Fluid Therapy in the Perioperative Setting, ed. Robert G. Hahn. Published by Cambridge University Press. © Cambridge University Press 2011.

overestimates the plasma volume and, therefore, the result is usually multiplied with a correction factor of 0.9.

Evans Blue is a dye that has been used as a substitute for the albumin method because the measurement does not involve exposure to radioactivity. The dye binds to albumin, just like iodine, and the concentration is measured by light absorption.

There are several possibilities for labeling *erythrocytes* with radioactive tracers to calculate red cell mass. Such tracers include *chromium* and *technetium*.

Carbon monoxide binds to hemoglobin and can also be used to measure red cell mass. Drawbacks are mainly safety issues, as carbon monoxide is toxic.

The size of the interstitial fluid space and the ICF volume cannot be measured by tracers. They have to be inferred as the difference between body fluid spaces that can be measured, i.e., the plasma volume, the ECF volume and the total body water.

These conventional tracer methods of measuring body fluid volumes have limited application in perioperative medicine. A comparison with standard values would indicate whether the patient is dehydrated or hyperhydrated before or after an operation. However, conventional tracers cannot be used to reflect what happens during surgery because the situation is too unstable. During the mixing period there must be steady state with regard to fluid shifts, a situation that is hardly ever met in the operating room. It might even be hard to fully accept that the results can be accurate in the early postoperative period.

If applied during steady state conditions the tracer methods have an accuracy of between 1% (total body water) and 10% (radioiodinated albumin).

Indocyanine green

Indocyanine green (ICG) is a dye that binds to plasma globulins. The half-life is only 3 min due to rapid uptake by the liver. Therefore, ICG can be used both to measure liver blood flow and plasma volume.

The method can apparently be applied during surgery, as steady state with regard to the fluid balance is required only for a few minutes [3].

Drawbacks include that the circulation time (about 1 min in normal humans) becomes crucial. Hence, ICG should be injected via a central venous catheter.

ICG concentration can be measured both in the blood and by pulse oximetry (pulse dye densitometry) [4]. The precision is claimed to be a few per cent.

Bioimpedance

Bioimpedance (BIA) means that a series of weak electrical currents of different frequency are run through the body, typically running between the arm to the foot [5]. The method is based on the fact that currents have more difficulty passing through large amounts of water than small. An estimate of both the ICF and ECF volumes can be made as various frequencies pass through and outside cells with varying ease.

Bioimpedance (BIA) is often applied while the patient is in bed before and after surgery, but rarely perioperatively due to the risk of mechanical and electrical interference. In the author's experience, BIA can provide useful data only for groups and has a place mainly as an adjunct to more precise methods.

Anthropometry

Empirical relationships may be used to estimate the size of the body fluid compartments at baseline.

The simplest ones state that the plasma volume corresponds to 4.5% of the body weight, the blood volume is 7% of the body weight and that the ECF volume makes up 20% of the body weight [1]. Total body water represents 50% of the body weight in the adult female. The percentage is 60% in young adult men and 50% in older men. Children have a higher percentage. Such rules are simple but useful for the clinician to remember.

More precise information can be obtained by *regression equations*. These are typically based on tracer measurements of body fluid volumes performed in a large number of humans, and usually employ the sex, body weight and height of the subject as predictors. Below is an example of such equations for estimation of the blood volume in women and men [6].

BV (L, female) = 0.03308 weight (kg) + 0.3561 height^3 (m) + 0.1833
BV (L, male) = 0.03219 weight (kg) + 0.3669 height^3 (m) + 0.6041

Sodium method

The distribution of infused fluid between the ICF and ECF may be estimated based on the use of serum sodium (SNa) as the marker. Sodium is then used as an endogenous tracer.

If all infused fluid and sodium, as well as all voided amounts are known, the change in ICF volume can be estimated based on the assumption that sodium is evenly distributed in the ECF volume, which makes up 20% of the body weight. From time 0 to time t, we get:

$$\Delta ICF = ECF + (\text{infused} - \text{voided}) \text{ volume} - \frac{(SNa*ECF - (\text{added} - \text{voided})\ Na)}{SNa(t)}$$

This *mass balance equation* has mostly been used to calculate the intracellular distribution of electrolyte-free irrigating fluids [7,8] but it can be used to estimate the intracellular distribution of any infusion fluid [9]. For example, the sodium method was used to demonstrate that acetated Ringer's solution does not expand the ICF volume in volunteers despite the fact that the fluid is slightly hypo-osmolar [10].

Translocation of fluid from the ICF space when infusing hypertonic saline can also be estimated without measuring serum sodium. This calculation is then based on the osmolar balance between the ECF and ICF spaces of which one space gradually becomes expanded and the other concentrated as more fluid is infused [11].

Central blood volume

Measurement of the *intrathoracic* or *central blood volume* is possible with certain modern hemodynamic monitoring systems, such as the PiCCO and LiDCO. These apparatuses are used mainly to measure central flow rates and blood pressures, while the central blood volume is provided as an adjunct output. A central venous pressure line or arterial catheterization is needed to obtain the data on body fluid volumes.

Measurement of the central blood volume is of interest because it is more clearly related to hypovolemia-related physiological responses than to total circulating blood volume. However, little has been published on intrathoracic blood volume in connection with infusion fluids.

Fluid "efficiency"

The *volume effect* of an infusion fluid implies how much of the infused volume that expands the blood volume. The strength and the duration of blood volume expansion are the properties that represent the *efficiency* of the fluid. One may also talk about *potency* when comparing the efficiency of various fluids.

For this purpose, physiological endpoints may be used. For example, a certain amount of blood can be withdrawn and the amount of fluid then required to restore baseline physiological parameters (such as cardiac output) can be taken to represent the "efficiency" [12].

Tracer methods (mostly radioiodinated albumin) have also been used to determine the efficiency of infusion fluids. This implies that the tracer method is applied twice and that the result before and after the infusion is compared. Assessment of colloid fluids is likely to work well by this approach, while the precision must be questioned if crystalloid fluids are studied. Most data relying on tracers refer to the period when distribution has already been completed and voiding has eliminated more than a negligible fraction of the infused crystalloid fluid volume.

Blood hemoglobin

A third and more simplistic approach to quantify the volume effect of an infusion fluid is to measure the hemoglobin (Hb) concentration before and after the infusion. Hemoglobin can be used as an endogenous tracer as it remains completely in the bloodstream and it is reasonable to assume that any dilution of its concentration is due to the infused fluid volume.

Radio-albumin, Evans blue and carbon monoxide may be used to measure the blood volume (BV) before an infusion is provided. Thereafter, changes in blood volume are calculated based on the changes in blood Hb. More frequently, one assumes the BV before the infusion based on some anthropometric equation.

The Hb concentration is measured before (Hb) and after (Hb(t)) the infusion [13]:

$$\Delta BV = BV(Hb/Hb(t)) - BV$$

The amount of fluid retained in the blood is then given by:

$$\text{Fluid retained (\%)} = 100 * \Delta BV / \text{infused volume}$$

The fraction of fluid retained over time is the *efficiency*.

If the urinary output is known, the difference between the infused volume and the sum of the urine and blood volumes represents the change in interstitial fluid volume [14].

Accounting for blood loss

The Hb dilution concept can be developed to account for blood loss, if known. This is (usually) necessary when calculating fluid shifts based on Hb during surgery. One then calculates the total Hb mass and subsequently subtracts all losses (or adds transfused erythrocytes):

$$\text{Hb mass} = BV * Hb$$

$$BV(t) = \frac{\text{Hb mass} - \text{loss of Hb mass}}{Hb(t)}$$

$$\Delta BV(t) = BV(t) - BV$$

These simple equations can be entered into a pocket calculator and may be helpful for the clinician when assessing whether a patient is hypervolemic or hypovolemic. The calculations can be applied repeatedly during surgery without loss of accuracy [15].

These basic relationships shown above can, in turn, be further elaborated upon to quantify the efficiency of infusion fluids during ongoing surgery. Another approach then uses a multiple regression equation to separate the effects of various factors that influence the blood volume.

$$\Delta BV(t) = A^*(\text{infused fluid volume}) - B^* (\text{blood loss})$$

Data may be entered for an entire operation or for shorter periods of time. For example, this approach was used to show that acetated Ringer's solution expands the blood volume by as much as 60% of the infused amount during transurethral resection of the prostate performed under general anesthesia [16].

The Hb method may be more difficult to apply in animals than in humans because several species (such as sheep and dogs) have reservoirs of erythrocytes in the spleen that are mobilized in stressful situations, including hemorrhage. In humans, such recruitment is very small [17].

Volume kinetics

Drug regimens are commonly based on pharmacokinetic analysis. For this purpose, the Hb mathematics presented above have been elaborated upon to create a pharmacokinetic system for the analysis and simulation of the distribution and elimination of infusion fluids [18]. Serial analyses of the Hb concentration in whole blood are then re-calculated to give the dilution of the plasma resulting from an infusion, the reason being that it is the plasma rather than whole blood that equilibrates with other body fluids.

From baseline at time 0 to time t, the dilution of the plasma can be expressed as:

$$\text{Plasma dilution}(t) = \frac{\dfrac{Hb - Hb(t)}{Hb(t)}}{(1 - \text{hematocrit})}$$

The plasma dilution data are then fitted to the solutions of differential equations describing the situation in a kinetic model that describes (reasonably well) what happens in the body. The distribution of fluid between a *central* and a *peripheral* compartment (V_c and V_t, respectively) is proportional to the difference in dilution between them multiplied by the intercompartment clearance, Cl_d. *Elimination* is proportional to the dilution of the central compartment multiplied by the elimination clearance, Cl (Figure 15.1). If urinary excretion is measured, the excreted volume divided by the area under the curve of the plasma dilution gives renal clearance. Accumulation of fluid in the body is given by the difference between Cl and renal clearance.

A complete volume kinetic analysis yields five parameters; the sizes of V_c and V_t along with three clearances (the intercompartmental clearance, elimination clearance and renal clearance).

The parameters in the models are estimated by a mathematical procedure called non-linear-least squares regression. This minimizes the difference between the experimental concentration–time data with theoretical values generated by a computer. When the parameters in the kinetic model have been estimated, the effect of various infusion regimens on the body fluid compartments can be predicted and compared by computer simulation.

The working process is very similar to drug pharmacokinetics, albeit there are certain differences with regard to underlying assumptions. One difference is that drugs are

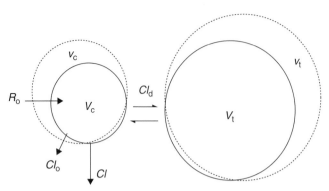

Figure 15.1. Schematic drawing of the two-compartment volume kinetic model that is applicable for analysis of the distribution and elimination of crystalloid infusion fluids during anesthesia and surgery. Note the expandable walls. *Cl*, elimination clearance; *Cl$_d$*, intercompartment–clearance; *Cl$_o$*, baseline fluid loss; *R$_o$*, infusion rate; *v$_c$*, volume expanded state of central compartment; *V$_c$*, central compartment; *v$_t$*, volume–expanded state of peripheral compartment; *V$_t$*, peripheral compartment.

not assumed to expand their volume of distribution, while infusion fluids exert their most important therapeutic effect by doing just that.

The body fluid spaces expanded by infused fluid are called "functional" as they may not correspond exactly to the physiological plasma volume and interstitial fluid volumes. However, studies performed in volunteers provide data in which the central body fluid space correlates closely with the expected size of the plasma volume, whereas the peripheral body fluid space is usually only twice as large as the central one, which is smaller than the interstitial fluid space as measured with tracers. This difference might be explained by the fact that volume kinetics only measures the size of spaces that can be expanded, which is not the case for all parts of the ECF.

Volunteer studies

Approximately 50 studies of volume kinetics have been performed [18].

Key findings show that distribution of *crystalloid fluids*, like the Ringer's solutions, results in a 50–75% larger plasma dilution during an infusion of crystalloid fluid than would be expected if distribution had been immediate. It is often claimed that only 20–25% of the fluids expand the plasma volume, but these figures are valid only some 25–30 min after the infusion is turned off.

The distribution effect of crystalloid fluid means that its efficiency is much better during an actual infusion than after it is completed.

The efficiency of the fluid is also much better, and the peripheral edema less pronounced, if Ringer's solution is infused slowly (Figure 15.2).

Comparisons between infusion fluids in volunteers have been made to quantify their relative efficiency to expand the plasma volume over time. This can be made both by an area method and by computer simulation to a target dilution [11].

Acetated and lactated Ringer's have a potency of 0.9 compared with the reference, which was normal saline. This difference is due to the slower elimination of normal saline as compared with Ringer's. Hypertonic (7.5%) saline is four times more potent, and hypertonic saline in 6% dextran (HSD) is seven times more potent, than normal saline [11].

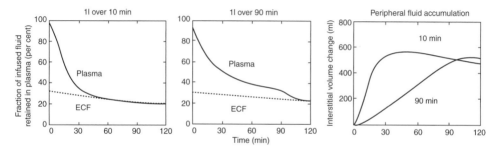

Figure 15.2. The effectiveness of Ringer's solution as a plasma volume expander is greater when given slowly. Computer simulation based on volume kinetic data from thyroid surgery [9], showing how much of the infusion that resides in the plasma when 1 l of acetated Ringer's solution is infused over 10 min (left) and 90 min (middle). The hatched lower line shows the theoretical percentage of the infused fluid that would remain in the the plasma if all fluid had been distributed over the ECF space immediately. Right panel: the expansion of the interstitial fluid space. Note the slow elimination of infused Ringer's during surgery.

Repeated infusions of crystalloid fluid are normally followed by a slightly higher Cl. In contrast, hemorrhage of up to 900 ml reduces Cl by 50% although the blood pressure is unchanged [19].

Colloid fluids differ from crystalloids in that they lack a marked distribution phase. The kinetics then become quite simple. The infused fluid only occupies one body fluid space, which has a size fairly similar to the expected plasma volume, from which elimination occurs according to a mono-exponential function.

Anesthesia and surgery

Anesthesia and surgery exert several effects on the distribution and elimination of crystalloid fluids. The distribution clearance drops by approximately 50% during the onset of spinal, epidural and general anesthesia [20], which increases the plasma volume expansion resulting from an ongoing infusion.

During surgery a reduction in arterial pressure promotes some additional fluid accumulation in the plasma volume, which is reflected by a small size of the central body fluid space.

The most significant finding during surgery is that the *renal clearance is very low*, which has been found during thyroid [9], laparoscopic [21] and open abdominal surgery [22]. One can expect that only 5–15% of a volume load would be excreted within 2 h during surgery, while this fraction is 40–75% in conscious subjects. Hormonal changes, such as aldosterone release, are probably responsible for much of this reduction, half of which can be seen also during experimental anesthesia [23]. Vasodilatation caused by the anesthetic drugs may also play a role by lowering the baseline for Hb concentration.

Low renal clearance increases plasma volume expansion in response to crystalloid fluid, and acts to retain infused fluid during surgery. Hence, it is a delicate balance to provide the patient with an optimal dose of crystalloid fluid as the normal mechanisms for elimination of excess fluid operate poorly. Low renal clearance also implies that monitoring of the urine flow can only indicate hypovolemia but not hypervolemia.

It is unknown whether colloid fluid is excreted more slowly during anesthesia and surgery as compared with the unstressed conscious state.

"Nonfunctional" fluid spaces

Volume kinetic studies performed in the perioperative setting indicate that a single clearance parameter is not always sufficient to describe the distribution of fluid between the central and the peripheral fluid space. A single constant would suffice if there is free flow of fluid between compartments, but fluid seems to accumulate in the periphery during surgery.

Fluid accumulation may be interpreted as allocation of fluid to non-functional spaces, a finding with similarities to the *third space* that was described in the 1960s [24]. In kinetic terms, accumulation implies that a fraction of the infused fluid is not available for excretion, at least not within the period of study. In patients undergoing thyroid surgery, such allocation to nonfunctional spaces amounted to 2 ml/min or approximately 20% of the infused fluid volume, regardless of whether anesthesia was performed with propofol or isoflurane [9].

Ongoing kinetic studies, and also other data [25], indicate that catecholamines play a role in creating such uneven distribution of crystalloid fluid.

Glucose solutions and hypertonic saline

Glucose and hypertonic saline contain molecules that govern the distribution of the accompanying fluid volume by virtue of osmosis. These fluid shifts may be included in volume kinetic analysis, and the forces due to osmosis and those due to the fluid volume alone can be separated [11,26].

The duration of plasma volume expansion by glucose solution is only partly governed by the half-life of infused glucose – renal elimination also operates alongside the osmotic-driven translocation of water to the ICF [26]. In contrast, renal capacity to excrete sodium strongly governs the rate of restoration of baseline plasma volume after infusion of 7.5% saline [27].

Possible clinical use

Volume kinetics can be used to simulate plasma dilution, volume expansion and fluid distribution resulting from infusion of any fluid. This provides insight about how fluid volume expands the body fluid compartments and can be employed for a number of research tasks.

There are two reasons why volume kinetics is not used clinically. The first problem is that the ideal volume expansion during surgery is not known. Such an ideal "target volume expansion" is likely to be dependent on the degree of preoperative dehydration. Patients who have an increase in cardiac output when receiving a crystalloid fluid load when surgery begins ("responders") retain much more of the infused fluid in plasma than those who have decreased cardiac output ("non-responders") [22]. Hence, an optimal Hb baseline is often not at hand at this time.

The second problem is that volume kinetic analysis requires a series of 25–40 very precise Hb measurements. Clinical utility could be greatly increased by noninvasive Hb monitoring, but the devices available for this purpose are not yet accurate enough [28].

References

1. Zdolsek J, Lisander B, Hahn RG. Measuring the size of the extracellular space using bromide, iohexol and sodium dilution. *Anesth Analg* 2005; **101**: 1770–7.

2. Norberg Å, Sandhagen B, Bratteby L-E, *et al.* Do ethanol and deuterium oxide distribute into the same water space in healthy volunteers? *Alcohol Clin Exp Res* 2001; **25**: 1423–30.

3. Henschen S, Busse MW, Zisowsky S, Panning B. Determination of plasma volume and total blood volume using indocyanine green: a short review. *J Med* 1993; **24**: 10–27.

4. Reekers M, Simon MJG, Boer F, *et al.* Puylse dye densitometry and indocyanine green plasma disappareanace in ASA physical status I-II-patients. *Anesth Analg* 2010; **110**: 466–72.

5. De Lorenzo A, Andreoli A, Matthie J, Withers P. Predicting body cell mass with bioimpedance by using theoretical methods. *J Appl Physiol* 1997; **82**: 1542–58.

6. Nadler SB, Hidalgo JU, Bloch T. Prediction of blood volume in normal human adults. *Surgery* 1962; **51**: 224–232.

7. Zhang WB, Hahn RG. Water and solute dynamics after intravenous infusion of new irrigating fluids in the rabbit. *Scand J Urol Nephrol* 1995; **29**: 241–7.

8. Sandfeldt L, Riddez L, Rajs J, *et al.* High-dose intravenous infusion of irrigating fluids containing glycine and mannitol in the pig. *J Surg Res* 2001; **95**: 114–25.

9. Ewaldsson C-A, Hahn RG. Kinetics and extravascular retention of acetated Ringer´s solution during isoflurane and propofol anesthesia for thyroid surgery. *Anesthesiology* 2005; **103**: 460–9.

10. Hahn RG, Drobin D. Rapid water and slow sodium excretion of Ringer´s solution dehydrates cells. *Anesth Analg* 2003; **97**: 1590–4.

11. Drobin D, Hahn RG: Kinetics of isotonic and hypertonic plasma volume expanders. *Anesthesiology* 2002; **96**: 1371–80.

12. Riddez L, Hahn RG, Brismar B, *et al.* Central and regional hemodynamics during acute hypovolemia and volume substitution in volunteers. *Crit Care Med* 1997; **25**: 635–40.

13. Hahn RG. Haemoglobin dilution from epidural-induced hypotension with and without fluid loading. *Acta Anaesthesiol Scand* 1992; **36**: 241–4.

14. Tollofsrud S, Elgo GI, Prough DS, *et al.* The dynamics of vascular volume and fluid shifts of lactated Ringer´s solution and hypertonic-saline-dextran solutions infused in normovolemic sheep. *Anesth Analg* 2001; **93**: 823–31.

15. Hahn RG. Blood volume at the onset of hypotension in TURP performed during epidural anaesthesia. *Eur J Anaesth* 1993; **10**: 219–25.

16. Hahn RG. Volume effect of Ringer solution in the blood during general anaesthesia. *Eur J Anaesth* 1998; **15**: 427–32.

17. Ebert RV, Stead EA. Demonstration that in normal man no reserves of blood are mobilized by exercise, epinephrine, and hemorrhage. *Am J Med Sci* 1941; **201**: 655–64.

18. Hahn RG. Volume kinetics of infusion fluids (review). *Anesthesiology* 2010; **113**: 470–81.

19. Drobin D, Hahn RG. Volume kinetics of Ringer´s solution in hypovolemic volunteers. *Anesthesiology* 1999; **90**: 81–91.

20. Li Y, Zhu S, Hahn RG. The kinetics of Ringer´s solution in young and elderly patients during induction of general and epidural anesthesia. *Acta Anaesth Scand* 2007; **51**: 880–7.

21. Olsson J, Svensén CH, Hahn RG. The volume kinetics of acetated Ringer´s solution during laparoscopic cholecystectomy. *Anesth Analg* 2004; **99**: 1854–60.

22. Svensén CH, Olsson J, Hahn RG. Intravascular fluid administration and hemodynamic performance during open abdominal surgery. *Anesth Analg* 2006; **103**: 671–6.

23. Norberg Å, Hahn RG, Husong Li, *et al.* Population volume kinetics predicts retention of 0.9% saline infused in awake and isoflurane-anesthetized volunteers. *Anesthesiology* 2007; **107**: 24–32.

24. Shires GT, Williams J, Brown F. Acute changes in extracellular fluids associated with major surgical procedures. *Ann Surg* 1961; **154**: 803–10.

25. Nygren A, Redfors B, Thorén A, Ricksten SE. Norepinephrine causes a pressure-dependent plasma volume decrease in clinical vasodilatory shock. *Acta Anaesthesiol Scand* 2010; **54**: 814–20.

26. Hahn RG, Edsberg L, Sjöstrand F. Volume kinetic analysis of fluid shifts accompanying intravenous infusions of glucose solution (review). *Cell Biochem Biophys* 2003; **39**: 211–22.

27. Svensén CH, Waldrop KS, Edsberg L, Hahn RG. Natriuresis and the extracellular volume expansion by hypertonic saline. *J Surg Res* 2003; **113**: 6–12.

28. Hahn RG, Li Y, Zdolsek J. Non-invasive monitoring of blood haemoglobin for analysis of fluid volume kinetics. *Acta Anaesthesiol Scand* 2010; **54**: 1233–40.

Chapter 16

Adverse reactions

Hengo Haljamäe

Intravenous infusion of any type of fluid (crystalloids as well as colloids) for correction of fluid and plasma volume disturbances in connection with surgical procedures includes a potential risk of adverse effects [1]. Such effects may be either local responses at the site of infusion or more generalized systemic reactions, which, in severe cases, may even be life-threatening. Safe clinical practice requires proper knowledge of possible iv fluid-associated risks so that optimal fluid choices and safe administration routines can be used for each individual patient.

In the present survey the iv fluids considered will be those regularly used for rehydration and plasma volume support in the perioperative period. Such fluids include different crystalloid types of solution (glucose solutions, normal saline, Ringer's type of solutions, hypertonic saline) and artificial/synthetic colloids (hydroxyethyl starches – HES, gelatins – GEL, dextrans – DEX). Specific concerns associated with transfusion/infusion of blood, plasma and plasma protein fractions (including human serum albumin, HSA) will not be discussed.

Local adverse effects

Isotonic crystalloid and colloid solutions are mainly non-toxic and do not adversely affect the vessel wall at the site of infusion, unless the fluid is extremely cold or warm, or the osmolality of the fluid is grossly non-physiological. Therefore, local concerns at the site of infusion are due to direct effects of improper fluid temperature or osmolality on the vessel wall causing pain and sometimes the occurrence of thrombophlebitis or thrombosis.

Intravenous infusion of glucose solutions with a glucose concentration of more than 10%, i.e., osmolality of more than 600 mOsm/kg H_2O, are considered to include a potential risk of local inflammatory reactions which may lead to the development of painful thrombophlebitis in the vessel. Solutions with such a high osmolality (> 600 mOsm/kg H_2O) should therefore preferably be infused via a central venous line so that the local osmolar load will be moderated by the rather high blood flow in the central vein.

Hypertonic (7.5%) saline (HS), used for acute fluid resuscitation in trauma situations or perioperatively in the management of patients undergoing major surgical procedures, has an osmolality of about 2400 mOsm/kg H_2O and may consequently induce local inflammatory responses. Therefore, it is not surprising that this type of hyperosmolar fluid has been reported to cause sensations of heat and compression around the arm at the site of infusion

---

Clinical Fluid Therapy in the Perioperative Setting, ed. Robert G. Hahn. Published by Cambridge University Press. © Cambridge University Press 2011.

Table 16.1. Systemic adverse effects caused by crystalloids and colloids commonly used perioperatively.

Temperature-and osmolality-associated sensations
Hypervolemia/hypertension
Excessive tissue hydration/edema formation
Hypothermia
Acid–base balance derangements
Hemostatic disturbances
Hypersensitivity/anaphylactoid /anaphylactic reactions
Tissue deposition/pruritus
Colloid-associated interference with organ function

[2]. These sensations seem to last during the ongoing infusion of the fluid and will disappear after completion of the infusion. Since usually a small volume (about 4 ml/kg) of HS is infused, it appears that these local adverse effects of HS fluid therapy are rather mild and well tolerated [2].

Temperature- and osmolality-associated sensations

Systemic adverse effects of perioperatively used infusion fluids are much more common and may, depending on the causative factors, be classified according to Table 16.1.

Infusion of cold fluid may sometimes cause shivering in response to the temperature change, while fluid of body temperature may cause an unpleasant feeling of "heaviness" in the chest [3]. Rather rapid iv infusion of hyperosmolar HS (7.5% NaCl + 6% dextran 70, HSD), at a dosage of 4 ml/kg within 10 min, has, in addition to previously mentioned local sensations [2], been reported also to cause a feeling of heat, starting in the upper part of the thorax and spreading upwards to the throat, face and head [4]. These sensations following infusion of HSD seem more pronounced in normovolemic than in hypovolemic individuals [4].

Hypervolemia/hypertension

The plasma volume-expanding capacity of colloid-containing iv plasma replacement solutions is dependent on the molecular size and concentration of the colloid and the extent to which the macromolecules remain in the intravascular compartment.

Colloids with a *colloid osmotic pressure* (COP) equal to or lower than that of plasma will, even at a rather high infusion rate, result in a mainly isovolemic plasma volume expansion.

Colloids with a COP higher than that of plasma will, in addition to the intravascular volume expansion, mobilize extravascular fluid from the interstitial compartment into the intravascular compartment. Therefore, the initial intravascular plasma volume-expanding capacity of such solutions will exceed the actual infused volume.

The COP of commonly used plasma replacement fluids varies from half that of normal human serum (4% HSA – about 14 mm Hg) up to a level about eight times higher (20% HSA – about 195 mm Hg) [1,5].

Dextran 70 (6%) has a COP more than twice that of serum and thereby it has a potential to increase plasma volume by about 1.4 times the infused volume. The corresponding plasma volume-expanding capacity of DEX 40 (10%) is about 1.8.

Colloid osmotic pressure variations between half and three times that of normal human serum, depending on molecular weight and concentration of colloid, have been observed for hydroxyethyl starch (HES). This indicates that 10% HES 200/0.5 solutions have the potential to expand the plasma volume considerably while the volume effect of 6% HES is about 1.1. The medium molecular weight HES 130/0.4 with a colloid concentration of 6% has a rather ideal volume effect of about 1.0, whereas that of GEL solutions (usually about 3.5%) is less pronounced and more difficult to assess due to a rather rapid leakage of the small GEL molecules out of the intravascular compartment [1,5].

Considering the rather high plasma volume-supporting efficacy of several of the clinically routinely used colloids, it is obvious that for the euvolemic or only moderately hypovolemic patient there is a potential risk of plasma volume overload and increased blood pressure. Consequently, rapid infusion of a colloid with a good plasma volume-supporting capacity may in a high-risk patient with latent or manifest cardiac failure cause *intravascular volume overload* resulting in circulatory deterioration. Proper measurement of the hemodynamic and cardiac functional consequences of iv volume load is consequently clinically indicated, especially in high-risk patients [1].

Infusion of HS (7.5% NaCl) is considered of value in the early resuscitation of shock and trauma patients, in connection with the perioperative management of surgical patients and in some specific intensive care unit situations [1]. The high osmolality (about 2400 mosm/kg H_2O) of HS will induce an efficient mobilization of fluid from extravascular sources into the intravascular compartment. Infusion of HS therefore includes a potential risk of transiently increased intravascular volume load and hypertension. Such a response pattern may be hazardous for a patient with critical cardiovascular disease and could include a risk of myocardial ischemia and cardiac failure. Therefore, it is of importance to have strict blood pressure criteria (documented hypotension due to hypovolemia) and proper monitoring of the hemodynamic response when HS fluid therapy is given [1].

Similar osmotic fluid mobilization from extravascular sources may be expected at the infusion of other types of hyperosmolar solutions (urea, mannitol, glucose). Infusion of hyperosmolar glucose solutions may in addition be associated with a risk of hyperglycemia and glycosuria, which in case of pronounced glycosuria may result in fluid losses leading to dehydration [1]. In order to avoid severe adverse responses proper monitoring of the patient during the infusion of hyperosmolar solutions is always indicated.

Excessive tissue hydration/edema formation

The choice of crystalloid solutions for plasma volume support in the hypovolemic patient necessitates infusion of a relatively large volume of fluid, about three to four or even up to five times the estimated intravascular volume deficit, in order to achieve normovolemia and hemodynamic stability [6]. This is explained by the rather rapid redistribution of crystalloid from the intravascular space throughout the whole extracellular fluid compartment. Most (60–80%) of the infused fluid will, within 20 to 40 min, lodge in the interstitial space. At the same time plasma COP will be reduced, and a new Starling equilibrium for transcapillary fluid exchange will be established between the intravascular and the interstitial compartments.

The leaking crystalloid fluid accumulates mainly in tissues with a *high compliance*, such as skin and connective tissue, but at the same time there is also an increased fluid content in vital organs, e.g., in the lungs and the gastrointestinal tract [1,5,6]. Therefore, it may be assumed that excessive crystalloid resuscitation could not only include a rather harmless cosmetic problem but also affect vital organ function.

Clinical experience indicates that a significant *weight gain* from fluid resuscitation includes a risk of impaired clinical outcome. A perioperative fluid overload may be more critical for elderly patients with reduced functional capacity of vital organs and therefore negatively affect the recovery process after surgery. Even late adverse effects on cardio-respiratory function after massive crystalloid fluid resuscitation may occur as a "third day" transient circulatory overload. This phenomenon may be explained by a redistribution of tissue edema back into the intravascular compartment [1,5,6]. Perioperative monitoring of body weight changes may be a valuable tool whereby crystalloid overload causing tissue edema can be assessed and monitored.

It is obvious that formation of tissue edema and overhydration-related problems can be moderated if a decrease of COP is avoided by early addition of a colloid with a good plasma volume-supporting capacity [7,8]. Consequently, a combination of fixed crystalloid administration to replace extravascular fluid losses and individualized goal-directed colloid administration to support intravascular volume and COP seems an advantageous approach to perioperative fluid therapy [9].

Hypothermia

The importance of *warming* of iv administered fluids in case of massive volume therapy has been recognized for many years. The deleterious effects caused by infusion of cold fluids and the development of hypothermia are risks of cardiac arrhythmias, impaired tissue perfusion, metabolic disturbances and coagulopathy [10].

Many of the coagulation reactions occur insufficiently at a temperature below 37 °C, and at reduced temperature platelet function is also impaired. Hypothermia will furthermore reduce the hepatic synthesis of coagulation factors. Therefore, in case of hypothermia induced by liberal perioperative infusion of cold fluids, there is an obvious risk of coagulopathy due to the temperature effect on the coagulation cascade.

Coagulopathy is further aggravated by the dilution of coagulation factors caused by the fluid infusion. These factors may consequently affect perioperative blood loss and thereby the need for blood transfusion.

The general clinical concept to be favored is that iv-administered fluids should be warmed, especially if massive volume therapy is needed, unless body temperature of the fluid recipient is increased in response to infectious complications/septic states.

Acid–base balance derangements

Perioperatively used crystalloid solutions may be acidotic due to a high chloride content. Infusion of such a fluid, e.g., physiological saline (0.9% NaCl; 154 mmol/l of Na and 154 mmol/l of Cl) may cause hyperchloremic acidosis and thereby worsen any prevailing acidosis due to tissue hypoperfusion prior to the fluid administration.

Prolonged surgery (≥ 4 h) has for instance been shown to result in increased chloride levels and negative effects on acid–base balance when perioperative fluid therapy is based on normal saline infusion [11]. It seems that the increase in the chloride concentration will cause a decrease in plasma strong ion difference (SID = $[Na^+]$ + $[K^+]$ + $[Ca^{2+}]$ + $[Mg^{2+}]$ – $[Cl^-]$ – [other strong anions]) and thereby induce acidosis. Hyperchloremic metabolic acidosis may cause hemostatic defects and impair renal function and urine output [12].

It should furthermore be remembered that in addition to saline administration the infusion fluid of several of the available colloids is based on 0.9% NaCl. Infusion of such a colloid will further increase the chloride load.

The use of Ringer's types of solution, having a lower chloride concentration (usually about 110 mmol/l), prevents the occurrence of the metabolic acidosis resulting from hyperchloremia. Ringer's solutions have, in addition, a buffering capacity of their own due to the content of either lactate or acetate [1,6]. In the metabolic breakdown of these substances bicarbonate will be formed. Therefore, new colloid (HES) preparations are also based on balanced electrolyte composition [13]. Such balanced colloid preparations seem to have fewer adverse effects on acid-base balance than saline based ones.

Hemostatic disturbances

Hemostatic disturbances may be caused by all types of available infusion fluids, i.e., crystalloids as well as colloids (Table 16.2). Basic mechanisms involved are dilution of endogenous circulating coagulation factors, hypothermia and acidosis (as considered above), and specific interactions of fluid components (usually colloid associated) with normal hemostatic mechanisms.

Crystalloid-associated

Crystalloid fluid therapy exerts only minor effects on coagulation and hemostasis. The plasma volume expansion achieved with crystalloids is rather small and balanced physiological Ringer's types of solution do not themselves exert any specific effects on hemostatic mechanisms. Therefore, crystalloid resuscitation does not significantly affect hemostatic competence unless extensive volume of fluid is infused.

The hemodilution achieved at more extensive plasma volume expansion will lower the concentration of coagulation factors and, in case of excessive chloride load (infusion of physiological saline), hemostatic defects may be caused by the ensuing hyperchloremic metabolic acidosis as discussed above [1]. Therefore, Ringer's types of fluid with a lower chloride content and a buffering capacity (lactate or acetate content) should be preferred to minimize the risk of hemostatic disturbances. The fluid should furthermore be warmed so that hypothermia-induced negative effects on hemostatic competence are prevented.

Colloid-associated

All colloidal plasma substitutes interfere with the physiological mechanisms of hemostasis either through a non-specific effect correlated to the degree of hemodilution or through specific actions of the macromolecules on platelet function, coagulation proteins and/or the fibrinolytic system [14,15]. The risk of coagulopathy associated with infusion of colloid differs between the different available artificial/synthetic colloids (Table 16.2).

Perioperative use of dextran and some of the older HES preparations has been recognized as more problematic than that of more recent HES preparations (tetrastarch) and gelatin [1,5,15,16].

Hydroxyethyl starches are widely used plasma substitutes for correcting perioperative hypovolemia. Hydroxyethyl starch preparations are defined by concentration, molar substitution (MS), mean molecular weight (M[w]), the C(2)/C(6) ratio of substitution, the solvent and the origin of the product (amylopectin from waxy maize or potato) [16].

Table 16.2. Influences of infusion fluids on blood coagulation and hemostasis.

Type of fluid	Factors influencing hemostatic mechanisms
Crystalloids	excessive dilution of coagulation factors
	hypothermia
	hyperchloremic metabolic acidosis following NaCl infusion
Colloids	*General effects*
	dilution of plasma-clotting proteins
	hypothermia
	Colloid-specific impairment of hemostatic competence
	Dose dependent but – DEX > HES > GEL
	• HES (high MW > medium or low MW)
	– decrease factor VIII/von Willebrand complex
	– inhibition of platelet function
	– accelerated fibrin clot formation
	• DEX (a general "antithrombotic" potency)
	– decrease in factor VIII/von Willebrand complex
	– enhanced fibrinolytic activity
	– moderation of molecular structure and tensile behaviour of fibrin
	• GEL (minor intrinsic effects)
	– a von Willebrand-like syndrome
	– impaired ristocetin-induced platelet aggregation

DEX, dextran; GEL, gelatin; HES, hydroxyethyl starch

The *first generation* of HES preparation (hetastarch) showing a high M(w) (> 450 kD) and a high MS (> 0.7) exerted negative effects on hemostasis. Bleeding complications associated with infusion of such high molecular HES were therefore all too uncommon [1,14,15,16]. A von Willebrand-like syndrome is induced by hetastarch, seen as decreased factor VIII coagulant activity and von Willebrand factor (vWF) antigen, and affecting factor VIII-related ristocetin cofactor [16]. Hydroxyethyl starch preparations also exert inhibiting effects on platelet function by reducing the availability of the functional receptor for fibrinogen on the platelet surface [16–18].

The effects of HES on coagulation are dose dependent. Infusion of moderate doses produces rather trivial and transient effects on blood clotting while the higher the initial dose, the molecular weight, the C2/C6 hydroxyethyl ratio and the degree of hydroxyethyl substitution, the more pronounced the effects are on factor VIII/von Willebrand complex.

The *third generation* of HES preparations (tetrastarch) are more rapidly degradable due to a lower M(w) (130 kD) and a lower MS (< 0.5) [14–16]. These HES 130/0.4 products are much safer to use and exert only negligibly negative effects on hemostasis [16].

The latest type of HES preparations are furthermore dissolved in balanced, plasma-adapted solutions that no longer contain nonphysiological amounts of sodium chloride [13,16,19]. These plasma-adapted HES solutions exert minor effects on clot formation, clot strength and platelet aggregation [16]. Additional beneficial effects of this type of HES include moderation of surgery-associated inflammatory reaction. Therefore, these new third-generation HES preparations seem much safer and more suitable for perioperative plasma volume support than the older heta- or pentastarch HES solutions [13,16]. An additional advantage is that a safe daily dosage as high as 50 ml/kg of HES 130/0.4 (6%) can be given routinely without risk of adverse effects on hemostasis.

Dextran (DEX) is known to exert antithrombotic effects by inducing hemodilution, enhancing microvascular blood flow and modulating the hemostatic system) [1,5,6]. Combined effects of dextran on the concentration of coagulation factors, red blood cell aggregation, platelet activity, plasma levels of von Willebrand factor (vWF) and associated factor VIII (VIII:c), plasminogen activation and plasma fibrinogen levels are all factors contributing to the reduced hemostatic competence induced by dextran [1,5]. The molecular structure and tensile behavior of fibrin is modulated by dextran so that clots formed in the presence of dextran are more fragile, which, together with the enhanced fibrinolytic activity, results in increased lysis of already formed clots.

Since dextran counteracts the hypercoagulable state induced by surgery and other types of trauma it has been considered a plasma substitute that may significantly reduce the risk of perioperative pulmonary embolism and adult respiratory distress syndrome [1]. However, interference with hemostatic mechanisms includes an increased risk of disturbed hemostasis and increased blood loss. Therefore, perioperative use of dextran has, to a large extent, been discontinued in most countries since safer colloids for plasma volume support are now available.

Gelatin solutions seem to affect hemostasis, in addition to direct dilutional effects, only to a limited extent. Binding of vWF to gelatin has been suggested to induce a von Willebrand-like syndrome with lengthening of bleeding time, impaired ristocetin-induced platelet aggregation and decreased levels of plasma vWF [16,20].

The clinical experience of volume replacement with gelatin in connection with major surgery is that platelet function usually remains within the normal range and, therefore, gelatin appears to be relatively safe from of hemostatic point of view [21]. This is also evident by the fact that no maximum dose is prescribed for gelatin preparations.

Hypersensitivity/anaphylactoid/anaphylactic reactions

All intravenous colloids can induce the anaphylactoid type of reactions but the available incidence numbers vary to a considerable extent between different countries depending on efficacy of official reporting systems, true local variations in predisposition or endemic antibody titers and use of prophylactic measures.

Hydroxyethyl starches

An extensive prospective study by Laxenaire *et al.* in 1994 reported a low frequency of anaphylactoid reactions to HES [22]. At this time the old types of HES products were used, but it is obvious that the antigenicity of new third-generation HES preparations is very low [16]. Therefore, the general concept is that the safety profile of modern HES preparations is rather optimal since it carries a very low risk for occurrence of anaphylactoid reactions.

Dextrans are associated with a potential risk of anaphylactoid/anaphylactic reactions (DIARs) that can range from mild skin manifestations to circulatory and respiratory deterioration, sometimes with fatal outcome [1,22]. Mild reactions were assumed to be either antibody dependent or unspecific. Patients reacting at the infusion of dextran have rather high titers of preformed, circulating dextran-reactive antibodies, predominately of IgG class. Infusion of dextran to such patients results in generation of large immune complexes leading to release of vasoactive mediators and clinical symptoms.

Safe use of dextran should include preinjection of low-molecular dextran-1 (1 kDa) prior to infusion of the plasma volume expander. By this hapten inhibition principle any anti-dextran antibodies present in the recipient will be inactivated since complexes too small to be reactive will be formed between the antibodies and dextran-1 [1,23].

Gelatin-based plasma substitutes consist of polydispersed polypeptides produced by degradation of bovine collagen. Three types of modified gelatin products are available: crosslinked or oxypolygelatins, urea-crosslinked and succinylated or modified fluid gelatin. Anaphylactic or anaphylactoid reactions to gelatin solutions may occur but are relatively uncommon.

The allergic/anaphylactoid potential of gelatin solutions probably differs considerably between the different gelatin preparations. The urea cross-linked polygeline preparation has been reported rather commonly to induce histamine release that may influence cardiorespiratory stability [25]. Although the modern gelofucine type of gelatin products is considered to be more safe, caution should still be practiced when used for patients with known allergic tendency.

Tissue deposition and pruritus

Dextran and gelatin seem to be fully metabolized to CO_2 and H_2O while high-molecular HES is not completely degraded or metabolized [1].

Insufficient metabolic breakdown and tissue deposition is a problem associated more commonly with older types of high-molecular weight variants of HES (450/0.7) than with medium-molecular weight HES preparations with a lower degree of substitution (130–200/0.4–0.5), which are more rapidly metabolized and eliminated. Some concern has been raised that HES residues may also irreversibly block the reticuloendothelial system (RES), but no concrete evidence of severe immunosuppression has emerged to date.

Pentastarch (HES 200/0.5) might persist in human lymph nodes and muscle biopsies for at least 10 months after a dose of only 1 g/kg, and HES residues can be found in human skin macrophages up to 19 months after HES administration [1,25].

The pathophysiological basis for HES-associated pruritus is considered to be a widespread tissue deposition of HES, prominently in macrophages, perineural cells, keratinocytes and Langerhans cells. Usually several weeks elapse between HES exposure and the onset of pruritus. This HES-associated pruritus is frequently severe and protracted with a serious negative impact on patient quality of life, including sleep disturbance, disruption of daily routine and mental distress, since it can persist for 12–24 months.

It is obvious that a rather large dose of HES is needed to induce pruritus. When relatively small volumes of HES are infused, it seems that the incidence of itching 8 weeks after surgery is similar to that seen after infusion of Ringer´s solution [1]. Since there is an obvious dose–response relationship, the patient at risk is the one receiving repeated HES infusions for several days, often infused for otological and neurological reasons in order to achieve hemodilution, improved microvascular blood flow and enhanced organ perfusion.

The chemical improvement of starch colloids that has taken place in recent years has affected metabolic degradation and tissue storage. The newer 130/0.4 HES preparations do not accumulate in plasma, not even in case of repeated application, and tissue storage is reduced by approximately 75%. Therefore, it may be assumed that the more efficient metabolic degradation in the body and reduced tissue deposition will influence the safety profile and considerably reduce the incidence of HES-induced pruritus previously seen after large-dose administration of older types of HES preparations.

Only a few reports on pruritus caused by HES 130/0.4 after high or repeated doses are available [16].

Colloid-associated interference with organ function

Renal failure has been reported following infusion of dextran 40 (10%) and HES, as well as gelatin [27]. There is an increased risk of renal failure developing in dehydrated patients with latent renal failure who receive repeated high doses of hyperoncotic colloid causing hyperviscosity of the urine and tubular obstruction in the kidney [27].

The patient at risk for renal failure after HES infusion is the critically ill trauma patient, or septic patient with severely disturbed hemodynamics and fluid imbalance [16]. For such high-risk patients administration of adequate amounts of crystalloid is essential to avoid the risk of hyperoncotic renal failure.

Effects of HES on organs are not only dose dependent and time related, but also dependent on the molecular characteristics of the HES infusion fluid administered. The medium-molecular type of HES with a lower degree of hydroxyethyl substitution, e.g., HES 130/0.4, seems to be much safer than high-molecular weight HES with a high degree of hydroxyethyl substitution.

In the perioperative period there is no evidence for HES-induced negative effects on renal function, not even in patients undergoing major surgical procedures. Compared with gelatin, volume expansion with HES during abdominal aortic aneurism surgery has been shown rather to improve renal function and reduce the risk of renal injury [28]. In patients undergoing coronary artery bypass surgery 6% HES 130/0.4 is a safe alternative colloid for priming the cardiopulmonary bypass circuit and for perioperative volume replacement [29].

Conclusions

All types of intravenous fluids, crystalloids as well as colloids, may induce adverse reactions in case of improper use or presence of patient-associated specific risk factors.

- Local adverse effects at the site of infusion can be avoided by appropriate control of fluid temperature and osmolarity.
- Systemic adverse responses to fluid therapy caused by too rapid infusion or excessive fluid administration resulting in hypervolemia, circulatory overload or, in case of fluid therapy with mainly crystalloids, formation of tissue edema or development of hyperchloremic acidosis, should be avoided by proper choice of a balanced type of fluid (Ringer's rather than saline) and by adequate monitoring of the physiological responses to the fluid therapy.
- Adverse effects of colloids on hemostasis can mainly be avoided if the choice of colloid for plasma volume support is based on a proper knowledge of the specific molecular characteristics of each available colloid, and the way in which and at what dosage the colloid compromises the hemostatic competence. Use of HES (preferably HES in balanced electrolyte solution) or gelatin rather than dextran will prevent negative effects on hemostasis.

- Colloid-associated problems due to tissue deposition resulting in adverse effects on organ function (renal failure, itching) seem to have reduced since newer types of colloids have been introduced that are more rapidly metabolized and eliminated.
- A key factor for the safe use of iv fluids is that the fluid therapy is always based on a proper knowledge of the specific needs of the individual patient and that the potential hazards associated with the infusion of the various available fluids are known so that safe practice can always be provided.

References

1. Haljamäe H. Adverse reactions to infusion fluids. In: Hahn RG, Prough DS, Svensen CH, eds. *Perioperative Fluid Therapy*. New York: Informa Healthcare USA, 2007, pp. 459–75.

2. Järvelä K, Kööbi T, Kauppinen P, *et al.* Effects of hypertonic 75 mg/ml (7.5%) saline on extracellular water volume when used for preloading before spinal anaesthesia. *Acta Anaesthesiol Scand* 2001; **45**: 776–81.

3. Tølløfsrud S, Bjerkelund CE, Kongsgaard U, *et al.* Cold and warm infusion of Ringer´s acetate in healthy volunteers: the effects on haemodynamic parameters, transcapillary fluid balance, diuresis and atrial peptides. *Acta Anaesthesiol Scand* 1993; **37**: 768–73.

4. Tølløfsrud S, Tønnessen T, Skraastad O, *et al.* Hypertonic saline and dextran in normovolaemic and hypovolaemic healthy volunteers increases interstitial and intravascular fluid volumes. *Acta Anaesthesiol Scand* 1998; **42**: 145–53.

5. Haljamäe H, Dahlqvist M, Walentin F. Artificial colloids in clinical practice: pros and cons. *Baillière´s Clin Anaesthesiol* 1997; **11**: 49–79.

6. Haljamäe H. Crystalloids versus colloids: The controversy. In: *NATA Textbook*. Paris: R & J Éditions Médicale, 1999, pp. 27–36.

7. Prien T, Backhaus N, Pelser F, *et al.* Effects of intraoperative fluid administration and colloid osmotic pressure on the formation of intestinal edema during gastrointestinal surgery. *J Clin Anesth* 1990; **2**: 317–23.

8. Lang K, Boldt J, Suttner S, *et al.* Colloids versus crystalloids and tissue oxygen tension in patients undergoing major abdominal surgery. *Anesth Analg* 2001; **93**: 405–9.

9. Bundgaard-Nielsen M, Secher NH, Kehlet H. "Liberal" vs "restrictive" perioperative fluid therapy – a critcal assessment of the evidence. *Acta Anaesthesiol Scand* 2009; **53**: 843–51.

10. Rohrer MJ, Natale AM. Effect of hypothermia on the coagulation cascade. *Crit Care Med* 1992; **20**: 1402–5.

11. Waters JH, Miller LR, Clack S, *et al.* Cause of metabolic acidosis in prolonged surgery. *Crit Care Med* 1999; **27**: 2142–6.

12. Stephens RC, Mythen MG. Saline based fluids can cause a significant acidosis that may be clinically relevant. *Crit Care Med* 2000; **28**: 3375–7.

13. Base EM, Standl T, Lassnigg A, *et al.* Efficacy and safety of hydroxyethyl starch 6% 130/0.4 in a balanced electrolyte solution (Volulyte) during cardiac surgery. *J Cardiothorac Vasc Anesth* 2011; Ahead of print.

14. de Jonge E, Levi M. Effects of different plasma substitutes on blood coagulation: a comparative review. *Crit Care Med* 2001; **29**: 1261–7.

15. van der Linden P, Ickx BE. The effects of colloid solutions on hemostasis. *Can J Anaesth* 2006; **53**: S30–9.

16. Boldt J. Modern rapidly degradable hydroxyethyl starches: current concepts. *Anesth Analg* 2009; **108**:1574–82.

17. Franz A, Braunlich P, Gamsjager T, *et al.* The effects of hydroxyethyl starches of varying molecular weights on platelet function. *Anesth Analg* 2001; **92**: 1402–7.

18. Huraux C, Ankri AA, Eyraud D, *et al.* Hemostatic changes in patients receiving

hydroxyethyl starch: the influence of ABO blood group. *Anesth Analg* 2001; **92**: 1396–1401.

19. Casutt M, Kristoffy A, Schuepfer G, *et al.* Effects on coagulation of balanced (130/0.42) and non-balanced (130/0.4) hydroxyethyl starch or gelatin compared with balanced Ringer´s solution: an in vitro study using two different viscoelastic coagulation tests ROTEMTM and SONOCLOTTM. *Br J Anaesth* 2010; **105**: 273–81.

20. de Jonge E, Levi M, Berends F, *et al.* Impaired haemostasis by intravenous administration of a gelatin-based plasma expander in human subjects. *Thromb Haemost* 1998; **79**: 286–90.

21. Hüttner I, Boldt J, Haisch G, *et al.* Influence of different colloids on molecular markers of haemostasis and platelet function in patients undergoing major abdominal surgery. *Br J Anaesth* 2000; **85**: 417–23.

22. Laxenaire MC, Charpentier C, Feldman L. Anaphylactoid reactions to colloid plasma substitutes: incidence, risk factors, mechanisms. A French multicentre prospective study. *Ann Fr Anesth Reanim* 1994; **13**: 301–10.

23. Ljungström K-G. Safety of dextran in relation to other colloids – ten years

experience with hapten inhibition. *Infusionsther. Transfusionsmed* 1993; **20**: 206–210.

24. Lorenz W, Duda D, Dick W, *et al.* Incidence and clinical importance of perioperative histamine release: randomised study of volume loading and antihistamines after induction of anaesthesia. *Lancet* 1994; **343**: 933–40.

25. Bork K. Pruritus precipitated by hydroxyethyl starch: a review. *Br J Dermatol* 2005; **152**: 3–12.

26. Moran M, Kapsner C. Acute renal failure associated with elevated plasma oncotic pressure. *N Engl J Med* 1987; **317**: 150–3.

27. Haskell LP, Tannenberg AM. Elevated urinary specific gravity in acute oliguric renal failure due to HES. *NY State J Med* 1988; **88**: 387–8.

28. Mahmood A, Gossling P, Vohra RK. Randomized clinical trial comparing the effects on renal function of hydroxyethyl starch or gelatine during aortic aneurysm surgery. *Br J Surg* 2007; **94**: 427–33.

29. Ooi JS, Ramzisham AR, Zamrin MD. Is 6% hydroxyethylstarch 130/0.4 safe in coronary artery bypass graft surgery? *Asian Cardiovasc Thorac Ann* 2009; **17**: 368–72.

Chapter 17

Irrigating fluids

Robert G. Hahn

A number of different sterile water solutions are employed for irrigation in connection with various operative procedures. Medical aspects of these are primarily of interest when used during endoscopy. Here, these solutions dilate the operating field and wash away debris and blood. A potential complication of such irrigation is absorption of the fluid by the patient, even to the extent that symptoms ensue. The rate and volume of fluid absorbed, as well as the type of fluid used, are of importance to the appearance of this iatrogenic complication.

Patients developing overt symptoms due to absorption of irrigating fluid were first described in connection with transurethral resection of the prostate (TURP). The complication was named "transurethral resection (TUR) syndrome" and was proved during the 1940s to be due to uptake of more than 3 l of sterile water used for irrigation. An intense effort started to add various non-electrolyte solutes to the sterile water for the purpose of preventing fluid absorption from causing hemolysis-induced renal failure. In the mid-1950s the hemolysis problem had disappeared but other types of adverse effects continued to appear. Since then, several hundred life-threatening and even fatal TUR syndromes have been reported [1].

The TUR syndrome might also develop in other operations, including transcervical resection of the endometrium (TCRE), transurethral resection of bladder tumors, cystoscopy, arthroscopy, rectal tumor surgery, vesical ultrasonic lithotripsy and percutaneous nephrolithotripsy.

The most common irrigating fluids used today contain one or two solutes, such as glycine, sorbitol or mannitol, to prevent hemolysis in case of absorption. These fluids are intended for *monopolar* electrocautery, i.e., when current travels between the tip of the resectoscope to an electrode placed on the patient's hip or back.

With *bipolar* electrocautery the current only travels cross the tip of the resectoscope, and electrolyte-containing solutions (most often normal saline) can then be used.

Sterile water is still often used during cystoscopy as it provides superior vision for the urologist.

Mechanisms

Irrigating fluid is most often absorbed directly into the vascular system during TURP and TCRE and implies that a vein has been severed by the electrosurgery. The event usually starts in the middle or at the end of the surgery, and continues until it is completed [2].

Clinical Fluid Therapy in the Perioperative Setting, ed. Robert G. Hahn. Published by Cambridge University Press. © Cambridge University Press 2011.

Extravasation occurs after perforations of anatomic structures with the resectoscope. The perforated tissue is the prostatic capsule in TURP, the uterine wall in TCRE and the bladder wall during cystoscopy and transurethral resection of bladder tumors. Extravasation is the predominant route of absorption during renal stone surgery [3].

Smoking is the only constitutional patient factor associated with large-scale fluid absorption during TURP [4], which is probably due to anoxia-induced enlargement of the prostate vessels. Transurethral resection in prostate cancer is associated with the same incidence of fluid absorption as those with benign tissue [2].

Fluid absorption increases with the extent of the resection since the exposure to the fluid then becomes prolonged [2].

During TCRE, fluid absorption occurs more often when fibroids are resected [5]. Some extravasation via the Fallopian tubes can be expected to occur as the fluid pressure used is much higher than during TURP [6].

Incidence and clinical presentation

Symptoms of fluid absorption occur in between 1% and 8% of TURPs performed [1]. Absorption in excess of 1 l of glycine solution is associated with a statistically increased risk of symptoms [7]. This has been reported in between 5% and 20% of TURPs performed [2,8]. Extravasation is the cause in about 20% of these patients [7].

Fluid absorption seems to be slightly more common during TCRE and percutaneous stone surgery than during TURP [9, 10].

The incidence and severity of symptoms for increasing amounts of absorbed fluid have been best established for glycine solution during TURP. Olsson et al. [7] recorded an average of 1.3 symptoms from the circulatory and nervous systems in each TURP during which very little or no fluid was absorbed (0–300 ml). This figure increased to 2.3 symptoms per operation when between 1 and 2 l of glycine 1.5% was taken up, while 5.8 symptoms developed when the absorption exceeded 3 l. The dose-dependent increase in the number of symptoms has been confirmed in later prospective studies [8,11].

During surgery, the patient may experience transient prickling and burning sensations in the face and neck, chest pain, become restless and complain of headache. Bradycardia and arterial hypotension are very common signs of volume overload, which occasionally progress to pulmonary edema.

Nausea and arterial hypotension followed by vomiting and low urinary output are typical symptoms in the postoperative period [7,8,11]. Absorption of a few hundred milliliters is associated with transient cognitive dysfunction [12], while apparent confusion might occur after absorption of 1–2 l [13], which, with larger absorption volumes, eventually results in coma [14].

Abdominal pain is a common first sign of extravasation, which is further associated with a higher incidence of arterial hypotension and poor urinary output [15].

Mild TUR syndromes are incomplete and easily overlooked. A drop in arterial pressure at the end of surgery and postoperative nausea is the most common presentation. The severe TUR syndrome is rare and occurs perhaps in 0.1–0.5% of operations. A French review of 24 severe TUR syndromes showed neurological (92%) and cardiovascular symptoms (54%), visual disturbances (42%), digestive symptoms (25%) and renal failure (21%). The mortality rate was 25% [16].

The irrigating solutions

Glycine is an amino acid with a dose-dependent half-life of between 40 min and several hours [17]. Glycine is an inhibitory neurotransmittor in the retina and absorption sometimes causes visual disturbances or transient blindness, which always resolve within 24 h.

Elimination occurs by direct cleavage in the liver, which is a process that yields ammonia. Those who absorb glycine may develop hyperammonemic encephalopathy, which is associated with blood ammonia concentrations > 100 µmol/l (normal range 10–35) [18]. A genetic disposition seems to be involved since only 15–20% of a group of volunteers had a rise in blood ammonia when challenged by glycine overload [19].

Absorption of glycine solution induces osmotic diuresis, whereby 5–10% of an excess dose becomes excreted along with electrolytes, including sodium. This creates an absolute loss of sodium from the body which undoubtedly prolongs the hyponatremia that always results from dilution of the extracellular fluid (ECF) with electrolyte-free irrigating fluid. Glycine is usually marketed in a 1.5% solution, which is slightly hypo-osmotic.

Mannitol is an isomer of glucose that is marketed as a 3% or 5% solution, of which the latter is iso-osmotic. The elimination half-life is 100–130 min but is markedly longer in patients with a raised serum creatinine concentration. Mannitol cannot be metabolized and is excreted unchanged in the urine. The lack of reabsorption causes osmotic diuresis.

Circulatory symptoms following absorption of mannitol 3% are as common as for glycine 1.5%, but neurological symptoms are rare [8].

Sorbitol is metabolized to fructose and glucose in the liver with a half-life of 30 min. Overload with sorbitol may be complicated by lactic acidosis [20], and intolerance to a metabolite, fructose, can be life-threatening. In commercial solutions sorbitol is often combined with mannitol in a 5:1 or 2:1 ratio.

A comparison between glycine 1.5% and a combination of sorbitol–mannitol solutions did not reveal any difference in symptomatology [21].

Sterile water causes hemolysis and renal damage if absorbed into the blood. Therefore this irrigating solution should only be used *without* electrocautery, i.e., for visual inspections.

These hypo-osmotic irrigating fluids hydrate the ECF space but also add water to the intracellular fluid (ICF). Volume expansion of the ICF becomes more apparent with time when glycine and sorbitol are used as solutes as they undergo intracellular metabolism [22].

Normal saline is used for irrigation with the bipolar resection technique. Infusion of 2 l of normal saline in volunteers was followed by mental changes and discomfort from swelling [23]. Normal saline also gives rise to hyperchloremic metabolic acidosis due to its high amount of chloride [24]. However, the classical symptoms of "TUR syndrome" seem to be absent [25].

Pathophysiology

The TUR syndrome induced by an electrolyte-free irrigating fluid has a complex pathophysiology [1]. Key elements comprise a two-stage cardiovascular disturbance, hyponatremia and cerebral edema.

The cardiovascular response to fluid absorption consists of transient hypervolemia with increased central hemodynamic pressures, which level off within 15 min. This phase might involve chest pain, dyspnea and acute pulmonary edema on the operating table.

Hypervolemia is followed by a hypokinetic phase with low cardiac output, hypovolemia and low arterial pressure [26]. Disturbances of heart function include bradycardia and depression of the ST segment and the T wave. The Frank–Starling mechanism of the heart is probably overwhelmed by the large amount of fluid, but cardiac function is also impaired by fluid-induced damage to the myocardium [22, 26–29]. Glycine causes more damage to the myocardium than other fluids [27].

Hyponatremia (< 120 mmol/l) is a feared but invariable consequence of absorption of electrolyte-free irrigating fluid [14]. Hyponatremia is aggravated by osmotic diuresis, which attracts sodium ions despite the presence of hyponatremia [22].

Hyponatremia is typically accompanied by hypo-osmolality (reduction by 10–25 mosmol/kg) since most irrigating fluids are hypo-osmolar. These changes promote brain edema, which lowers consciousness a few hours after the surgery.

Serum potassium often increases transiently by 15–25% and a moderately severe metabolic acidosis develops. The risk of urosepsis is increased [8].

The kidneys ultimately swell in response to large amounts of irrigating fluid, which is followed by poor urinary output and ultimately by renal damage and anuria. Absorption of sterile water exerts a more direct toxic effect on the kidneys due to the accompanying hemolysis.

Death from the TUR syndrome is caused by cardiovascular collapse and shock during the hypokinetic hemodynamic phase, or else by cerebral herniation resulting from brain edema.

Comparisons between the different irrigating fluids show that mannitol solution appears to be better than glycine with respect to tissue damage [27] and mortality [30] (animals) and symptoms (volunteers [31] and patients [8]).

Normal saline does not cause brain edema, but the experience of this fluid with regard to other symptoms is limited. Besides abdominal discomfort and nausea [23], large amounts of normal saline promote the development of pulmonary edema.

Animal experiments show that replacing electrolyte-free irrigating fluids with normal saline reduces, but does not eliminate, tissue damage [29] and mortality [32]. In any event, symptoms of the TUR syndrome are a smaller issue when using normal saline as the irrigant as compared with glycine 1.5% [25], which usually rates worst in comparison with other fluids [27,30,31].

Measuring fluid absorption

Absorption of electrolyte-free irrigating fluid can be estimated by measuring *serum sodium* at the very end of surgery. The correlation between the decrease in serum sodium from the preoperative value and volume of irrigant absorbed is somewhat dependent on the period of time during which absorption has occurred. However, a good estimate can be obtained by taking a decrease of 5–6 mmol/l to represent absorption of 1 l of fluid during TURP, and that 10–12 mmol/l corresponds to absorption of twice as much volume [31,33].

The hyponatremic response to fluid absorption in females undergoing TCRE is stronger, and 1 l of fluid corresponds to a reduction of approximately 10 mmol/l in serum sodium. In both groups of patients, the drop in serum sodium is only 1/3 as large at the end of surgery in response to fluid that has been absorbed by extravasation [33] (Figure 17.1a).

The possibility to assess fluid absorption by serum sodium does not exist when using normal saline, although the addition of glucose to a concentration of 0.5% in the saline solution can serve as replacement [34].

The *volumetric fluid balance* is based on a calculation of the difference between the amount of irrigating fluid used and the volume recovered. Positive values are regarded as

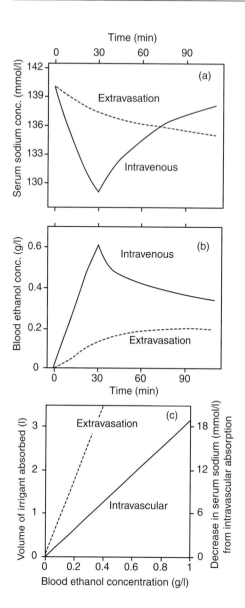

Figure 17.1. Expected course of serum sodium (a) and blood ethanol concentration (b) (the latter measured in the expired breath) during and after TURP during which absorption of 2 l of irrigating fluid containing glycine 1.5% and ethanol 1% has occurred over 30 min depending on the route of absorption. (c) Nomogram correlating blood ethanol and serum sodium cocentrations with the volume of irrigant absorbed during TURP. For intravascular absorption, the nomogram is valid at any time during the operation. For extravasation, the correlation with fluid absorption relates to the steady state ethanol level, which usually occurs after the surgery has ended. TURP, transurethral resection of the prostate.

absorption. The accuracy is moderately good, and errors up to 1 l can be made due to variations in bag-to-bag content, spillage on the floor and the addition of blood and urine to the irrigating fluid returns. The volumetric fluid balance is less prone to error during TCRE.

Ethanol has been added to the irrigating fluid to a concentration of 1% and the body concentration measured used an index of fluid absorption. Measurements of the ethanol level in exhaled breath can be made during surgery with relatively little effort. The sensitivity is superior to the other two methods (approximately 100 ml is detected) and has the benefit of being non-invasive (Figure 17.1b). Ethanol monitoring has been well evaluated worldwide and is an excellent educational tool for urologists-in-training [33]. The method might also be used during TCRE [9].

Measuring serum sodium has the purpose of confirming that fluid absorption is the cause of the symptoms. On the other hand, non-invasive methods that can be repeated perioperatively, like volumetric balance and the ethanol method, open up the possibility to prevent large-scale fluid absorption from occurring. Once data indicate that 1 l of fluid has been absorbed it is suggested that the operation should be concluded earlier than planned, and after 2 l it becomes even more important to stop surgery. An early indication that irrigating fluid has been absorbed allows the optimal level of postoperative care to be chosen and also that earliest possible treatment can be initiated.

Prevention

Fluid absorption and blood loss is reduced, but not eliminated, by vaporizing rather than resecting tissue.

The irrigating fluid used during TURP might be evacuated through a suprapubic trocar. This allows the use of continuous irrigation at a low fluid pressure, which speeds up the operation but increases the use of irrigating fluid. Low-pressure irrigation limits or prevents fluid absorption as long as the outflow is not obstructed by debris and blood clots.

Fluid absorption varies between surgeons and depends on their skill in avoiding prostatic capsule perforations and the opening up of venous sinuses.

There is a belief among urologists that dangerous fluid absorption during TURP can be prevented by limiting the operating time to 1 h. However, the odds for having absorption involve a similar likelihood over time, which accumulates to a gradually increased total risk [2]. Hence, massive fluid absorption might already be at hand after 20 min of surgery.

Placing the irrigating fluid bag at low height above the operating table is of little help because urologists tend to operate at a much lower fluid pressure than made possible by the bag height [35,36].

The bipolar resection technique allows the use of normal saline for irrigation, and is often claimed to prevent the TUR syndrome. Experience with fluid overload during bipolar resection is still limited. There is no reason to believe that fluid absorption will be less frequent, but the TUR syndrome is likely to have a different appearance.

Treatment

The TUR syndrome requires general *supportive measures* if breathing and/or consciousness is affected. Severe hypotension should be treated promptly with colloid volume loading, intravenous calcium and adrenergic drugs.

Hypertonic saline should be infused when the hemodynamics is under control. The indication requires either that symptoms have developed or that the serum sodium concentration has fallen to below 120 mmol/l, which corresponds to absorption of approximately 3.5 l of fluid (Figure 17.1c).

Hypertonic saline combats cerebral edema and expands plasma volume, reduces cellular swelling and increases urinary excretion.

Both experimental [37] and clinical [14,38] studies support the usefulness of treating the TUR syndrome with hypertonic saline. Above all, raising the serum sodium level is most essential in menstruating women because they are more prone to develop brain damage from hyponatremia than other patients.

Rapid correction of chronic hyponatremia might induce pontine myelinolysis but this is not the experience with acute hyponatremia. An infusion of 250 ml of 7.5% NaCl can be started slowly and another bag added later if necessary. Raising the serum sodium level by 1 mmol/l per hour has been suggested as a safe rate [39], but hypertonic saline has not been reported to induce pontine myelinolysis when given faster. Treatment should stop when serum sodium has reached 130 mmol/l as there is a risk of over-correction.

Diuretic treatment is imperative in case pulmonary edema or renal failure develops. However, such drugs aggravate hypotension and hyponatremia and should therefore be withheld until the hemodynamic situation is under control and a drip of hypertonic saline is ongoing. The value of diuretics has not been evaluated in randomized clinical studies, but without diuretics absorbed electrolyte-free irrigating fluid in excess of 1 l is strongly associated with a positive fluid balance 24 h after TURP [40]. Hypertonic mannitol might be superior to furosemide if used early on after the surgery [41].

Massive extravasation to the periprostatic or intraperitoneal spaces can be treated with surgical drainage. Here, electrolytes from the ECF enter the pool of irrigating fluid more quickly than the pool is absorbed by the circulation [42]. Hence, surgical drainage removes electrolytes from the body and they need to be replaced. Special attention should be given to the high risk of arterial hypotension and associated oliguria [15].

Large-scale fluid absorption with normal saline is a possibility during bipolar resection. Treatment should probably be limited to general supportive measures and diuretics. Hypertonic saline is not indicated.

References

1. Hahn RG. Fluid absorption in endoscopic surgery (review). *Br J Anaesth* 2006; **96**: 8–20.

2. Hahn RG, Ekengren J. Patterns of irrigating fluid absorption during transurethral resection of the prostate as indicated by ethanol. *J Urol* 1993; **149**: 502–6.

3. Gehring H, Nahm W, Zimmermann K, *et al*. Irrigating fluid absorption during percutaneous nephrolithotripsy. *Acta Anaesthesiol Scand* 1999; **43**: 316–21.

4. Hahn RG. Smoking increases the risk of large-scale fluid absorption during transurethral prostatic resection. *J Urol* 2001; **166**: 162–5.

5. Istre O. Transcervical resection of the endometrium and fibroids: the outcome of 412 operations performed over 5 years. *Acta Obstet Gynecol Scand* 1996; **75**: 567–74.

6. Olsson J, Berglund L, Hahn RG. Irrigating fluid absorption from the intact uterus. *Br J Obstet Gynaecol* 1996; **103**: 558–61.

7. Olsson J, Nilsson A, Hahn RG. Symptoms of the transurethral resection syndrome using glycine as the irrigant. *J Urol* 1995; **154**: 123–8.

8. Hahn RG, Sandfeldt L, Nyman CR. Double-blind randomized study of symptoms associated with absorption of glycine 1.5% or mannitol 3% during transurethral resection of the prostate. *J Urol* 1998; **160**: 397–401.

9. Olsson J, Hahn RG. Ethanol monitoring of irrigating fluid absorption in transcervical resection of the endometrium. *Acta Anaesthesiol Scand* 1995; **39**: 252–8.

10. Istre O. Transcervical resection of the endometrium and fibroids: the outcome of 412 operations performed over 5 years. *Acta Obstet Gynecol Scand* 1996; **75**: 567–74.

11. Hahn RG, Shemais H, Essén P. Glycine 1.0% versus glycine 1.5% as irrigating fluid during transurethral resection of the prostate. *Br J Urol* 1997; **79**: 394–400.

12. Nilsson A, Hahn RG. Mental status after transurethral resection of the prostate. *Eur Urol* 1994: **26**: 1–5.

13. Tuzin-Fin P, Guenard Y, Maurette P. Atypical signs of glycine absorption following transurethral resection of the prostate: two case reports. *Eur J Anaesth* 1997; **14**: 471–4.

14. Henderson DJ, Middleton RG. Coma from hyponatraemia following transurethral

resection of the prostate. *Urology* 1980; **XV**: 267–71.

15. Hahn RG. Transurethral resection syndrome from extravascular absorption of irrigating fluid. *Scand J Urol Nephrol* 1993; **27**: 387–94.

16. Radal M, Jonville Bera AP, Leisner C, Haillot O, Autret-Leca E. Effets indésirables des solutions d´irrigation glycollées. *Thérapie* 1999; **54**: 233–6.

17. Hahn RG. Dose-dependent half-life of glycine. *Urol Res* 1993; **21**: 289–91.

18. Hoekstra PT, Kahnoski R, McCamish MA, Bergen W, Heetderks DR. Transurethral prostatic resection syndrome – a new perspective: encephalopathy with associated hyperammonaemia. *J Urol* 1983; **130**: 704–7.

19. Hahn RG, Sandfeldt L. Blood ammonia levels after intravenous infusion of glycine with and without ethanol. *Scand J Urol Nephrol* 1999; **33**: 222–7.

20. Treparier CA, Lessard MR, Brochu J, Turcotte G. Another feature of TURP syndrome: hyperglycaemia and lactic acidosis caused by massive absorption of sorbitol. *Br J Anaesth* 2001; **87**: 316–19.

21. Inman RD, Hussain Z, Elves AWS, *et al.* A comparison of 1.5% glycine and 2.7% sorbitol-0.5% mannitol irrigants during transurethral prostate resection. *J Urol* 2001; **166**: 2216–20.

22. Hahn RG. Irrigating fluids in endoscopic surgery (review). *Br J Urol* 1997; **79**: 669–80.

23. Williams EL, Hildebrand KL, McCormick SA, Bedel MJ. The effect of intravenous lactated Ringer´s solution versus 0.9% sodium chloride solution on serum osmolality in human volunteers. *Anesth Analg* 1999; **88**: 999–1003.

24. Scheingraber S, Rehm M, Sehmisch C, Finsterer U. Rapid saline infusion produces hyperchlorekic acidosis in patients undergoing gynecologic surgery. *Anesthesiology* 1999; **90**: 1265–70.

25. Yousef AA, Suliman GA. Elashry OM, *et al.* A randomized comparison between three types of irrigating fluids during transurethral resection in benign prostatic hyperplasia. *BMC Anesthesiology* 2010; **10**: 7.

26. Sandfeldt L, Riddez L, Rajs J, *et al.* High-dose intravenous infusion of irrigating fluids containing glycine and mannitol in the pig. *J Surg Res* 2001; **95**: 114–25.

27. Hahn RG, Nennesmo I, Rajs J, *et al.* Morphological and X-ray microanalytical changes in mammalian tissue after overhydration with irrigating fluids. *Eur Urol* 1996; **29**: 355–61.

28. Hahn RG, Zhang W, Rajs J. Pathology of the heart after overhydration with glycine solution in the mouse. *APMIS* 1996; **104**: 915–20.

29. Hahn RG, Olsson J, Sótonyi P, Rajs J. Rupture of the myocardial histoskeleton and its relation to sudden death after infusion of glycine 1.5% in the mouse. *APMIS* 2000; **108**: 487–95.

30. Olsson J, Hahn RG. Survival after high-dose intravenous infusion of irrigating fluids in the mouse. Urology 1996; **47**: 689–92.

31. Hahn RG, Stalberg HP, Gustafsson SA. Intravenous infusion of irrigating fluids containing glycine or mannitol with and without ethanol. *J Urol* 1989; **142**: 1102–5.

32. Olsson J, Hahn RG. Glycine toxicity after high-dose i.v. infusion of glycine 1.5% in the mouse. *Br J Anaesth* 1999; **82**: 250–4.

33. Hahn RG. Ethanol monitoring of irrigating fluid absorption (review). *Eur J Anaesth* 1996; **13**: 102–15.

34. Piros D, Fagerström T, Collins JW, Hahn RG. Glucose as a marker of fluid absorption in bipolar transurethral surgery. *Anesth Analg* 2009; **109**: 1850–5.

35. Hahn RG, Ekengren J. Absorption of irrigating fluid and height of the fluid bag during transurethral resection of the prostate. *Br J Urol* 1993; **72**: 80–3.

36. Ekengren J, Zhang W, Hahn RG. Effects of bladder capacity and height of fluid bag on the intravesical pressure during transurethral resection of the prostate. *Eur Urol* 1995; **27**: 26–30.

37. Bernstein GT, Loughlin KR, Gittes RF. The physiologic basis of the TUR syndrome. *J Surg Res* 1989; **46**: 135–41.

38. Ayus JC, Krothapalli RK, Arieff AI. Treatment of symptomatic hyponatremia and its relation to brain damage. *New Engl J Med* 1987; **317**: 1190–5.

39. Ayus JC, Arieff AI. Glycine-induced hypo-osmolar hyponatremia. *Arch Intern Med* 1997; **157**: 223–6.

40. Hahn RG. Total fluid balance during transurethral resection of the prostate. *Int Urol Nephrol* 1996; **28**: 665–71.

41. Crowley K, Clarkson K, Hannon V, McShane A, Kelly DG. Diuretics after transurethral prostatectomy: a double-blind controlled trial comparing frusemide and mannitol. *Br J Anaesth* 1990; **65**: 337–41.

42. Olsson J, Hahn RG. Simulated intraperitoneal absorption of irrigating fluid. *Acta Obstet Gynecol Scand* 1995; **74**: 707–13.

Severe sepsis and septic shock

Palle Toft and Else Tønnesen

Patients subjected to infections, trauma, burns or surgery are characterized by *systemic inflammatory response syndrome* (SIRS) or *sepsis* in cases with suspected or documented infection. These complex syndromes are defined as the presence of at least two of the following criteria:

- Temperature < 36°C or > 38°C
- Heart rate > 90 beats/min
- Respiratory rate > 20 breaths/min or $PaCO_2$ < 4.3 kPa (32 mmHg)
- White blood cell count > 12 000 mm^{-3} or < 4000/mm^3 or 10% immature (band) forms

Severe sepsis is defined as sepsis associated with hypoperfusion or dysfunction of at least one organ system, and s*eptic shock* is associated with acute circulatory failure defined as persistent hypotension despite "adequate" volume resuscitation [1]. Severe sepsis and septic shock carry mortality rates of 30% and 40–70%, respectively.

Sepsis is a systemic disorder with a protean clinical picture and a complex pathogenesis characterized by the release of both pro- and anti-inflammatory elements. The organ dysfunction and organ failure occurring in the early phase of severe sepsis is believed to result from an excessive inflammatory response.

The critically ill patient

The development of septic complications is usually prolonged, taking days to develop into organ dysfunction and, in the worst cases, multi-organ dysfunction and septic shock. The acute phase is different from the prolonged phase with respect to the inflammatory and hemodynamic response.

In severe sepsis and septic shock, all organ systems are affected, although acute kidney injury is especially frequent. The etiology of organ dysfunction in response to critical illness is multifactorial and may include hypoperfusion, ischemia-reperfusion injuries, a dysfunctional immune system and coagulopathies. The microcirculation is compromised by massive vasodilatation, making the clinical picture of the patient with septic shock (*warm* shock) quite different from the patient with cardiogenic or hemorrhagic shock (*cold* shock).

Central in the pathogenesis of sepsis is *capillary leakage*, i.e., transudation of fluid from the vascular space into extravascular tissue. The capillary leakage contributes to a generalized edema in the lungs, heart, gut, brain and other tissues, and it contributes to the impairment

Clinical Fluid Therapy in the Perioperative Setting, ed. Robert G. Hahn. Published by Cambridge University Press. © Cambridge University Press 2011.

of organ function and sometimes to excessive weight gain. Capillary leakage may also make the patient hypovolemic.

Critically ill patients are often elderly with significant comorbidity, with the presence of disorders such as ischemic heart disease, diabetes, cancer and alcohol-related organ dysfunction in addition to the acute illness.

Another complicating factor that influences fluid and electrolyte therapy is acute renal dysfunction/failure, meaning that fluid therapy must be restricted until renal replacement therapy has been initiated. Ongoing intravenous treatments in the intensive care unit comprise nutrition, sedatives, analgesics, vasoactive drugs and insulin infusion – all contributing to a considerable fluid administration, which must be included in the calculation of intraoperative fluid management.

The principles of perioperative fluid therapy have traditionally been based on the assumption that preoperative deficit, maintenance, third-space losses and blood loss require replacement by crystalloids or colloids. However, the principles of fluid therapy used for patients undergoing elective surgery are not applicable in critically ill patients.

Anesthesia for septic patients

Surgery performed on critically ill septic patients is often acute, and fluid therapy is fundamentally different from fluid treatment in relation to elective surgery [2]. Perioperative fluid therapy in patients with severe sepsis and septic shock must follow the principles applied for critically ill patients in general.

Deep general anesthesia should also be avoided in patients with severe sepsis or septic shock. Patients are often more or less sedated to tolerate ventilator therapy, and even without sedation, they may not be fully awake due to septic encephalopathy. Even a smaller amount of anesthetic agents may have a detrimental effect on their hemodynamic stability. Postoperative patient-controlled analgesia may be an approach in some septic patients. Reducing the amount of postoperative sedation improves fluid balance, increases diuresis and improves renal function [4].

Early vs. late septic shock

The fluid therapy used in septic patients undergoing surgery depends on where in the course of the septic disease the patient is. Moreover, fluid management in the early course of sepsis or septic shock should be modified if organ failure has already developed.

As described by Cuthbertson nearly 60 years ago, the inflammatory response in the very early ebb-phase is characterized by low cardiac output, reduced tissue perfusion and profound peripheral vasoconstriction. According to Cuthbertson, this phase is followed by a flow phase characterized by increased cardiac output and normalization of tissue perfusion.

Early fluid resuscitation

During the initial phase of sepsis or inflammation, adequate volume replacement is a cornerstone in management as restoration of flow is a key component in avoiding tissue ischemia or reperfusion injury. In 2001, Rivers *et al.* [5] performed a randomised study and described the beneficial effect of early, aggressive, goal-directed therapy (EGDT) in the acute treatment of severe sepsis and septic shock.

The Principles of EGDT

- Within the first 6 h after admission to hospital, patients with severe sepsis or septic shock were hemodynamically optimized. All the patients were intubated, mechanically ventilated and had a central venous line and arterial catheter.
- When the central venous pressure (CVP) was < 8 mmHg, crystalloids and colloids were infused to achieve CVP between 8 and 12 mmHg (The "Surviving Sepsis Campaign" recommends an even higher target CVP of 12–15 mmHg).
- If the mean arterial pressure (MAP) was > 65 mmHg, fluid resuscitation alone would be enough while patients with MAP < 65 mmHg were also treated with vasoactive agents to obtain MAP > 65 mmHg.
- The central venous oxygen saturation ($ScvO_2$) was monitored. If $ScvO_2$ was < 70%, a blood transfusion was initiated until a hematocrit > 30% was achieved. In case the $ScvO_2$ was below 70%, inotropic agents were given.

A clinically important finding was that the beneficial effect of EGDT was not related to the total amount of fluid given. It was the *speed* with which the septic patients were fluid resuscitated that made the difference. The importance of rapid and early fluid resuscitation has also been confirmed in pediatric septic shock cases. Hence, early fluid optimization, before organ failure is manifested, is of major importance.

The goal-directed approach to stabilization of the hemodynamics resulted in a mortality of only 30.5% in the intervention group compared with 46% in the control group receiving "standard therapy." The EGDT also resulted in a lower serum lactate concentration, a smaller base deficit, higher pH and a significantly lower APACHE II score.

Rivers' study has been the subject of much discussion, but there is no doubt that implementation of the principles of EGDT have improved and optimized the acute treatment of patients with severe sepsis and septic shock. Later work has confirmed the beneficial effects [6] (Figure 18.1).

Fluid resuscitation of a patient with severe sepsis and septic shock must start as early as possible. The tissue perfusion will suffer for every minute or hour that the resuscitation is delayed, and cellular dysfunction and cell death will develop. It is unclear when the transition from reversible to irreversible cell dysfunction occurs, but it might be different in various tissues.

Other studies of EGDT

In 2002, Kern & Shoemaker reviewed 21 randomized clinical trials that described hemodynamic optimization in acutely ill patients [7]. They included different types of high-risk patients: those undergoing elective surgery and trauma and septic patients. *Early* optimization was defined as that occurring 8–12 h postoperatively or before organ failure, and *late* was defined as later than 12 h after surgery, 24 h after injury or after organ failure had developed.

There was a significantly lower mortality in those cases where early optimization was completed before organ failure occurred.

Survival did not improve significantly in six of the studies where optimization was instituted *after* organ failure was manifested. A confidential inquiry was made concerning the quality of care before admission to intensive care in the group of patients where care was

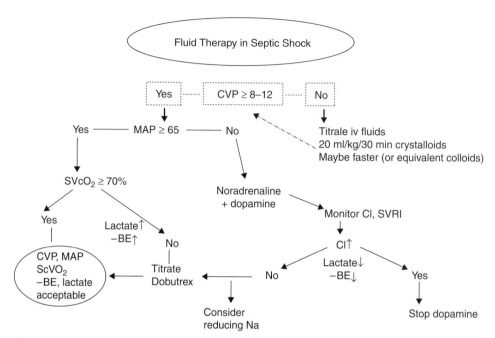

Figure 18.1. Fluid therapy in septic shock. BE, base excess; CI, cardiac index; CVP, central venous pressure; MAP, mean arterial pressure; NA, noradrenaline; ScVO$_2$, central venous oxygen saturation; SVRI, systemic vascular resistance index.

assessed as suboptimal. This inquiry showed that circulatory support and monitoring most often were suboptimal.

Results from animal studies show that, in early septic shock, autoregulation of the microcirculatory blood flow is largely intact [8]. Videomicroscopy of the sublingual microcirculation of humans has shown that increased microcirculatory flow during resuscitation is associated with reduced organ failure without substantial differences in global hemodynamics [9].

While aggressive fluid resuscitation is beneficial early in the course of sepsis, it is of minor importance when organ dysfunction has occurred. It has been demonstrated that early fluid resuscitation in septic patients reduces the secretion of pro- and anti-inflammatory cytokines and the amount of apophtotic biomarker [10].

Later course of sepsis

The EGDT principles focus on the initial fluid resuscitation within the first six hours. Severe sepsis and septic shock are, however, characterized by venous dilation and ongoing capillary leakage. Therefore, most patients require continuous aggressive fluid resuscitation during the first 24 h of management. In most septic patients, early resuscitation transforms a hypovolemic and hypodynamic circulation into a hyperdynamic, low-resistance circulation where oxygen delivery/transport is normal or high, at least in the macrocirculation.

In the course of sepsis, unnecessary fluid might aggravate edema due to capillary leakage and not enhance perfusion. A continuous positive fluid balance lasting for days is a significant predictor of mortality [11]. However, it is possible that a positive fluid balance is only a marker of the severity of illness.

In "fluids and catheter treatment trial," 1000 patients with acute lung injury or acute respiratory distress syndrome were randomized to a conservative fluid administration strategy compared with a more liberal strategy [12]. The trial lasted for 7 days, and the liberal group was brought into a positive fluid balance of 1 l/day. In the conservative group, the fluid balance was nearly 0. The conservative strategy improved oxygenation, increased the number of ventilator-free days and reduced the length of stay in the intensive care unit (ICU). Patients were relatively young (approximately 50 years old), and those with overt renal failure were excluded from the trial. However, fluid therapy in this trial was started on average 43 h after admission to the ICU and 24 h after the establishment of acute lung injury. These patients were, in other words, already optimized with early fluid administration.

This study underlines that what is beneficial in the early course of sepsis might not be beneficial later. In the later course of the disease, between 2 and 7 days, a more *restricted* fluid management strategy should be instituted. Thus, it is prudent to treat patients with severe sepsis or septic shock with EGDT during the first 6–24 h only.

Crystalloids vs. colloids

Overall, there is no evidence to support using one type of fluid over another. The "Surviving Sepsis Campaign" recommends administering either crystalloids or colloids as the initial fluid [13]. Subgroup analysis of meta-analyses has demonstrated that crystalloid resuscitation was associated with a lower mortality in trauma patients. In contrast, colloid resuscitation in some subgroup analysis has been associated with a better outcome in septic patients [14]. The same tendency was observed in a large prospective randomized trial, the SAFE study [15].

Fluid resuscitation with colloids results in a greater and faster increase in cardiac filling and cardiac output than crystalloid resuscitation in septic hypovolemia. Colloids remain in circulation for a longer time than the crystalloids, and crystalloids require that more fluid is used in a patient to attain the same goals, whereby more edema might develop [16]. As an initial resuscitation in septic patients, colloids as well as crystalloids can be used. In clinical practice, crystalloids and colloids are often used simultaneously.

Blood transfusions

Anemia is a common problem in critically ill patients. Harmful effects of anemia include increased risk of cardiac-related morbidity and mortality as well as a general decrease in oxygen-carrying capacity [17].

The consequences of anemia may be deleterious in this population because critical illness is often associated with increased metabolic demands. A surgical procedure will accentuate metabolic demands and intraoperative blood loss reduces oxygen delivery. Therefore, an optimal hemoglobin level must be maintained. However, the criteria for an optimal hemoglobin level in critical illness are not clearly defined. A Canadian study indicated that a liberal use of transfusions (10–12 g/dl) may result in increased hospital mortality rates compared with a more restrictive transfusion regime (7–9 g/dl) [18]. A later observational multicenter study confirmed that there is an association between transfusions and diminished organ function as well as between transfusions and mortality [19].

The use of blood transfusions for the treatment of anemia in critically ill patients warrants further evaluation. There seems to be a very delicate balance between the harmful effects of anemia on organ function and the harmful effects of transfusion.

Fluid responsiveness in septic shock

It is important that the critically ill patient is hemodynamically stable and normovolemic before being transported from the ICU or emergency room to the operation theatre. This is not always possible in, for example, patients with ongoing and uncontrolled bleeding.

Patients with severe sepsis or septic shock are often resuscitated with *fluid challenges*. In this process, a large amount of fluid is administered under close monitoring to evaluate the hemodynamic response. The "Surviving Sepsis Campaign" recommends an initial fluid challenge of 20 ml/kg of crystalloids or an equivalent amount of colloids administered over 30 min. If the patient is in severe shock, a more rapid infusion might be necessary. Repeated fluid challenges are performed as long as the patient improves hemodynamically. Clinical signs of hemodynamic improvement might be increasing arterial pressure, decreasing heart rate, increasing urine output or improvement in capillary refill time.

Adequate fluid resuscitation cannot, however, be based only on normalization of vital signs. Traditionally, physicians have used static hemodynamic values such as CVP or the pulmonary artery occlusion pressure (PAOP) to evaluate whether the patient would benefit from further fluid challenge. There is increasing evidence that estimates of intravascular volume based on CVP or PAOP do not reliably predict the patient's response to a fluid challenge [11,20].

In addition to the Swan–Ganz (SG) catheter, cardiac output can be measured by pulse contour analysis. This method also estimates the global end-diastolic volume and intrathoracic blood volume. These new static preload parameters correlate better with cardiac index than the traditionally measured CVP. However, static preload measurements are inaccurate and must be supplemented with more dynamic measures.

Functional hemodynamic parameters, such as systolic pressure variation (SPV) and pulse pressure variation (PPV), are more sensitive indices of fluid responsiveness. SPV and PPV can be used only in sedated, mechanically ventilated patients with rather large tidal volumes. With more invasive monitoring, cardiac output can be measured and used as an adjunct when evaluating the response to a fluid challenge. Cardiac output measurement may also help to identify the minority of patients who have a low cardiac output despite adequate fluid resuscitation.

After fluid resuscitation, septic shock is often hyperdynamic with high cardiac output, low systemic vascular resistance (SVR) and reduced MAP. This hyperdynamic state is, however, often confined to the large vessels, whereas the regional microcirculation is compromised.

As there is no perfect hemodynamic parameter, the patient's response to fluid administration must be evaluated together with other parameters, such as the $ScvO_2$. A multimodal monitoring approach has to be instituted. The goal of fluid resuscitation in the study by Rivers *et al.* [5] was a $ScvO_2$ greater than 70%. If a SG catheter was used, a mixed venous oxygen saturation (SvO_2) greater than 65% could be the goal.

SvO_2 has been considered to be the gold standard to monitor whole-body perfusion. This might be true in hemorrhagic shock, but in septic shock the SvO_2 is often normal or even supernormal owing to reduced oxygen extraction at the microvascular level. In contrast, serum lactate is a useful measure of anaerobic metabolism, and base excess is often negative if the organs are not adequately perfused [21]. Monitoring serum lactate as well as the base excess improves the overall evaluation of the patient's response to fluid challenge.

Treatment with vasopressors and inotropic agents

The "Surviving Sepsis Campaign" recommends that noradrenaline or dopamine are used as the initial vasopressor agents [13]. There has been some concern that dopamine is associated with increased mortality. However, a new, large multicenter study was not able to show any significant difference in mortality in septic patients treated with noradrenaline compared with dopamine, although those treated with dopamine had more arrhythmic events [22]. There has also been some concern that the use of noradrenaline in patients who are inadequately fluid resuscitated would increase blood pressure due to vasoconstriction, and thereby reduce the blood flow to the organs.

It might be necessary to use noradrenaline to restore MAP during the early course of septic shock, before the patient is adequately fluid resuscitated. Animal studies have shown that noradrenaline-masked hypovolemia is associated not only with renal failure but also with cardiomyocyte necrosis [23]. To avoid this complication, the "Surviving Sepsis Campaign" recommends the combined use of noradrenaline and dopamine while the patient is not adequately monitored. In this way noradrenaline increases MAP and dopamine ensures cardiac output.

When the patient is monitored with a SG catheter or pulse contour analysis, cardiac output can be measured and SVR calculated. When this monitoring is instituted, the vasoconstrictor noradrenalin should be used to increase MAP guided by SVR, whereas dobutamine can be used to increase cardiac output, if necessary. When adequately fluid-resuscitated, the septic patient most often has hyperdynamic shock with high cardiac output and low SVR. Only in a minority of fluid-resuscitated septic patients is it necessary to administer dobutamine to increase cardiac output. In the study by Rivers *et al.* 15.4% of the patients who received EGDT were treated with dobutamine [5].

Epinephrine is not used very often in septic patients as it can impair the splanchnic circulation in septic shock. Compared with noradrenaline there was no difference in mortality, but epinephrine was associated with more adverse effects [24].

Key messages

Surgery performed on critically ill septic patients is often acute, and fluid therapy is fundamentally different from fluid treatment in relation to elective surgery.

Perioperative fluid therapy in patients with severe sepsis and septic shock must follow the principles applied for critically ill patients in general.

In septic patients, the institution of fluid therapy at an early stage is of vital importance to the outcome.

Early resuscitation might transform a hypovolemic and hypodynamic circulation into a hyperdynamic, low-resistance circulation where oxygen delivery/transport is normal or high.

The "Surviving Sepsis Campaign" recommends the combined use of noradrenaline and dopamine while the patient is not adequately monitored.

When full monitoring is instituted, noradrenaline can be used to increase MAP guided by SVR whereas dobutamine can be used to increase cardiac output, if necessary.

If the patient is anesthetized, the anesthetic agents will nearly always induce some vasodilatation, and it might be necessary to increase an ongoing noradrenaline infusion during the anesthesia, but the anesthetist should always be aware of the danger of noradrenaline-masked hypovolemia.

References

1. Levy MM, Fink MP, Marshall JC, *et al.* 2001 SCCM/ESICM/ACCP/ATS/ SIS International Sepsis Definitions Conference. *Crit Care Med* 2003; **31**: 1250–6.

2. Brandstrup B, Tonnesen H, Beier-Holgersen R, Hjortso E, Ording H, Lindorff-Larsen K *et al.* Effects of intravenous fluid restriction on postoperative complications: comparison of two perioperative fluid regimens: a randomized assessor-blinded multicentre trial. *Ann Surg* 2003; Nov; **238**(5): 641–8

3. Joshi GP. Intraoperative fluid restriction improves outcome after major elective gastrointestinal surgery. *Anesth Analg* 2005; Aug; **101**(2): 601–5.

4. Strom T, Martinussen T, Toft P. A protocol of no sedation for critically ill patients receiving mechanical ventilation: a randomised trial. *Lancet* 2010; **375**: 475–80.

5. Rivers E, Nguyen B, Havstad S, *et al.* Early goal-directed therapy in the treatment of severe sepsis and septic shock. *N Engl J Med* 2001; **345**: 1368–77.

6. Lin SM, Huang CD, Lin HC, *et al.* A modified goal-directed protocol improves clinical outcomes in intensive care unit patients with septic shock: a randomized controlled trial. *Shock* 2006; **26**: 551–7.

7. Kern JW, Shoemaker WC. Meta-analysis of hemodynamic optimization in high-risk patients. *Crit Care Med* 2002; **30**: 1686–92.

8. Hiltebrand LB, Krejci V, tenHoevel ME, Banic A, Sigurdsson GH. Redistribution of microcirculatory blood flow within the intestinal wall during sepsis and general anesthesia. *Anesthesiology* 2003; **98**: 658–69.

9. Trzeciak S, McCoy JV, Phillip DR, *et al.* Early increases in microcirculatory perfusion during protocol-directed resuscitation are associated with reduced multi-organ failure at 24 h in patients with sepsis. *Intensive Care Med* 2008; **34**: 2210–7.

10. Rivers EP, Kruse JA, Jacobsen G, *et al.* The influence of early hemodynamic optimization on biomarker patterns of severe sepsis and septic shock. *Crit Care Med* 2007; **35**: 2016–24.

11. Durairaj L, Schmidt GA. Fluid therapy in resuscitated sepsis: less is more. *Chest* 2008; **133**: 252–63.

12. Wiedemann HP, Wheeler AP, Bernard GR, *et al.* Comparison of two fluid-management strategies in acute lung injury. *N Engl J Med* 2006; **354**: 2564–75.

13. Dellinger RP, Levy MM, Carlet JM, *et al.* Surviving Sepsis Campaign: international guidelines for management of severe sepsis and septic shock: 2008. *Crit Care Med* 2008; **36**: 296–327.

14. Velanovich V. Crystalloid versus colloid fluid resuscitation: a meta-analysis of mortality. *Surgery* 1989; **105**: 65–71.

15. Finfer S, Bellomo R, Boyce N, French J, Myburgh J, Norton R. A comparison of albumin and saline for fluid resuscitation in the intensive care unit. *N Engl J Med* 2004; **350**: 2247–56.

16. Trof RJ, Sukul SP, Twisk JW, Girbes AR, Groeneveld AB. Greater cardiac response of colloid than saline fluid loading in septic and non-septic critically ill patients with clinical hypovolaemia. *Intensive Care Med* 2010; **36**: 697–701.

17. Rao SV, Jollis JG, Harrington RA, *et al.* Relationship of blood transfusion and clinical outcomes in patients with acute coronary syndromes. *JAMA* 2004; **292**: 1555–62.

18. Hebert PC, Wells G, Blajchman MA, *et al.* A multicenter, randomized, controlled clinical trial of transfusion requirements in critical care. Transfusion Requirements in Critical Care Investigators, Canadian Critical Care Trials Group. *N Engl J Med* 1999; **340**: 409–17.

19. Vincent JL, Baron JF, Reinhart K, *et al.* Anemia and blood transfusion in critically ill patients. *JAMA* 2002; **288**: 1499–507.

20. Michard F, Teboul JL. Predicting fluid responsiveness in ICU patients: a critical analysis of the evidence. *Chest* 2002; **121**: 2000–8.

21. Antonelli M, Levy M, Andrews PJ, *et al.* Hemodynamic monitoring in shock and implications for management. International Consensus Conference, Paris, France, 27–28 April 2006. *Intensive Care Med* 2007; **33**: 575–90.

22. De BD, Biston P, Devriendt J, *et al.* Comparison of dopamine and norepinephrine in the treatment of shock. *N Engl J Med* 2010; **362**: 779–89.

23. Hinder F, Stubbe HD, Van AH, *et al.* Early multiple organ failure after recurrent endotoxemia in the presence of vasoconstrictor-masked hypovolemia. *Crit Care Med* 2003; **31**: 903–9.

24. Myburgh JA, Higgins A, Jovanovska A, Lipman J, Ramakrishnan N, Santamaria J. A comparison of epinephrine and norepinephrine in critically ill patients. *Intensive Care Med* 2008; **34**: 2226–34.

Chapter 19

Hypovolemic shock

Niels H. Secher and Johannes J. van Lieshout

Second only to control of ventilation, intravenous volume administration is the cornerstone physiological treatment modality for anesthesia and intensive care medicine. Providing fluid to patients supports their blood volume but, as revealed 65 years ago by Barcroft *et al.* [1] and Gordh [2], in regard to anesthesia, cardiovascular integrity depends on the central (CBV) rather than on the total blood volume.

Hypovolemic shock is characterized by a critically reduced CBV, as illustrated when CBV is restrained by actual or simulated gravitational pooling of blood during head-up tilt (HUT) and lower body negative pressure (LBNP), respectively, or by limiting venous return by pressure breathing. Such interventions evaluate the influence of CBV on various physiological variables but they are also relevant to surgery. For example, surgery on the shoulder is carried out with the patient sitting up and during upper laparoscopic procedures, the anesthetized patient is tilted at the same time as the caval vein is compressed by inflation of CO_2 and venous return further limited by positive pressure ventilation. Notably, pressure breathing is a lung recruitment manoeuver following thoracic surgery.

For surgical patients volume treatment corrects a preoperative volume deficit and attenuates negative influences on CBV caused by, e.g., hemorrhage, positioning of the patient, anesthesia and ventilation [3,4]. Volume treatment is most often planned according to an albeit somewhat arbitrary fixed volume regime [5] and to compensate for an eventual blood loss. The treatment is further adjusted by recordings of heart rate and arterial pressure, as introduced for surgery by Cushing in 1903 [6].

Heart rate and arterial pressure

Interpretation of the heart rate (HR) and arterial pressure responses to a reduced CBV is complex. Cardiovascular variables are regulated and affected by influences other than CBV, including surgical stress and anesthesia [7]. It is unlikely that accurate volume treatment can be based on HR and blood pressure alone, and the most accurate recording of fluid balance is probably obtained by physical rather than by physiological variables. For example, thoracic electrical impedance changes in close relation to hemorrhage, and subsequent administration of the withdrawn amount of blood [8] and thoracic electrical impedance is similarly accurate for monitoring fluid balance during and after cardiac surgery [9].

To identify hypovolemic shock and to specify volume treatment to patients in shock, as well as to surgical patients in general, we address the cardiovascular responses to a reduced

Clinical Fluid Therapy in the Perioperative Setting, ed. Robert G. Hahn. Published by Cambridge University Press. © Cambridge University Press 2011.

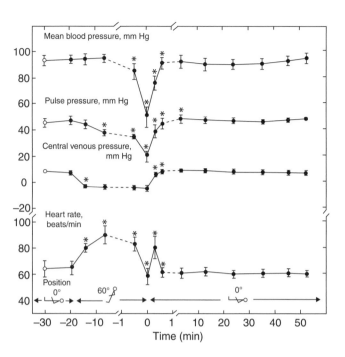

Figure 19.1. Circulatory dynamics in seven subjects at rest and during passive head-up tilt until the onset of (pre)syncopal symptoms, and return to the horizontal position. Values are mean and SE * Different from rest. (Reproduced from Sander-Jensen et al., 1986 [18], with permission from the American Physiological Society.)

CBV followed by a definition of normovolemia as reference for volume treatment. Finally, considerations on the fluid administered to restore the blood volume are mentioned. For an historical account of hypovolemic shock the texts by Beecher [10] and Wiggers [11] or a more recent summary [12] should be consulted.

Pre-shock

The cardiovascular response to a reduced CBV is illustrated during tilt table experiments (Figure 19.1). In response to a progressively reduced CBV, cardiovascular variables vary with activation of the autonomic nervous system and, accordingly, are divided into three stages among which regulation follows the textbook description only in the first stage [13].

With a moderate reduction of the CBV (< 30%), mean arterial pressure (MAP) is maintained by total peripheral resistance compensating for an approximate 20% reduction in cardiac output (CO) [1]. As demonstrated during gravitational stress, MAP is stable at the level of the carotid baroreceptors and reduced distension of the carotid sinus elicits sympathetic excitation. In support, and as an extreme example, the approximately two fold elevated blood pressure of the giraffe [14] is related to the height of the animal making its cerebral perfusion pressure similar to that of humans.

In addition, volume and/or pressure receptors within the central circulation that transmit through myelinated nerve fibres respond to a reduced CBV and initiate sympathetic activation. Enhanced sympathetic activity results not only in a relatively stable MAP but also in an elevated HR [15], albeit the increase is modest with values typically being lower than 100 bpm (Figure 19.1). Values above 100 bpm can occasionally be seen (Figure 19.2) and yet the HR response to (central) hypovolemia depends on age and does not always reach a statistical significant level [16].

v Systolic arterial pressure (mm Hg)
o Heart rate (bpm)
∧ Diastolic arterial pressure (mm Hg)

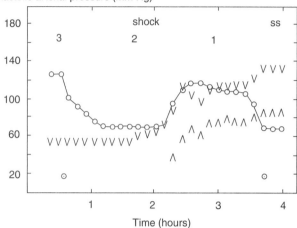

Figure 19.2. Heart rate and systolic and diastolic pressures during surgery for a ruptured abdominal aortic aneurysm. Stages III-I of shock indicated as 3, 2 and 1. (Reproduced from Jacobsen and Secher, 1992 [35], with permission from John Wiley and Sons.). ss, steady state.

Stage II of hypovolemic shock

For volume treatment it is important to recognize that the *second stage* of hypovolemic shock represents a *reversal* of the autonomic response (Figure 19.1). While sympathetic activation dominates the first stage, parasympathetic activity is prevalent during the second stage, which is entered when CBV is reduced by 30% [17].

Only sympathetic activity to the adrenal gland is maintained, as identified by a progressive increase in plasma adrenaline [18]. In contrast, plasma noradrenaline reaches a plateau or decreases when central hypovolemia progresses to provoke cerebral hypoperfusion with loss of consciousness. Reduced sympathetic activity, as indicated by plasma noradrenaline, explains the fall in total peripheral resistance that lowers MAP, and the rise in plasma adrenaline is not important in regard to loss of vascular tone [19]. During central hypovolemia, elevated peripheral resistance is replaced by a decrease since muscle sympathetic activity is eliminated [20].

Bradycardia

With the decrease in HR provoked by a significant reduction in CBV, there is usually a concomitant decrease in HR in consequence of parasympathetic activity as identified by an elevated plasma pancreatic polypeptide level [18,21] and confirmed by blocking the bradycardic response by glycopyrron [15]. The bradycardia developed during central hypovolemia may be so profound that no ECG is detected on a monitor and, accordingly, hypovolemia should be suspected whenever "cardiac arrest" manifests in trauma patients, as in patients within the perioperative period. Conversely, initiation of cardiac resuscitation, including external cardiac compression by applying pressure to the chest besides positive pressure ventilation, to patients in hypovolemic shock further reduces their CBV and could provoke an irreversible stage of shock.

Immediate restoration of CBV leads to recovery of both cardiovascular and ventilatory functions, within seconds, as exemplified in the cardiovascular laboratory by the termination of HUT (Figure. 19.1), LBNP or pressure breathing, and indeed by providing ample volume to the patient in shock [21](Figure 19.2). For surgical patients, therefore, cardiac resuscitation procedures are counterproductive until it is verified that rapid infusion of at least one liter is proven without an effect. If it is not possible to administer such a volume immediately when the patient becomes ill, CBV can, at least partly, be restored by elevating the legs and/or placing the patient head-down (Trendenenburg's position) and only after such measures are found futile; a failing circulation should be considered of cardiac origin and appropriate resuscitation initiated.

Accordingly, it remains questionable why the bradycardic response to hemorrhage is not included in textbook descriptions (see, for example, Mair [22]), but the texts seem in general to be based on observations derived from acute animal experiments rather than from observations in chronically instrumented conscious animals [7] or in awake humans [23]. Also it may be that vagal activity in response to a reduced CBV is not considered theologically rational, although there is evidence for a beneficial effect of vagal activity during hemorrhage. It has been demonstrated that vagal activity promotes hemostasis to an extent that it limits blood loss and, conversely, that administration of atropine to block vagal activity maintains bleeding and can, eventually, be fatal [24]! Accordingly, the second stage of hypovolemic shock may be seen as an attempt by the body to stop bleeding by lowering blood pressure, at the same time as coagulation competence is enhanced by combined increase in both vagal activity and plasma adrenaline.

Yet it is has to be accepted, obviously, that not all patients in hypovolemic shock present with a low HR. The bradycardic response to a significantly reduced CBV carries the prerequisite that vagal activity is intact and that may not be the case for all patients, as exemplified by those suffering from atrial fibrillation or autonomic dysfunction, e.g., in consequence of diabetes mellitus. Of more general relevance to the patient in hypovolemic shock is the observation that vagal tone to the heart is overruled by pain-related sympathetic activity [25], and many trauma patients are in pain due to crushed tissue and similarly, e.g., ileus is associated with pain and an elevated HR during hemorrhage [26].

Pale skin and sympathetic activity

Besides the bradycardic response to stage II hypovolemic shock, it is also a characteristic for the manifestations associated with significant hemorrhage that the skin is *pale*, as can be observed during a vasovagal syncope, a condition that shares most (if not all) of the pathophysiology of stage II of hypovolemic shock. Perhaps the pale skin has inspired the notion that total peripheral resistance is elevated in response to enhanced baroreceptor activity as the arterial pressure becomes low although it, as mentioned, decreases in reflection of ceased sympathetic activity.

Ceased sympathetic activity reflects that baroreceptor control of blood pressure and HR is eliminated at this stage of shock [27]. Rather than being caused by sympathetic activity, during (central) hypovolemia, pale skin is a result of a marked (about 25-fold) increase in the plasma vasopressin level [28], while a similar reduction in cutaneous blood flow by the increase in plasma angiotensin II is irrelevant to the colour of the patient [29]. The marked increase in plasma vasopressin, together with lowering of the plasma atrial natiuretic peptide (ANP) level, also explains the prolonged low urine production following hypovolemic shock and, conversely, conforms to maintained CO during surgery promoting diuresis. Similarly, cardiac afferent nerves provoke vomiting and inhibit gastric mobility [30], which explains why maintained stroke volume of the heart (SV) during surgery reduces postoperative nausea and vomiting (PONV) [31].

The Bezold–Jarish reflex

Collectively, the appearance of bradycardia, low vascular resistance, increase in plasma vasopressin, etc., during hemorrhage conforms to a critically reduced CBV being characterized by responses that are similar to those described in the pharmacologic literature as a *Bezold–Jarish reflex*, but it remains somewhat controversial why the reflex is elicited. Öberg & White [32] demonstrated in 1970 that the Bezold–Jarish-like reflex in response to hemorrhage appears by activation of unmyelinated nerve fibres from the left ventricle, and suggested that it is provoked when the heart is emptied of blood. The second stage of hypovolemic shock is associated with only a 10%–25% reduction in the diastolic filling of the heart [33] and yet, it remains possible that the most densely innervated apical part of the left ventricle is emptied by a significant reduction in CBV.

A concomitant reduction in HR and blood pressure can, however, also be provoked by hemorrhage following cardiac denervation [34]. Therefore, the specific trigger for the reflex in response to hemorrhage remains in some doubt, or it might vary depending on circumstances. The common and clinically relevant finding is however that the reflex originates from the central circulation.

Stage III of hypovolemic shock

Although stage II of hypovolemic shock may be fatal, there is also a third stage. If the reduction in HR in response to a low CBV is not a terminal event, HR increases again, typically to 120–130 bpm (Figure 19.2) [35], conforming to the tachycardia most textbooks hold as a key feature of hypovolemic shock [22]. As demonstrated in animals, sympathetic activity is resumed during severe hemorrhage as indicated by the plasma catecholamine level [26]. Maybe cerebral ischemia, in consequence of prolonged hypotension and a low CO, is important for reactivation of sympathetic activity, and a critically reduced cerebral perfusion could perhaps indicate that the third stage may represent a transition to an irreversible stage of shock [12]. However, in contrast to the common description indicating an increase in total peripheral resistance during severe hemorrhage, total peripheral resistance in fact decreases or does not change [26].

Central vascular pressures during hypovolemic shock

Cardiovascular monitoring of critically ill patients is supplemented by recording of central vascular pressures. In experimental studies, central venous pressure decreases (Figure 19.1) together with mean pulmonary artery and wedge pressures with increasing levels of HUT or LBNP [17,18].

Yet, for clinical evaluation of the circulation during progressive hypovolemia, it is a problem that the reduction in central vascular pressures relates to the intervention rather than to the subject's well-being. Central vascular pressures are similar when the level of HUT or LBNP is established as when the subject faints. During sustained HUT or LBNP, the reduction in CBV progresses with accumulation of fluid in the legs [36] and, consequently, CO also decreases although there is a tendency for the pulmonary artery wedge pressure to increase [37].

Stable "filling pressures" of the heart do not secure that CO is sufficient to maintain cerebral blood flow and oxygenation, and there are no clinical data to support volume treatment based on central vascular pressure [38]. In fact, for patients CO is not related to the filling pressures of the heart, although there exists a relationship between CO and the diastolic filling of the heart [39].

Normovolemia

It is agreed that patients need volume supplementation during anesthesia and intensive care medicine, but the strategy remains debated both in regard to the amount that should be provided and to the preferred solutions. What seems established is that for surgery not associated with a significant blood loss, patients should be administered 1 l of crystalloid [5]. Otherwise, it can be stated only that it, intuitively, is difficult to defend a volume treatment regime that keeps the patient hypovolemic or one that provides the patient with a volume overload and yet, there is no agreement in regard to the volume load that defines "normovolemia."

With the importance of a limited CBV for circulatory shock, a definition of normovolemia may be derived from individualized goal-directed volume therapy, not only to the patient in shock but also to patients throughout the perioperative period, and to patients in general. It appears important that monitoring of the circulation allows for intervention well before cerebral blood flow and oxygenation become affected, and evidence is provided for a volume administration strategy that is accurate within 100 and 200 ml.

Cerebral blood flow and oxygenation become affected with a blood loss corresponding to 30% of the (central) blood volume [40] or a blood loss of 1.0–1.5 l. The proposed volume administration strategy thereby allows volume administration within approximately one tenth of the volume loss that is significant for brain function.

CBV is important for filling the heart. The impact of a reduced CBV for SV, CO and thus central and mixed (from the pulmonary artery) venous oxygen saturation (SvO_2) offers monitoring modalities for evaluating the functional consequence of a reduced CBV.

Tilt table experiments

The influence of CBV on flow-related variables is readily illustrated during *tilt table experiments*. As mentioned, SV, CO and thus SvO_2 decrease during HUT, while maximal values are obtained during supine rest. Furthermore, with the increase in central pressures and also filling of the heart during head-down tilt, there is no further increase in SV, CO or SvO_2 [37,41] and SV decreases only during extreme (90°) head-down tilt [42].

Similarly, healthy non-fastening healthy supine subjects are not volume responsive with regard to SV [43] and together these observations indicate that for supine humans, maximal flow-related variables define normovolemia.

The surgical patient

In contrast to supine healthy subjects, the preoperative patient [3,4] and many patients under intensive care are volume responsive. To supplement volume is important since any limitation to CO has consequences for all vascular beds, independent of an eventually large metabolic demand as exemplified by muscle blood flow during exercise [44], and cerebral blood flow and oxygenation become affected already with the moderate reduction of CO that is associated with standing up [40]. Even more so skin, muscle and notably splanchnic and renal blood flow decrease in response to the elevated sympathetic activity provoked by a limited CBV and thereby CO. Conversely, a volume strategy that secures CO preserves not only splanchnic and renal flows of relevance for surgical healing and diuresis, respectively, but also for cerebral oxygenation, which is widely independent of MAP (Figure 19.3) [45].

Thus, it seems evident that the primary focus of volume therapy is to prevent episodes of hypovolemia, and on line monitoring of flow-related variables makes that a possible consequence of postoperative complications [31].

For individual patients, maintenance of cerebral oxygenation may require a MAP of 90 mmHg, probably because of arteriosclerosis in the vessels that serve the cerebral circulation. Monitoring of cerebral blood flow and/or oxygenation is advocated for older and vascular surgical patients, also considering that cerebral autoregulation might be compromised by the inhalation agents used for general anesthesia (Figure 19.3).

Evaluation of cerebral oxygenation is relevant especially to cardiac surgery during which the heart–lung machine determines CO. Maintaining cerebral oxygenation, e.g., by increasing the pump speed of the machine, reduces postoperative complications and secures the mental well-being of the patient [46]. Similarly, maintained cerebral oxygenation is important for reducing complications following other types of surgery, and maintained cerebral oxygenation may be taken as an index for whether handling of the circulation has been adequate [47].

Titration to establish normovolemia

A problem with directing volume treatment by flow-related variables is their individual variability. For example, the trained athlete has a low resting HR and a compensating large SV that makes it difficult to evaluate whether a given filling of the heart is sufficient to secure a maximal SV.

For CO and SvO_2 the inter-individual variation is smaller, but there remain significant differences among subjects/patients, and only some of the variation can be explained. Notably, there are inter-individual differences in CO according to beta-adrenergic polymorphism with the "Gly-Gly" carrying an approximate one liter per minute larger CO than the "Arg-Arg" phenotype [48]. In other words, there is a genetic background for why accurate volume administration based on flow-related variables should be individualized [31]. More importantly, however, is the fact that CO (and thereby SvO_2) varies depending on circumstances including type of anesthesia, temperature and notably disease.

Choice of volume treatment

Volume treatment is usually with a crystalloid, eventually supplemented by a (typically synthetic) colloid, considering that administration of blood is an independent risk factor for the surgical patient. Accordingly, initial volume treatment is associated with hemodilution that itself increases CO because of the inverse relationship between CO and hematocrit [49]. Volume treatment, thereby, becomes a self-promoting strategy that leaves little indication for when it should be terminated. To circumvent that limitation to flow-directed volume therapy, a common algorithm requires that SV be increased by 10% in response to a 200 ml bolus of colloid to justify further administration of volume [31].

An alternative approach to individualized goal-directed fluid therapy is to take advantage of the observation that *SvO_2 rather than CO is the regulated variable* [50]. Thus variation in SvO_2 is independent of the fluid used for volume administration (a crystalloid, a colloid or blood products) (Figure 19.4).

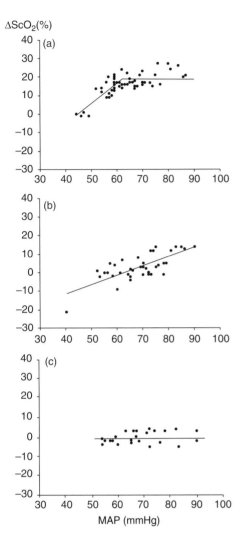

Figure 19.3. Changes in frontal lobe ScO_2 and MAP during anesthesia. Illustrated are three patients of whom one patient demonstrated a lower limit of cerebral autoregulation (a), for another patient no cerebral autoregulation was found (b) and also illustrated is a patient for whom no lower limit of cerebral autoregulation was detected (c) (derived from Nissen et al., 2009 [45]). ScO_2, cerebral oxygenation; ScO_2, venous oxygen saturation; MAP, mean arterial pressure.

Clinical outcome

For patients in hypovolemic shock the chosen transfusion strategy may be decisive. An attempt may be made to stop bleeding by administration of a pro-hemostatic agent [51], but the chosen fluid is also important. Synthetic colloid suspensions possess a high intravascular volume expansion effect, but also attenuate coagulation competence and that may lead to uncontrollable hemorrhage [52]. Alternatively, crystalloids enhance, when administered in a moderate amount, coagulation competence and are recommended for trauma patients. It remains that patients exposed to a massive blood loss require administration of plasma and platelets in addition to red blood cells in order to maintain coagulation competence and, if such balanced administration of blood products is established, survival of the trauma patient is enhanced.

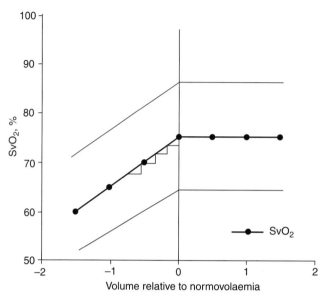

Figure 19.4. Venous oxygen saturation (SvO$_2$) during volume administration. With infusion of 100 ml of volume, SvO$_2$ increases by approximately 1% and the administration of volume is continued until SvO$_2$ does not increase further. For individual patients there are established markedly different relationships between SvO$_2$ and the volume load, but the administration of volume is continued until a maximal value is reached and that may be high, e.g., in a patient with liver disease or fever.

References

1. Barcroft H, Edholm OG, McMichael J, Sharpey-Schafer EF. Posthaemorrhagic fainting; study by cardiac output and forearm flow. *Lancet* 1944; **1**: 489–91.

2. Gordh T. Postural circulatory and respiratory changes during ether and intravenous anesthesia. *Acta Chir Scand* 1945; Suppl. **92**.

3. Jenstrup M, Ejlersen E, Mogensen T, Secher NH. A maximal central venous oxygen saturation (SvO$_{2max}$) for the surgical patient. *Acta Anaesthesiol Scand* 1995; **39** (Suppl. 107): 29–32.

4. Bundgaard-Nielsen M, Jørgensen CC, Secher NH, Kehlet H. Functional intravascular volume deficit in patients before surgery. *Acta Anaesthesiol Scand* 2010; **54**: 464–9.

5. Bundgaard-Nielsen M, Secher NH, Kehlet H. "Liberal" vs. "restrictive" perioperative fluid therapy – a critical assessment of the evidence. *Acta Anaesthesiol Scand* 2009; **53**: 843–51.

6. Cushing HW. On routine determination of arterial tension in operating room and clinic. *Boston Med Surg J* 1903; **148**: 250–6.

7. Schadt JC, Ludbrook J. Hemodynamic and neurohormal responses to acute hypovolaemia in conscious animals. *Am J Physiol* 1991; **260**: H305–18.

8. Krantz T, Laurizen T, Cai Y, Warberg J, Secher NH. Accurate monitoring of a blood loss: thoracic electrical impedance during haemorrhage in the pig. *Acta Anaesthesiol Scand* 2000; **44**: 598–604.

9. Perko M, IL Jarnvig IL, Højgaard-Rasmussen N, Eliasen K, Arendrup H. Electric impedance for evaluation of body fluid balance in cardiac surgery patients. *J Cardiothorac Vasc Anesth* 2001; **15**: 44–8.

10. Beecher HK. *Resuscitation and Anesthesia for Wounded Men. The Management of Traumatic Shock.* Springfield, IL: CC Thomas, 1949.

11. Wiggers CJ. *Physiology of Schock.* New York: The Commonwealth Fund, 1950.

12. Secher NH, Pawelczyk JA, Ludbrook J (eds.) *Blood Loss and Shock*. London: Edward Arnold, 1994.

13. Secher NH, Jacobsen J, Friedman DB, Matzen S. Bradycardia during reversible hypovolaemic shock: associated neural reflex mechanisms and clinical implications. *Clin Exp Pharm Physiol* 1992; **19**: 733–43.

14. Brøndum E, Hasenkam JM, Secher NH, *et al.* Jugular venous pooling during lowering of the head affects blood pressure of the anesthetised giraffe. *Am J Physiol* 2009; **297**: R1058–65.

15. Pedersen M, Madsen P, Klokker M, Olesen HL, Secher NH. Sympathetic influence on cardiovascular responses to sustained head-up tilt in humans. *Acta Physiol Scand* 1995; **155**: 435–44.

16. Murrell C, Cotter JD, George K, *et al.* Influence of age on syncope following prolonged exercise: differential responses but similar orthostatic intolerance. *J Physiol* 2009; **587**: 5959–69.

17. Murray RH, Thomson LJ, Bowers JA, Albreight CD. Hemodynamic effects of graded vasodepressor syncope induced by lower body negative pressure. *Am Heart J* 1968; **76**: 799–811.

18. Sander-Jensen K, Secher NH, Astrup A, *et al.* Hypotension induced by passive head-up tilt: endocrine and circulatory mechanisms. *Am J Physiol* 1986; **251**: R742–8.

19. Matzen S, Secher NH, Knigge U, Bach FW, Warberg J. Pituitary-adrenal responses to head-up tilt in humans: effect of H_1- and H_2- receptor blockade. *Am J Physiol* 1992; **263**: R156–63.

20. Jacobsen TN, Jost CMT, Converse Jr. RL, Victor RG. Cardiovascular sensors: the bradycardic phase in hypovolaemic shock. In *Blood Loss and Shock* (eds Secher NH, Pawelczyk JA, Ludbrook J). London: Edward Arnold, 1994, pp. 3–10.

21. Sander-Jensen K, Secher NH, Bie P, Warberg J, Schwartz TW. Vagal slowing of the heart during haemorrhage: observations from 20 consecutive hypotensive patients. *Br Med J* 1986; **292**: 364–6.

22. Mair RV. Hypovolemic shock. In *Harrison's Online* 17th edn. (eds Fauci AS, E Braunwald E, Kasper DL, *et al.*) New York: McGraw-Hill, 2010..

23. Secher NH, Bie P. Bradycardia during reversible haemorrhagic shock – a forgotten observation? *Clin Physiol* 1985; **5**: 315–23.

24. Guarini S, Cainazzo MM, Giuliani D, *et al.* Adrenocorticotropin reverses hemorrhagic shock in anesthetized rats through the rapid activation of a vagal anti-inflammatory pathway. *Cardiovasc Res* 2004; **63**: 357–65.

25. Sawdon M, Ohnishi M, Little RA, Kirkman E. Naloxone does not inhibit the injury-induced attenuation of the response to severe haemorrhage in the anaesthetized rat. *Exp Physiol* 2009; **94**: 641–7.

26. Jacobsen J, Hansen OB, Sztuk F, Warberg J, Secher NH. Enhanced heart rate response to haemorrhage by ileus in the pig. *Acta Physiol Scand* 1993; **149**: 293–301.

27. Ogoh S, Volianitis S, Raven PB, Secher NH. Carotid baroreflex function ceases during vasovagal syncope. *Clin Autonom Resch* 2004; **14**: 30–33.

28. Bie P, Secher NH, Astrup A, Warberg J. Cardiovascular and endocrine responses to head-up tilt and vasopressin infusion in man. *Am J Physiol* 1986; **251**: R735–41.

29. Sander-Jensen K, Secher NH, Astrup A, *et al.* Angiotensin II attenuates reflex decrease in heart rate and sympathetic activity in man. *Clin Physiol* 1988; **8**: 31–40.

30. Abrahamsson H, Thorén P. Vomiting and reflex vagal relaxation of the stomach elicited from heart receptors in the cat. *Acta Physiol Scand* 1973; **88**: 8–22.

31. Bundgaard-Nielsen M, Holte K, Secher NH, Kehlet H. Monitoring of perioperative fluid administration by individualized goal-directed therapy. *Acta Anaesthesiol Scand* 2007; **51**: 331–40.

32. Öberg B, White S. The role of vagal cardiac nerves and arterial barorectors in the circulatory adjustments to hemorrhage in the cat. *Acta Physiol Scand* 1970; **80**: 395–403.

33. Jacobsen J, Søfelt S, Fernandes A, et al. Reduced left ventricular size at onset of bradycardia during epidural anaesthesia. *Acta Anaesthesiol Scand* 1992; **36**: 831–6.

34. Morita H, Vatner SF. Effects of hemorrhage on renal nerve activity in conscious dogs. *Circ Research* 1985; **57**: 788–93.

35. Jacobsen J, Secher NH. Heart rate during haemorrhagic shock. *Clin Physiol* 1992; **12**: 659–66.

36. Matzen S, Perko GE, Groth S, Friedman DB, Secher NH. Blood volume distribution during head-up tilt induced central hypovolaemia in man. *Clin Physiol* 1991; **11**: 411–22.

37. van Lieshout JJ, Harms MPM, Pott F, Jenstrup M, Secher NH. Stoke volume and central vascular pressures during tilt in humans. *Acta Anaesthesiol Scand* 2005; **49**: 1287–92.

38. Marik PE, Baram M, Vahid B. Does central venous pressure predict fluid responsiveness? A systemic review of the literature and the tale of seven mares. *Chest* 2008; 134: 172–8.

39. Thys DM, Hillel Z, Goldman ME, Mindich BP, Kapland JA. A comparison of hemodynamic indices derived by invasive monitoring and two-dimensional echocardiography. *Anesthesiology* 1987; 67: 630–4.

40. van Lieshout JJ, Wieling W, Karemaker JM, Secher NH. Syncope, cerebral perfusion and oxygenation. *J Appl Physiol* 2003; **94**: 833–48.

41. Jans Ø, Tollund C, Bundgaard-Nielsen M, et al. Goal-directed fluid therapy: stroke volume optimization and cardiac dimensions in healthy humans. *Acta Anaesthesiol Scand* 2008; **52**: 536–40.

42. Bundgaard-Nielsen M, Sørensen H, Dalsgaard M, Rasmussen P, Secher NH. Relationship between stroke volume, cardiac output and filling of the heart during tilt. *Acta Anaesthesiol Scand* 2009; 53: 1324–8.

43. Bundgaard-Nielsen M, Jørgensen CC, Kehlet H, Secher NH. Normovolaemia defined in relation to stroke volume in humans. *Clin Physiol Func Imang* 2010; 30: 318–22.

44. Secher NH, Volianitis S. Are the arms and legs in competition for cardiac output? *Med Sci Sports Exerc* 2006; **38**: 1797–803.

45. Nissen P, Pacino H, Frederiksen HJ, Novovic S, Secher NH. Near-infrared spectroscopy for evaluation of cerebral autoregulation during orthotopic liver transplantation. *Neurocrit Care* 2009; **11**: 235–41

46. Murkin JM, Adams SJ, Novick RJ, et al. Monitoring brain oxygen saturation during coronary bypass surgery: a randomized, prospective study. *Anesth Analg* 2007; **104**: 51–8.

47. Murkin JM, Arango M. Near-infrared spectroscopy as index of brain and tissue oxygeation. *Br J Anaesth* 2009; **103** (Suppl. 1): 3–13.

48. Snyder EM, Beck HC, Diez NM, et al. Arg16Gly polymorphism of the ß2-adrenergic receptor is associated with differences in cardiovascular function at rest and during exercise in humans. *J Physiol* 2006; **571**: 121–30.

49. Krantz T, Warberg J, Secher NH. Venous oxygen saturation during normovolaemic haemodilution in the pig. *Acta Anaesthesiol Scand* 2005; **49**: 1149–56.

50. González-Alonso J, Mortensen S, et al. Erythrocyte and the regulation of human skeletal muscle blood flow and oxygen delivery: Role of erythrocyte count and oxygenation state of haemoglobin. *J Physiol* 2006; **572**: 295–305.

51. Zaar M, Secher NH, Johansson PI, et al. Effects of a recombinant FVIIa analogue, NN1731, on blood loss and survival after liver trauma in the pig. *Br J Anaesth* 2009; **103**: 840–7.

52. Zaar M, Lauritzen B, Secher NH, et al. Initial administration hydroxyethyl starch vs. lactated Ringer after liver trauma in the pig. *Br J Anaesth* 2009; **102**: 221–6.

Chapter 20

Uncontrolled hemorrhage

Richard P. Dutton

Fluid therapy in the face of ongoing hemorrhage is a challenging clinical situation, because the strategy and tactics of resuscitation can strongly influence the patient's outcome. While anatomic control of open blood vessels is critical (i.e., the surgeon's part of the job), the choice of resuscitation fluid and the rate and timing of administration can mean the difference between uneventful recovery and death from the "lethal triad" of acidosis, hypothermia and coagulopathy. Improved understanding of the pathophysiology of uncontrolled hemorrhage has led to significant changes in resuscitation in the past two decades. This chapter will review those developments and present the author's recommendations for clinical management.

The pathophysiology of uncontrolled hemorrhage

Cardiac output, and thus organ perfusion, is a function of the quantity of intravascular fluid and the size (capacity) of the intravascular fluid compartment. This relationship is shown in Figure 20.1.

Hemorrhage causes an immediate reduction in circulating blood volume. While the majority of fluid in the body is extravascular, only a limited quantity is available for recruitment into the blood stream. In the unanesthetized trauma patient, in whom bleeding occurs prior to medical intervention, reduced blood volume leads to collapse of small vessels and arteriolar closure of less essential vascular beds. Cardiac contractility would be reduced in accordance with the Frank–Starling relationship, although this effect is initially offset by increased sympathetic stimulation leading to elevated heart rate and increased inotropic state.

The body acts to preserve blood flow to essential organs: the heart and the brain. Peripheral vasoconstriction and increased sympathetic tone lead to the signs and symptoms of hemorrhagic shock: pallor, diaphoresis, agitation, oliguria, tachycardia and narrowed pulse pressure. In young healthy adults, core perfusion and systolic blood pressure can be temporarily maintained despite loss of up to 50% of blood volume (Figure 20.1, point 1).

As the limits of physiologic compensation are reached cardiac output will fall, and the late and ominous signs of shock will develop: hypotension, anuria, lethargy and then vascular system failure [1] (Figure 20.1, point 2). Death from hemorrhagic shock is characterized by profound acidosis, complete loss of vascular tone, irreversible coagulopathy and coma.

Clinical Fluid Therapy in the Perioperative Setting, ed. Robert G. Hahn. Published by Cambridge University Press. © Cambridge University Press 2011.

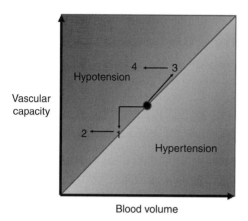

Figure 20.1. The physiologic relationship between vascular (bloodstream) capacity and the quantity of blood that fills it. In the normal state (the center dot) volume and capacity are matched. Hemorrhage reduces blood volume and compensatory vasoconstriction preserves blood pressure (point 1). Bleeding in excess of compensation leads to hypotension (point 2). Anesthesia increases vascular capacity through vasodilation, compensated by fluid administration (point 3). Bleeding while under anesthesia leads to hypotension (point 4).

In the perioperative setting, bleeding can also occur in patients who are already under general anesthesia. This is the normal state of affairs during major surgery or when unexpected hemorrhage occurs during a routine case. It is important to note that anesthesia will block some of the normal compensatory mechanisms described above, but that hypotension is typically offset by ongoing fluid administration (Figure 20.1, point 3). In particular, vasoconstriction is inhibited. This means that blood pressure will fall earlier, and in a more linear relationship to blood volume (Figure 20.1, point 4). On the one hand, this prevents the development of shock because tissue perfusion is preserved for a given blood pressure (low pressure but high flow), but on the other hand it removes some of the signs and symptoms of impending hemodynamic collapse.

Maintenance of hypotension

Clot formation early after injury occurs on the outside of damaged vessels [2]. The effectiveness of early clotting is determined by the size of the injury, but also by blood pressure, platelet and clotting factor concentration, temperature, acidosis and preexisting patient factors such as genetic abnormalities (factor deficiency diseases) and the use of anticoagulant medications such as aspirin, warfarin or thienopyridines (e.g., clopidogrel). Of these factors, the easiest to manage is blood pressure.

Deliberate hypotension – usually achieved by increasing the concentration of volatile anesthetic – has been in use for many decades as a strategy for reducing blood loss in elective surgeries where transfusion is a risk [3]. This includes hip and spine surgery, major facial surgery and prostate resections. A lower blood pressure directly reduces blood lost from open vessels and is typically associated with lower transfusion requirements, more rapid surgery and no demonstrable increase in postoperative complications.

One caveat to this approach is a reduced margin for error should uncontrolled hemorrhage occur, a risk that is managed by obtaining abundant intravenous access ahead of time, increasing the intensity of monitoring (e.g., using continuous arterial pressure measurement) and keeping a ready supply of blood products available for immediate transfusion if deterioration occurs. In this way an unexpected increase in bleeding can be immediately met with an increase in fluid administration, allowing for continued perfusion and preventing the onset of shock.

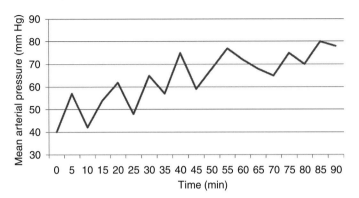

Figure 20.2. Mean arterial blood pressure vs. time during uncontrolled hemorrhage, managed with fluid and anesthesia loading. Bleeding and anesthetic administration cause a decrease in pressure; fluid administration causes an increase. Variability in response to fluid or anesthetic administration is decreased once hemostasis is achieved.

In contrast, the *trauma patient* begins hemorrhaging before induction of anesthesia, and is thus fully vasoconstricted and deeply in shock before therapy begins. This makes rapid infusion of fluid much more dangerous. The benefit of deliberate hypotensive resuscitation during uncontrolled hemorrhage has been demonstrated in numerous laboratory studies of mammals ranging from mice to swine [4,5].

Clinically, the danger of rapid fluid administration to bleeding casualties has been noted since World War I in the military medicine literature [6]. The efficacy of this approach in civilian trauma patients was demonstrated in one large clinical trial in the early 1990s [7] and its safety was further addressed in a smaller study published in 2002 [8]. Targeting a lower than normal blood pressure during early resuscitation is the standard of care today in most major trauma centers.

One barrier to deliberate hypotensive management during early resuscitation, even in centers that desire to do so, is the patient's brittle hemodynamic state. As illustrated in Figure 20.1 above, compensatory vasoconstriction may allow a hemorrhaging patient to preserve a near normal blood pressure even in the face of substantial blood loss. When the potential for physiologic compensation is exceeded the patient will become hypotensive very rapidly, because each further drop of blood lost represents a much greater per cent of blood in the remaining blood volume. The same is true in reverse: a 500ml fluid bolus represents 10% of the blood volume of a euvolemic patient, but 20% or more of the circulating volume of a patient in severe hemorrhagic shock.

In the uncontrolled situation of prehospital and Emergency Department care it is common for the blood pressure of trauma patients to oscillate wildly as they bleed, receive fluids and re-bleed. Blood pressure over the course of resuscitation is often oscillatory (Figure 20.2), with variability not damping out until hemostasis is achieved, and both blood volume and bloodstream capacity are restored to normal through administration of fluids and anesthesia.

The choice of resuscitation fluid

As important as managing the rate and timing of resuscitation is the choice of fluid. In the long run – after hemostasis is achieved – fluid administration will be required to make up the deficit produced by hemorrhage and by extravasation of fluids into the physiologically non-functioning "third space" [9].

Isotonic crystalloid solutions (lactated Ringer's solution and Plasma-Lyte A) are adequate to restore total body fluids over time, are inexpensive and logistically easy to work with and do not produce or exacerbate metabolic derangements. Laboratory evidence of ill effects from crystalloid administration is present, but the clinical significance appears to be relatively mild: rapid administration of normal saline (which is mildly hypertonic) will cause a subsequent hyperchloremic acidosis which must be managed [10], while various isotonic solutions have been associated with changes in inflammatory state [11]. The significance of this finding, especially in patients with major trauma or surgical wounds, is not yet clear.

Hypertonic and/or colloidal solutions have been advocated for resuscitation from hemorrhagic shock for several decades. By drawing free fluid in from the extravascular space, these solutions will increase intravascular volume more rapidly than isotonic crystalloid solutions, and will require a significantly lower volume of administration to produce a similar improvement in cardiac output.

The other side of this coin, however, is the potential to raise the blood pressure prematurely in patients still at risk for hemorrhage, thus disrupting early coagulation and contributing to ongoing or recurrent blood loss. Colloids have also been associated with more and more varied, negative effects on inflammatory state and coagulation than crystalloid solutions [12,13]. The largest prospective evaluation of crystalloids vs. colloids was the SAFE trial, conducted in Australia and New Zealand, which demonstrated absolutely no difference in outcome between albumin and lactated Ringer's solution as the primary resuscitative fluids used for intensive care patients [14].

Given this lack of clinical support for either type of solution, as well as the realities of clinical management during active hemorrhage, the author's preferred answer to the crystalloid vs. colloid question is: *"Blood!"*

Uncontrolled hemorrhage is a dynamic process with the potential for rapid and fatal deterioration at any moment. Clinical decision making cannot wait for laboratory assays or sophisticated monitoring (although these diagnostic steps should be undertaken as time and personnel allow). Empiric therapy is often required, and the most sensible approach is to emphasize fluids that either carry oxygen (red blood cells [RBC]) or promote coagulation (plasma or platelets). The ideal resuscitative fluid would be ABO- and HLA-matched fresh whole blood, and this is why preoperative autologous donation is a useful option when contemplating major elective surgery.

In the vast majority of uncontrolled hemorrhage cases, however, this option is not available. Random-donor fresh whole blood has been used successfully in trauma patients in Israel [15] and in selected military hospitals [16], but is not available in civilian hospitals in the US and Europe. This is due to stringent requirements for antiviral testing (which can take up to 72 h to complete – meaning that the blood product is no longer "fresh") and to the economic realities of transfusion medicine, which must fractionate units in order to match a precarious supply with an ever-increasing demand.

Most major trauma centers have made uncrossmatched Type-O RBC available for rapid administration to hemorrhaging patients, and this procedure is both safe and effective [17]. Transfusion with RBC will improve hemodynamics rapidly (potentially too rapidly, as above) and will support both perfusion and coagulation. Whereas banked blood has its own potential negatives, especially as it approaches the allowable limit of 42 days old, RBC are the first fluid that should be administered to any hemodynamically unstable patient with ongoing hemorrhage.

Recent clinical studies have demonstrated that the combination of shock and tissue injury will impair the clotting system even prior to any dilutional effects from resuscitation [18]. Indeed, abnormal admission prothrombin time is one of the most sensitive predictors

Table 20.1. Recommendations for management of resuscitation during active, uncontrolled hemorrhage in trauma patients or those with unexpected surgical bleeding.

Expedite anatomic control of bleeding (e.g., surgery or angiographic embolization), if not already in the operating room
Limit crystalloid infusion
Maintain systolic blood pressure at 80–90 mmHg
Administer fluid in titrated, small increments (100–200 ml per dose)
Resuscitate primarily with units of RBC, plasma and platelets in a 1:1:1 ratio
Monitor ionized calcium and lactate levels
Maintain normothermia
Achieve or maintain a deep anesthetic level, using titrated small increments of medication
When hemostasis is achieved, assess all laboratory and hemodynamic variables and complete resuscitation as needed

of mortality in trauma patients [19]. Early administration of plasma, in equal proportion to RBC, has been postulated as a management strategy for trauma patients in the past, and has now been retrospectively studied in both civilian and military practice [20,21].

Raw data show a strong association between survival and the early administration of plasma in trauma patients receiving a massive transfusion, although part of this effect is due to the confounding bias of patients with very rapid bleeding who die before plasma is available from the Blood Bank [22]. Prospective studies are now under way in centers that can supply plasma quickly to trauma patients, in an effort to more rigorously assess the potential benefit of this strategy.

In the meanwhile, it is reasonable, based on what is currently known about hemorrhagic shock and the pathophysiology of uncontrolled bleeding, to use RBC, plasma and platelet units in a 1:1:1 ratio as the primary resuscitative fluid prior to achieving hemostasis.

Because of the well-documented negative impact of transfusion on outcomes in critically ill patients [23], it is also reasonable to stop this empiric approach as soon as anatomic control of the source of uncontrolled bleeding is achieved. At that point, resuscitation should be continued in a more evidence-driven fashion based on laboratory assessment and hemodynamic and organ-function monitoring.

Clinical guidance for resuscitation

Table 20.1 shows the author's recommendations for management of the patient with uncontrolled hemorrhage. The overall strategic goal should be to facilitate and maintain hemostasis while simultaneously providing the best possible tissue perfusion.

Physiologically, the goal is to achieve the *high-flow, low-pressure state* that characterizes the use of deliberate hypotension in elective surgical cases and is associated with decreased blood loss without development of metabolic acidosis or coagulopathy.

If the patient is already anesthetized when hemorrhage occurs this will require fluid administration to keep up with blood loss, while maintaining a constant depth of anesthesia. The temptation to reduce the anesthetic dose because "the patient is not tolerating it" is a trap which should be avoided if at all possible, especially in a patient who has shown a normal response to anesthesia earlier in the case.

In the *trauma* patient, who begins in a vasoconstricted state, the paradoxical challenge is to administer fluid without increasing blood pressure, and administer anesthesia without exacerbating hypotension. Continuous arterial pressure monitoring and modern rapid infusion equipment make this possible in all but the most desperate cases. The key is to use small increments of fluid alternating with small doses of anesthesia, titrating the dose and timing to the patient's response and the progress of the surgery. When an adequate total dose of anesthesia is achieved (greater than 1 MAC equivalent in most patients) vasoconstrictive reflexes will be ablated, and increasing fluid administration will lead to increased tissue perfusion and reversal of shock. Skillfully performed, this transition from vasoconstricted to vasodilated physiology, without allowing an increase in systolic blood pressure, will create optimal conditions for surgical control of hemorrhage and subsequent resuscitation.

Table 20.1 makes note of some important adjuvant therapies in early resuscitation. Although laboratory studies have demonstrated a benefit to hypothermia in resuscitation, there have been no confirmatory clinical trials to date. Hypothermia will impair coagulation and imposes an additional metabolic burden on the patient during rewarming, and for this reason maintenance of normothermia is the current standard.

Rapid administration of blood products will include the unintended administration of citrate, which binds free calcium [24]. This will lead to the predictable development of hypocalcemia, which is easily managed with intravenous supplementation guided by frequent laboratory assays of ionized calcium level. If the patient is hypotensive and fails to respond to a fluid bolus then empiric administration of 500–1000 mg of calcium gluconate is reasonable, while awaiting laboratory results.

The other laboratory value of most ongoing utility is the serum *lactate* level. As the primary product of anaerobic metabolism, this provides a rough guide to the "dose" of shock sustained (i.e., the depth of hypoperfusion multiplied by the duration). In early resuscitation the goal should be to prevent lactate from increasing. Once hemostasis is achieved, the goal is to achieve a normal lactate level as rapidly as possible, by restoring both vascular capacity (reversing vasoconstriction) and blood volume. Survival following hemorrhagic shock is strongly associated with the rate of clearance of lactate from the circulation [25].

Conclusion

Successful fluid therapy during uncontrolled hemorrhage requires an understanding of the pathophysiology of shock and the ways in which survival can be improved. These include early support of the coagulation system, maintenance of deliberate hypotension and prevention or reversal of vasoconstriction. An empiric approach to early resuscitation, based on these principles, will facilitate hemostasis and provide the best possible conditions for survival.

References

1. Dutton RP. Current concepts in hemorrhagic shock. In: Weiss, Shamir (eds) *Anesthesiology Clinics of North America*, Vol. 25. Philadelphia, PA: Elsevier, 2007, pp. 23–34.

2. Shaftan GW, Chiu C, Dennis C, Harris B. Fundamentals of physiologic control of arterial hemorrhage. *Surgery* 1965; **58**: 851–6.

3. Sollevi A. Hypotensive anesthesia and blood loss. *Acta Anaesthesiol Scand* (Suppl.) 1988; **89**: 39–43.

4. Shoemaker WC, Peitzman AB, Bellamy R, *et al.* Resuscitation from severe hemorrhage. *Crit Care Med* 1996; **24**: S12–23.

5. Riddez L, Johnson L, Hahn RG. Central and regional hemodynamics during fluid therapy after uncontrolled intra-abdominal bleeding. *J Trauma* 1998; **44**: 433–9.

6. Cannon WB, Fraser J, Cowell EM. The preventive treatment of wound shock. *JAMA* 1918; **70**: 618–21.

7. Bickell WH, Wall MJ, Pepe PE, *et al.* Immediate versus delayed resuscitation for hypotensive patients with penetrating torso injuries. *N Engl J Med* 1994; **331**: 1105–9.

8. Dutton RP, Mackenzie CF, Scalea TM. Hypotensive resuscitation during active hemorrhage: impact on in hospital mortality. *J Trauma* 2002; **52**: 1141–6.

9. Shires T, Coln D, Carrico J, Lightfoot S. Fluid therapy in hemorrhagic shock. *Arch Surg* 1964; **88**: 688–93.

10. Kaplan LJ, Cheung NH, Maerz L, *et al.* A physicochemical approach to acid-base balance in critically ill trauma patients minimizes errors and reduces inappropriate plasma volume expansion. *J Trauma* 2009; **66**: 1045–51.

11. Rhee P, Wang D, Ruff P, Austin B, *et al.* Human neutrophil activation and increased adhesion by various resuscitation fluids. *Crit Care Med* 2000; **28**: 74–8.

12. Krausz MM, Bashenko Y, Hirsh M. Crystalloid and colloid resuscitation of uncontrolled hemorrhagic shock following massive splenic injury. *Shock* 2001; **16**: 383–8.

13. van Rijen EA, Ward JJ, Little RA. Effects of colloidal resuscitation fluids on reticuloendothelial function and resistance to infection after hemorrhage. *Clin Diagn Lab Immunol* 1998; **5**: 543–9.

14. Finfer S, Bellomo R, Boyce N, *et al.* SAFE Study Investigators. A comparison of albumin and saline for fluid resuscitation in the intensive care unit. *N Engl J Med* 2004; **350**: 2247–56.

15. Mohr R, Martinowitz U, Lavee J, Amroch D, Ramot B, Goor DA. The hemostatic effect of transfusing fresh whole blood versus platelet concentrates after cardiac operations. *J Thorac Cardiovasc Surg* 1988; **96**: 530–4.

16. Spinella PC. Warm fresh whole blood transfusion for severe hemorrhage: U.S. military and potential civilian applications. *Crit Care Med* 2008; **36**: S340–5.

17. Dutton RP, Shih D, Edelman BB, Hess JR, Scalea TM. Safety of uncrossmatched Type-O Red cells for resuscitation from hemorrhagic shock. *J Trauma* 2005; **59**: 1445–9.

18. Brohi, K., *et al.*, Acute traumatic coagulopathy. *J Trauma* 2003; **54**: 1127–30.

19. Hess JR, Lindell AL, Stansbury LG, Dutton RP, Scalea TM. The prevalence of abnormal results of conventional coagulation tests on admission to a trauma center. *Transfusion* 2009; **49**: 34–9.

20. Duchesne JC, Hunt JP, Wahl G, *et al.*, Review of current blood transfusions strategies in a mature level I trauma center: were we wrong for the last 60 years? *J Trauma* 2008; **65**: 272–6.

21. Borgman MA, Spinella PC, Perkins JG, *et al.* The ratio of blood products transfused affects mortality in patients receiving massive transfusions at a combat support hospital. *J Trauma* 2007; **63**: 805–13.

22. Stansbury LG, Dutton RP, Stein DM, *et al.* Controversy in trauma resuscitation: do ratios of plasma to red blood cells matter? *Transfus Medi Rev* 2009; **23**: 255–65.

23. Napolitano LM, Kurek S, Luchette FA, *et al.* Clinical practice guideline: red blood cell transfusion in adult trauma and critical care. *Crit Care Med* 2009; **37**: 3124–57.

24. Sihler KC, Napolitano LM. Complications of massive transfusion. *Chest* 2010; **137**: 209–20.

25. Abramson D, Scalea TM, Hitchcock R, Trooskin SZ, Henry SM, Greenspan J. Lactate clearance and survival following injury. *J Trauma* 1993; **35**: 584–8.

Fluids or blood products?

Oliver Habler

The transfusion dilemma

Although safer than ever, allogeneic transfusion is still associated with risks for the recipient (clerical error, hemolysis, infection, immunomodulation, transfusion-related acute lung injury [TRALI]) [1]. Unnecessary transfusion has been repeatedly demonstrated to increase mortality of intensive care and cardiac risk patients [2]. Moreover, the costs for allogeneic blood products are expected to rise in the future [3] due to an increasing imbalance between blood donors and potential recipients – particularly elder patients undergoing major surgery.

To control both the imminent risks as well as the increasing costs, allogeneic transfusion should either be completely avoided or at least minimized during surgical procedures. This can be achieved by:

1. the intraoperative transfusion of autologous blood collected preoperatively (autologous blood donation, acute normovolemic hemodilution) or intraoperatively (red blood cell salvage);
2. the reduction of the amount of blood loss; and
3. the tolerance of low perioperative hemoglobin (Hb) concentrations (anemia tolerance).

Management of intraoperative blood losses

An acute surgical blood loss will not immediately be compensated by the transfusion of red blood cells (RBC) and/or plasma. More likely the shed blood will initially be replaced by infusion of RBC-free crystalloidal and/or colloidal solutions.

This procedure is intended to maintain a normal circulating intravascular volume (i.e., normovolemia) while, at the same time, the dilution of all circulating blood components (normovolemic hemodilution) is tolerated.

Tolerance of dilutional anemia

Under general anesthesia "normovolemic hemodilution" is tolerated down to very low Hb concentrations and hematocrit (Hct) values, without any risk for tissue perfusion, tissue oxygenation and organ function. This reflects the large natural anemia tolerance of the human body.

Clinical Fluid Therapy in the Perioperative Setting, ed. Robert G. Hahn. Published by Cambridge University Press. © Cambridge University Press 2011.

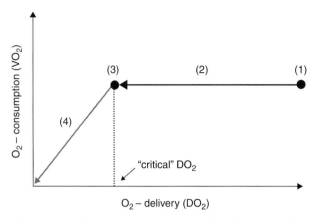

Figure 21.1. Schematic depicting the course of whole body O_2 delivery (DO_2) and O_2 consumption (VO_2) during normovolemic hemodilution (e.g., replacement of intraoperative blood loss with red blood cell-free infusion solutions); modified according to Cain, 1977 [11]). The graphic has to be read from the right side (starting with normal DO_2) to the left side (increasing dilutional anemia). Explanations in text.

The physiologic mechanisms enabling this anemia tolerance consist in [4]:

1. the increase of cardiac output (CO) – initially via the increase of ventricular stroke volume and, later on, via additional tachycardia – depending on the degree of hemodilution;
2. an increase of total body oxygen (O_2) extraction;
3. the physiologic difference between macro- and microvascular (capillary) Hct ("luxury Hct"). The microvascular Hct falls below its normal value only after a 30–50% reduction of the macrovascular Hct;
4. the physiologic over supply of organ tissues with O_2 ("luxury DO_2"). Under normal conditions, DO_2 exceeds tissue O_2 requirements by a factor of three to four (Figure 21.1, segment 1). Thus DO_2 can be reduced over a wide range without impairment of tissue oxygenation. Tissue O_2 demand is satisfied and tissue O_2 consumption (VO_2) remains constant (so called O_2 supply-independency of VO_2) (Figure 21.1, segment 2).

The compensatory mechanisms described above are decisive for the extent of anemia tolerance and likewise exist in infants [5], children [6,7], elderly patients [8], patients with cardiopulmonary disease [9] and patients under pharmacologic beta receptor blockade [10].

Limits of the natural anemia tolerance – concept of the "critical DO_2"(DO_{2crit})

At an extreme degree of hemodilution, O_2 demand will finally equal DO_2 (Figure 21.1, segment 3). The corresponding DO_2 is called "critical" (DO_{2crit}).

With ongoing hemodilution DO_2 falls below DO_{2crit} and the amount of O_2 delivered to the tissues becomes insufficient to further meet their O_2 demand. As a consequence VO_2 – stable by then – starts to decline (so-called O_2 supply-dependency of VO_2) (Figure 21.1, segment 4) [11]. This sudden decrease of VO_2 indirectly reflects the limit of anemia tolerance and the onset of tissue hypoxia. Energy needs of the body are now mainly met by anaerobic glycolysis and as a consequence the serum lactate concentration starts to rise.

In analogy to DO_{2crit}, the Hb or Hct values corresponding to the inflection point of VO_2 are called the "critical" Hb, Hb_{crit} and "critical" Hct, Hct_{crit}, respectively. Without treatment (transfusion, hyperoxic ventilation) the persistence of the "critical" DO_2, Hb or Hct finally leads to death within a short period of time [12,13].

The whole body's anemia tolerance may assume impressive proportions: in healthy awake volunteers DO_{2crit} was not met even after hemodilution to Hb 4.8 g/dl [14]. In healthy anesthetized animals and patients the limit of dilutional anemia was reported at Hct values between 12% and 3% (Hb 3.3 and 1.1 g/dl, respectively) (Table 21.1). Infants (1–7 months) [5] and children (12.5 years) [7] tolerated Hb of 3 g/dl and lower without falling below their DO_{2crit}. In pregnant sheep fetal tissue oxygenation was preserved down to a maternal Hct of 15% (Hb 5 g/dl) [15].

Unfortunately it is impossible to provide clinicians with universal numerical values for the aforementioned critical O_2 transport parameters.

DO_{2crit}, Hb_{crit} and Hct_{crit} vary inter- and intra-individually, and depend on a variety of determining factors: anesthesia in adequate depth, hyperoxemia, muscular relaxation and mild hypothermia *increase* anemia tolerance (see below); hypovolemia, restricted coronary reserve, heart failure, profound anesthesia, multiple trauma and sepsis *reduce* anemia tolerance.

Moreover it cannot be excluded that single organs meet their DO_{2crit} at a higher Hb (Hct) than the whole organism and develop tissue hypoxia prior to the drop of global VO_2. This would challenge whole body global VO_2 as a global monitoring parameter for tissue oxygenation.

In anesthetized subjects the anemia tolerance of the whole body and the brain [16], the myocardium with intact coronary perfusion [17,18] or the splanchnic system [16] could be demonstrated equal. However, the situation is different for the compromised heart with restricted coronary reserve. In anesthetized dogs with an experimental 50–80% coronary artery stenosis, signs of myocardial ischemia and/or functional deterioration appeared at Hb 7–10 g/dl [19].

In a retrospective cohort analysis of cardiac risk patients undergoing non-cardiac surgery and refusing allogeneic transfusion for religious reasons (affiliation to Jehovah's Witnesses), a significantly higher 30-day mortality was found if the postoperative Hb fell below 8 g/dl [20]. In otherwise healthy anesthetized rats the limit of renal anemia tolerance was identified to be between Hb 4 and 7 g/dl [21] and in patients undergoing cardiac surgery at between 7 and 8 g/dl [22,23].

In clinical practice it is difficult to identify the limit of the individual anemia tolerance of a single patient. Continuous measurement of VO_2 is technologically complex, costly and therefore restricted to scientific questions. Indirect clinical signs reflecting DO_{2crit} are uncertain but may consist in ECG-changes (ST-segment deviation, arrhythmia), echocardiographic regional myocardial wall motion disturbance, lactacidosis and a decrease of mixed-venous or central-venous O_2 saturation.

Support in estimating the significance of perioperative dilutional anemia *quoad vitam* is provided with the results of large clinical studies (generally performed in Jehovah's Witnesses) investigating the relation between postoperative anemia and mortality. Until a postoperative Hb of 8 g/dl no statistical relation between anemia and mortality could be detected even in elderly patients with preexisting cardiopulmonary disease [20,24] and intensive care patients with multiple morbidity [25–27]. In anemic patients (Hb < 8 g/dl), whose death was causally related to anemia, the Hb was always found to be below 5 g/dl [28]. Nevertheless, individual cases with much lower Hb level (1.5 g/dl and lower) could survive without transfusion.

Table 21.1. The limit of anemia tolerance. Overview of critical O_2 transport parameters determined in different species during extreme normovolemic hemodilution.

Reference	Species	Anesthesia	FiO_2	Blood exchange fluid	Identification of DO_{2crit}	Hct_{crit} (%)	Hb_{crit} (g/dl)
Fontana et al. [7]	human (child)	isoflurane sufentanil vecuronium	1.0	albumin	ST-segment depression		2.1
van Woerkens et al. [12]	human (84 years)	enflurane fentanyl pancuronium	0.4	gelatin	drop of VO_2	12	4
Zollinger et al. [42]	human (58 years)	propofol fentanyl pancuronium	1.0	gelatin	ST-segment depression		~1.1
Cain [11].	dog	pentobarbital	0.21	dextran	drop of VO_2	9.8	3.3
Perez-de-Sá et al. [43]	pig	isoflurane fentanyl midazolam cecuronium	0.5	dextran	drop of VO_2		2.3 ± 0.2
Meier et al. [13]	pig	propofol fentanyl	0.21	HES	drop of VO_2		3.1 ± 0.4
Pape et al. [44]	pig	propofol fentanyl pancuronium	0.21	HES	drop of VO_2		2.4 ± 0.4
Kemming et al. [18]	pig	midazolam morphine pancuronium	0.21	HES	ST-segment depression	7.2 ± 1.2	2.6 ± 0.3
Meisner et al. [45]	pig	diazepam morphin pancuronium	0.21	albumin	ST-segment depression	6.1 ± 1.8	2.0 ± 0.8
Meier et al. [46]	pig	propofol fentanyl pancuronium	0.21	HES	drop of VO_2		2.4 ± 0.5

DO_2, whole body oxygen delivery; FiO_2, inspiratory oxygen fraction; Hb_{crit}, critical hemoglobin concentration; Hct_{crit}, critical hematocrit; HES, hydroxyethyl starch; VO_2, oxygen consumption.

Therapeutic increase of anemia tolerance

In case of unexpected massive blood losses and/or logistic difficulties impeding an immediate start of transfusion, the anemia tolerance of the patient can be effectively increased by the following measures [29].

1. *Restoration and/or maintenance of normovolemia*: the basic prerequisite for the effective compensation of dilutional anemia is normovolemia. In case of "*hypovolemic hemodilution*" the whole body's O_2 demand *increases* – mediated by catecholamines. Under hypovolemic conditions DO_{2crit} is met at higher values than under normovolemia and anemia tolerance is reduced.

2. *Myocardial function*: another basic prerequisite for optimal cardiac compensation of dilutional anemia is the increase of myocardial blood flow realized by maximal coronary dilation as well as by the maintenance of an adequate coronary perfusion pressure (CPP). Situations accompanied by an increase of myocardial O_2 demand (tachycardia, increase of ventricular wall tension, increase of myocardial contractility) have to be avoided. The same applies for a decrease of diastolic aortic pressure due to reduction of systemic vascular resistance. Continuous application of norepinephrine increases whole body anemia tolerance. Sympathicolysis via betareceptor blockade or thoracic epidural anesthesia leaves anemia tolerance unaffected (author's unpublished data).

3. *Inspiratory oxygen fraction* (FiO_2): ventilation with supranormal FiO_2 (hyperoxic ventilation) increases the physically dissolved part of arterial O_2 content. Physically dissolved plasma O_2 is biologically highly available and covers up to 75% of the whole body's O_2 demand in conditions of extreme dilutional anemia. Experimental and clinical studies clearly demonstrate that hyperoxic ventilation effectively increases anemia tolerance and creates an important margin of safety for global, myocardial, gastrointestinal and cerebral tissue oxygenation.

4. *Muscular relaxation*: striated skeletal muscles amounts to about 30% of the total body mass. Muscular relaxation significantly reduces the whole body's O_2 demand and increases anemia tolerance.

5. *Body temperature*: hypothermia reduces the whole body's O_2 demand. In an animal experiment anesthetized hypothermic pigs died at lower Hb than normothermic control animals. Due to the negative impact of hypothermia on coagulation, however, the intentional induction of hypothermia in bleeding patients in order to increase anemia tolerance can not be recommended.

6. *Choice of the anesthetic drugs and depth of anesthesia*: almost all anesthetic drugs investigated suppress the CO response to dilutional anemia. In animal experiments a dose-related reduction of anemia tolerance could be demonstrated for halothane, enflurane, isoflurane, ketamine, propofol, etomidate and pentobarbital. Inadequately profound anesthesia has to be avoided to the same extent as inadequately flat anesthesia (increased sympathetic tone and O_2 consumption).

7. *Choice of the infusion solution*: the choice of the solution infused to compensate blood losses seems to influence anemia tolerance. While 3% gelatine and 6% hydroxyethylstarch (HES) 200.000/0.5 did not affect anemia tolerance in animals, an advantage of 6% HES 130.000/0.4 could be demonstrated over 3.5% gelatine, 6% HES 450.000/0.7 and lactated Ringer's. Application of infusion solutions with intrinsic O_2 transport capacity (artificial O_2 carriers based on human or bovine Hb; perfluorocarbons) increased anemia tolerance in animals and patients [30]. Unfortunately no artificial O_2 carrier is actually approved in USA or Europe.

Coagulation management

In analogy to dilutional anemia, the replacement of blood losses with crystalloid and/or colloid infusion fluids dilutes all components of the coagulatory and fibrinolytic systems. Finally, this results in "dilutional coagulopathy."

It could be demonstrated in animal experiments and patients that the first pro-coagulatory factor decreasing below a level requiring substitution is fibrinogen (i.e., < 150 mg/dl), followed by the activity of coagulation factors of the prothrombin complex and finally the platelet count [31,32]. Fibrinogen and fibrin are elementary for clot formation at the site of the vessel damage.

The lack of fibrinogen results in the formation of unstable clots unable to resist blood flow and to stop bleeding [33]. The plasma fibrinogen concentration is further reduced by infusion of HES-based colloidal infusion solutions [34]. Due to problems related to its processing fresh frozen plasma (FFP) contains factors of the coagulation system only in a reduced concentration. This implicates that FFP has to be infused in large quantities to stabilize or improve coagulation, often resulting in transfusion-related cardiac overload (TACO).

In the situation of the massively bleeding patient it is difficult, or even impossible, to monitor and detect the "critical" reduction of the different components of the coagulation system. While moderate dynamics of blood losses allow a differentiated coagulation management on the basis of the results obtained with thrombelastography [35], the lack of this analytic measure and/or the presence of more severe blood losses require the early and calculated administration of fibrinogen concentrate [36], prothrombin complex concentrate (PCC) [37], fresh frozen plasma and antifibrinolytic drugs (e.g., tranexamic acid) [38].

The administration of desmopressin [39] mobilizes stocks of factor VIII, increases the activity of von Willebrand factor and stimulates aggregatory platelet function. Clot stability may be additionally increased by application of factor XIII concentrate [40]. In case of massive bleeding the early administration of recombinant human factor VIIa ("off-label-use") may be taken into consideration [41] (Table 21.2). However, the maximum effectiveness of this substance depends on stable general conditions for coagulation, in particular on normothermia, normal pH and an adequate platelet count.

Summary

Thanks to the impressive anemia tolerance of the human body RBC transfusion may be often avoided despite even important blood losses – provided that normovolemia is maintained. While a Hb of 6–7 g/dl can be considered safe in young, healthy patients, elderly patients with pre existing cardiopulmonary morbidity should be transfused at Hb 8–10 g/dl.

Physiologic transfusion triggers (e.g., decrease of VO_2, ST-segment-depression in the ECG, arrhythmia, continuous increase in catecholamine needs, echocardiographic wall motion disturbances, lactacidosis) appearing prior to the aforementioned Hb necessitate immediate RBC transfusion.

In case of dilutional coagulopathy – often reflected by an intraoperatively upcoming diffuse bleeding tendency – a differentiated coagulation therapy can either be directed on the basis of thrombelastography or empirically replacing the different components in the order of their developing deficiency (i.e., starting with fibrinogen followed by factors of the prothrombin complex and platelets).

Table 21.2. Dosage of procoagulatory drugs in massive blood loss.

Fresh frozen plasma	> 30 ml/kg target: quick-value > 30–40%
Fibrinogen-concentrate	2–4 g target: plasma fibrinogen concentration > 150 mg/dl
Prothrombin complex concentrate	20–25 IU/kg target: quick-value > 30–40%
Tranexamic acid	initial bolus 10–15 mg/kg, then 1–5 mg/(kg h)
Desmopressin	0.3 µg/kg over 30 min
Factor XIII-concentrate	10–20 IU/kg
Recombinant human factor VIIa	90 µg/kg

The "global" stabilization of coagulation with fresh frozen plasma requires the application of high volumes and bears the risk of cardiac overload (TACO) and immunologic lung injury (TRALI).

References

1. Goodnough LT. Risks of blood transfusion. *Anesthesiology Clin N Am* 2005; **23**: 241–52.

2. Vamvakas EC, Blajchman MA. Transfusion-related mortality: the ongoing risks of allogeneic transfusion and the available strategies for their prevention. *Blood* 2009; **113**: 3406–17.

3. Shander A, Goodnough LT. Why an alternative to blood transfusion? *Crit Care Clin* 2009; **25**: 261–77.

4. Habler O, Messmer K. The physiology of oxygen transport. *Transfus Sci* 1997; **18**: 425–35.

5. Schaller RT, Schaller J, Furman EB. The advantages of hemodilution anesthesia for major liver resection in children. *J Pediatr Surg* 1984; **19**: 705–10.

6. Aly Hassan A, Lochbuehler H, Frey L, Messmer K. Global tissue oxygenation during normovolaemic haemodilution in young children. *Paediatr Anaesth* 1997; **7**: 197–204.

7. Fontana JL, Welborn L, Mongan PD, *et al.* Oxygen consumption and cardiovascular function in children during profound intraoperative normovolemic hemodilution. *Anesth Analg* 1995; **80**: 219–25.

8. Spahn DR, Zollinger A, Schlumpf RB, *et al.* Hemodilution tolerance in elderly patients without known cardiac disease. *Anesth Analg* 1996; **82**: 681–6.

9. Licker M, Ellenberger C, Sierra C, *et al.* Cardiovascular response to acute normovolemic hemodilution in patients with coronary artery disease: assessment with transoesophageal echocardiography. *Crit Care Med* 2005; **33**: 591–7.

10. Spahn DR, Schmid ER, Seifert B, Pasch T. Hemodilution tolerance in patients with coronary artery disease who are receiving chronic beta-adrenergic blocker therapy. *Anesth Analg* 1996; **82**: 687–94.

11. Cain SM. Oxygen delivery and uptake in dogs during anemic and hypoxic hypoxia. *J Appl Physiol* 1977; **42**: 228–34.

12. Woerkens van ECSM, Trouwborst A, Van Lanschot JJB. Profound hemodilution: What is the critical level of hemodilution at which oxygen delivery-dependent oxygen consumption starts in an anesthetized human. *Anesth Analg* 1992; **75**: 818–21.

13. Meier J, Kemming GI, Kisch-Wedel H, Wölkhammer S, Habler OP. Hyperoxic

ventilation reduces 6-hour mortality at the critical hemoglobin concentration. *Anesthesiology* 2004; **100**: 70–6.

14. Lieberman JA, Weiskopf RB, Kelley SD, *et al*. Critical oxygen delivery in conscious humans is less than 7.3 ml O$_2$ x kg^{-1} x min^{-1}. *Anesthesiology* 2000; **92**: 407–13.

15. Paulone ME, Edelstone DI, Shedd A. Effects of maternal anemia on uteroplacental and fetal oxidative metabolism in sheep. *Am J Obstet Gynecol* 1987; **156**: 230–7.

16. van Bommel J, Trouwborst A, L. Schwarte L, *et al*. Intestinal and cerebral oxygenation during severe isovolemic hemodilution and subsequent hyperoxic ventilation in a pig model. *Anesthesiology* 2002; **97**: 660–70.

17. Habler OP, Kleen M, Hutter J, *et al*. Iv Perflubron emulsion versus autologous transfusion in severe normovolemic anemia: effects on left ventricular perfusion and function. *Research in Experimental Medicine* 1998; **197**: 301–18.

18. Kemming GI, Meisner FG, Kleen M, *et al*. Hyperoxic ventilation at the critical hematocrit. *Resuscitation* 2003; **56**: 289–97.

19. Levy PS, Kim SJ, Eckel PK, *et al*. Limit to cardiac compensation during acute normovolemic hemodilution: influence of coronary stenosis. *Am J Physiol* 1993; **265**: H340–9.

20. Carson JL, Duff A, Poses RM, *et al*. Effect of anaemia and cardiovascular disease on surgical mortality and morbidity. *Lancet* 1996; **348**: 1055–60.

21. Johannes T, Mik EG, Nohe B, Unertl KE, Ince C. Acute decrease in renal microvascular pO2 during acute normovolemic hemodilution. *Am J Physiol Renal Physiol* 2007; **292**: F796–803.

22. Habib RH, Zacharias A, Schwann TA, *et al*. Role of hemodilutional anemia and transfusion during cardiopulmonary bypass in renal injury after coronary revascularization: implications on operative outcome. *Crit Care Med* 2005; **33**: 1749–56.

23. Ranucci M, Romitti F, Isgro G, *et al*. Oxygen delivery during cardiopulmonary bypass and acute renal failure after coronary operations. *Ann Thorac Surg* 2005; **80**: 2213–20.

24. Carson JL, Duff A, Berlin JA, *et al*. Perioperative blood transfusion and postoperative mortality. *JAMA* 1998; **279**: 199–205.

25. Hebert PC, Wells G, Blajchman MA, *et al*. A multicenter, randomized, controlled clinical trial of transfusion requirements in critical care. *N Engl J Med* 1999; **340**: 409–17.

26. Vincent JL, Baron JF, Reinhart K, *et al*. Anemia and blood transfusion in critically ill patients. *JAMA* 2002; **288**: 1499–507.

27. Carson JL, Noveck H, Berlin JA, Gould SA. Mortality and morbidity in patients with very low postoperative Hb levels who decline blood transfusion. *Transfusion* 2002; **42**: 812–8.

28. Viele MK, Weiskopf RB. What can we learn about the need for transfusion from patients who refuse blood? The experience with Jehovah's Witnesses. *Transfusion* 1994; **34**: 396–401.

29. Habler O, Meier J, Pape A, H. Kertscho H, Zwissler B. Perioperative anemia tolerance – mechanisms, influencing factors, limits. *Anaesthesist* 2006; **55**: 1142–56.

30. Habler O, Pape A, Meier J, Zwißler B. Artificial oxygen carriers as an alternative to red blood cell transfusion. *Anaesthesist* 2005; **54**: 741–54.

31. McLoughlin TM, Fontana JL, Alving B, Mongan PD, Bünger R. Profound normovolemic hemodilution: hemostatic effects in patients and in a porcine model. *Anesth Analg* 1996; **83**: 459–65.

32. Hiippala ST, Myllylä GJ, Vahtera EM. Hemostatic factors and replacement of major blood loss with plasma-poor red cell concentrates. *Anesth Analg* 1995; **81**: 360–5.

33. Fries D, Haas T, Salchner V, Lindner K, Innerhofer P. Management of coagulation after multiple trauma. *Anaesthesist* 2005; **54**: 137–44.

34. De Lorenzo C, Calatzis A, Welsch U, Heindl B. Fibrinogen concentrate reverses dilutional coagulopathy induced in vitro by

saline but not by hydroxyethyl starch 6%. *Anesth Analg* 2006; **102**: 1194–200.

35. Grashey R, Mathonia P, Mutschler W, Heindl B. Perioperative coagulation management controlled by thrombelastography. *Unfallchirurg* 2007; **110**: 259–63.

36. Weinkove R, Rangarajan S. Fibrinogen concentrate for acquired hypofibrinogenaemic states. *Transfusion Medicine* 2008; **18**: 151–7.

37. Samama CM. Prothrombin complex concentrates: a brief review. *Eur J Anaesth* 2008; **25**: 784–9.

38. Brown JR, Birkmeyer N, O'Connor GT. Meta-analysis comparing the effectiveness and adverse outcomes of antifibrinolytic agents in cardiac surgery. *Circulation* 2007; **115**: 2801–13.

39. Franchini M. The use of desmopressin as a hemostatic agent: a concise review. *Am J Hematol* 2007; **82**: 731–5.

40. Gödje O, Gallmeier U, Schelian M, Grünewald M, Mair H. Coagulation factor XIII reduces postoperative bleeding after coronary surgery with extracorporeal circulation. *Thorac Cardiovasc Surg* 2006; **54**: 26–33.

41. Franchini M, Franchi M, Bergamini V, *et al.* A critical review on the use of recombinant factor VIIa in life-threatening obstetric postpartum hemorrhage. *Semin Thromb Hemost* 2008; **34**: 104–12.

42. Zollinger A, Hager P, Singer T, Friedl HP, Pasch T, Spahn D. Extreme hemodilution due to massive blood loss in tumor surgery. *Anesthesiology* 1997; **87**: 985–7.

43. Perez-de-Sá V, Roscher R, Cunha-Goncalves D, Larsson A, Werner O. Mild hypothermia has minimal effects on the tolerance to severe progressive normovolemic anemia in swine. *Anesthesiology* 2002; **97**: 1189–97.

44. Pape A, Meier J, Kertscho H, *et al.* Hyperoxic ventilation increases the tolerance of acute normovolemic anemia in anesthetized pigs. *Crit Care Med* 2006; **34**: 1475–82.

45. Meisner FG, Kemming GI, Habler OP, *et al.* Diaspirin crosslinked hemoglobin enables extreme hemodilution beyond the critical hematocrit. *Crit Care Med* 2001; **29**: 829–38.

46. Meier J, Pape A, Loniewska D, Lauscher P, *et al.* Norepinephrine increases tolerance to acute anemia. *Crit Care Med* 2007; **35**: 1484–92.

Index

Abbreviations
AAA – abdominal aortic aneurysm
ANH – acute normovolemic hemodilution
EGDT – early, aggressive goal-directed therapy
GDT – goal-directed therapy
HES – hydroxyethylstarch
PVI – pleth variability index
TUR – transurethral resection

Note: All index entries pertain to fluid therapy, unless otherwise noted. "Fluid therapy" is not listed in the index, and readers are advised to seek more specific topics.

4/2/1 rule, 66

abdominal aortic aneurysm
    (AAA), hypovolemic
    shock, 168
abdominal aortic surgery
    heart rate and blood
        pressures, 168
    HES and renal function, 145
    hypovolemic shock, 168
    "rules-of-thumb" for fluids,
        25–6
acetate, in Ringer's solution, 3
acute normovolemic
        hemodilution (ANH),
        112, 184–5
    advantages, 112, 117
    anesthesia effects, 113, 114,
        115
    definition/description, 112,
        117
    efficacy, 116–17
        studies/literature reports,
            117
        theoretical, 116–17
    limits, 113–16, 187
        cardiac conditions,
            115–16
        hemostasis and, 116, 141
        physiological compensatory
            mechanisms, 112–13,
            117
    tolerance to, 115, 185
    see also anemia, dilutional;
        hemodilution
acute respiratory distress
        syndrome (ARDS), 74,
        75, 123

"fluids and catheter
    treatment trial", 161
adrenaline see epinephrine
    (adrenaline)
adverse reactions of iv fluids,
    137–47
    acid-base imbalance, 140–1
    excess tissue hydration and
        edema, 139–40
    hemostatic see hemostatic
        disturbances, fluid-
        associated
    hypersensitivity and
        anaphylaxis, 13, 123,
        143–4
    hypervolemia and
        hypertension, 138–9
    see also fluid overload
    hypothermia, 140, 141
    local effects, 137–8, 145
    organ function impairment,
        145
    summary, 145–6
    systemic, 138, 145
    temperature-/osmolality-
        associated, 138
    tissue deposition and
        pruritus, 144–5
Aesculon system, 99
albumin, 11, 123
    adverse effects, 12, 123
    clinical use, 12, 123
    in infants and neonates, 69
    iodated, 127–8, 130
    pharmacokinetics, 11–12
    plasma volume expansion,
        123, 124
"albumin debate," 12

ammonia, 150
analgesia, multimodal, day
    surgery, 56
anaphylactoid reactions,
    143–4
anaphylaxis, 143–4
    dextran associated, 13, 123,
        143–4
anemia
    in critically ill patients, 161
    preoperative, 20
anemia, dilutional
    tolerance, 184–5, 189
        in anesthetized subjects,
            186
        indirect signs for, 186
        limits, 185–6, 187, 189
        physiological
            mechanisms, 184–5
        therapeutic increase, 188
    see also hemodilution
anesthesia
    compensatory mechanisms
        in hemorrhage and, 178
    depth, dilutional anemia
        tolerance, 188
    effects on ANH response,
        113, 114, 115
    number of procedures, 103
    physiologic adjustments
        to, 113
    "rules of thumb" for
        perioperative fluids,
        21–2
    in severe sepsis/septic
        shock, 158
    in trauma, hemorrhage
        resuscitation and, 182

anesthesia (*cont.*)
　uncontrolled hemorrhage,
　　management, 181
　volume kinetics affected by,
　　133
anesthetic drugs, dilutional
　anemia tolerance, 188
anthropometry, 128–9
aortic reconstruction,
　hypertonic fluids,
　outcome, 78
aortic surgery
　abdominal *see* abdominal
　　aortic surgery
　hypertonic fluid benefits, 78
"Arg-Arg" phenotype, 172
arterial pressure, 103
　AAA surgery, 168
　hypovolemic shock, 166
　plasma volume expansion
　　and, 124
　reduced during surgery, 133
　　blood loss reduction, 178
　target in trauma
　　resuscitation, 179
　in uncontrolled hemorrhage,
　　178, 179
　see also mean arterial
　　pressure (MAP)
arterial pressure waveform
　analysis
　dynamic indices from, 85–6,
　　97, 98, 104
　limitations, 106
　PPV *see* pulse pressure
　　variation (PPV)
　respiratory systolic
　　variation test, 86
　SVV *see* stroke volume
　　variation (SVV)
　systolic pressure variation,
　　86, 162
　goal-directed therapy, 97–8,
　　108
　limitations, 98
arterial waveform pulse
　contour cardiac output
　see pulse contour
　analysis
atrial natriuretic peptide
　(ANP), 46, 124, 169

bariatric surgery, 61
baroreceptors, 167
basal fluid requirements, 18–19
Bezold–Jarish reflex, 170

bioimpedance (BIA), 128
BioZ system, 99
bleeding
　in hepatic surgery, 39
　see also blood loss (surgical);
　　hemorrhage
blood
　preoperative autologous
　　donation, 180, 184
　random-donor fresh whole,
　　180
blood–brain barrier (BBB), 122
　disrupted, 122, 123
　normal functions, 122
blood flow
　cerebral, in hypovolemic
　　shock, 171–2, 173
　microcirculatory,
　　autoregulation, early
　　septic shock, 160
　microvascular, enhancement,
　　20, 24
　by colloids, 20, 24, 97
　by hypertonic solutions,
　　73
　redistribution, hemodilution
　　effect, 113
blood fluidity, 112–13
blood groups, coagulation
　response to
　hemodilution, 116
blood loss (surgical), 92
　children, 67
　fluid "efficiency"
　　measurement, 130
　GDT using esophageal
　　Doppler, 94–5
　management, 184
　reduction in hepatic surgery,
　　39
　"rules of thumb," 21
　see also hemorrhage
blood pressure *see* arterial
　pressure
blood products, fluids vs.,
　184–92
blood transfusions
　antiviral testing, 180
　costs, 184
　deliberate hypotension in
　　hemorrhage and, 178
　hemorrhagic shock and
　　hypertonic fluid trials,
　　75
　indications, 20
　minimization strategies, 184

blood loss management,
　184
　dilutional anemia
　　tolerance *see* anemia,
　　dilutional
　intraoperative autologous,
　　184
　rapid, in hemorrhage, 182
　reduced by ANH, 112
　risk/benefits dilemma, 184
　in septic shock/severe sepsis,
　　161
　side effects, 125
　in uncontrolled hemorrhage,
　　180
　uncrossmatched type-O
　　RBC, 180
blood viscosity, 13, 115
blood volume
　central *see* central blood
　　volume (CBV)
　expansion *see* plasma volume
　　expansion
　intrathoracic *see* central
　　blood volume (CBV)
　reduced by hemorrhage, 177,
　　178
body temperature, reduced
　see hypothermia
body volume, 127–36
　calculation, using tracers,
　　127
　normal, 127
　see also fluid volumes;
　　volume kinetics
bowel preparation, 23, 29,
　52–3
bradycardia, in stage II of
　hypovolemic shock,
　168–9
brain injury
　hypertonic fluid
　　benefits, 73, 74
　clinical trials, 75–8
　Ringer's solution in, 5
bromide, extracellular fluid
　volume, 127

calories, requirements by
　children, 66
capillary fluid exchange
　see transcapillary fluid
　exchange
capillary leak, 12, 15, 19
　in sepsis, 157–8
carbohydrates, preoperative, 58

carbon monoxide, 128, 130
cardiac index, 91
  improvement by hypertonic
    fluids, 78
cardiac output, 177
  aortic blood flow velocity
    and, 39
  continuous, determination,
    83–5
  dilutional anemia tolerance
    mechanism, 185
  hypovolemic shock, 170,
    171–2
  increased, hemodilution
    effect, 112–13
  infants, 65
  inter-individual variation,
    172
  maximization in surgery, 103
  measurement/calculation
    arterial waveform pulse
      contour, 84
    esophageal Doppler
      monitoring, 88
    fluid responsiveness in
      septic shock, 162
    transesophageal
      echocardiography, 87
  monitoring, preload
    dependence and, 105
  reduced, in hemodilution,
    anesthesia effects, 113,
    114
  spinal anesthesia effect,
    46–7
  surrogate parameters for
    monitoring, 104, 105
  see also pulse pressure
    variation (PPV); stroke
    volume variation (SVV)
  thermodilution
    see thermodilution
    cardiac output
cardiac resuscitation,
    hypovolemic shock and,
    168, 169
cardiac surgery
  acute normovolemic
    hemodilution, 115–16
  dilutional anemia tolerance,
    186
  GDT using esophageal
    Doppler, 94
cardiopulmonary bypass
  surgery, hypertonic
    fluids, 78

cardiovascular response,
    absorption of irrigating
    fluids, 150–1
carotid baroreceptors, 167
catecholamines, 134
  see also specific catecholamines
cell membrane, 1
central blood volume (CBV),
    38, 166
  heart rate and arterial
    pressure response, 166
  in hypovolemic shock, 166,
    170, 171
    Bezold–Jarish reflex and,
      170
    pre-shock, 167
    stage II, 168–9
    stage III, 170
    surgical patients, 171–2,
      173
    tilt table experiments, 171
  measurement, 129
  reduced, impact, 171
central venous oxygen saturation
    (ScvO$_2$), 159, 162
central venous pressure (CVP),
    38
  in EGDT, 159
  fluid resuscitation in septic
    shock, 162
  hepatic surgery, blood loss
    reduction, 39
  in hypovolemic shock
    see hypovolemic shock
  in liver transplantation, 39
  volume status assessment,
    93, 104
cerebral blood flow, in
    hypovolemic shock,
    171–2, 173
cerebral capillaries, 122
cerebral damage, glucose
    solutions worsening, 6
cerebral edema
  absorption of irrigating
    fluids and, 151
  reduction by hypertonic
    fluids, 74
  vasogenic, 122, 123
cerebral oxygenation
  evaluation and maintaining,
    172
  in hypovolemic shock,
    171–2, 173
Cesarean section, 45, 46, 54
children, 65–72

acute hyponatremia, 70
blood loss (surgical), 67
dehydration, 67
  fluid therapy for, 67
fasting fluid deficit, 67
fasting guidelines, 66
fluid losses, 67, 68
fluid volumes and renal
    function, 65
intraoperative fluid
    management, 67–8
  clinical guidelines, 68
  glucose debate, 67–8
  isotonic hydrating
    solutions, 68
  quantity, 67
metabolic requirements,
    66
oral fluid intake, 70
perioperative hyperglycemia
    danger, 67–8
postoperative fluid therapy,
    70
  clinical guidelines, 70
  consensus on, 70
  controversies, 70
postoperative hyponatremia,
    70
preoperative assessments,
    66–7
preoperative hypoglycemia,
    67
resuscitation, hydroxyethyl
    starch (HES), 69
septic shock, 67, 69
volume replacement
    crystalloids, 67
    hydroxyethyl starch
      (HES), 69
  see also infants
chloride ion levels, 140
cholecystectomy, laparoscopic
  liberal fluids and outcome,
    37
  perioperative fluids, 58
  postoperative nausea and
    vomiting, 24
  "rules-of-thumb" for fluids,
    25
circulation, function, 103
citrate, 182
coagulation
  cascade activation
    prevention in trauma,
    20
  colloids affecting, 15

coagulation (*cont.*)
  HES effect on in children, 69
  crystalloids effect, 141
  hemodilution effect, 116, 189
  management, after fluid replacement, 189
  procoagulatory drugs, 190
  temperature for, hypothermia avoidance, 140, 141
  in uncontrolled hemorrhage, 189
coagulopathy
  colloid infusion-associated, 141
  dilutional, 189
  hypothermia-associated, 140, 141
  see also hemostatic disturbances, fluid-associated
colloid fluids (colloids), 11–17
  adverse reactions, 11, 137, 138, 146
    hemostatic disturbances, 141–3
    local, 137
    organ function impairment, 145
    renal failure, 145
    tissue deposition, 144–5, 146
    in uncontrolled hemorrhage, 180
  albumin *see* albumin
  based on balanced electrolyte fluids, 141
  clinical use, 11
  crystalloids comparison *see under* crystalloid fluids (crystalloids)
  dextran *see* dextran
  elimination, 133
  fluid overload, 139
  in gastrointestinal surgery, 24
  gelatin *see* gelatin
  goal-directed therapy, 97
    intra-abdominal surgery, 40
  in hypovolemic shock, 172, 173
  indication, 11, 97
  in massive fluid requirements, 20

  for microvascular blood flow enhancement, 20, 24, 97
  miscellaneous effects, 15
  plasma volume expansion, 122–4, 138
    colloid osmotic pressure effect, 138
    reducing need for, 124–5
  preloading, in spinal anesthesia, 47, 48
  saline base, effect on chloride load, 141
  in severe sepsis/septic shock, 161
  starch *see* hydroxyethyl starch (HES); starch
  synthetic, plasma volume expansion, 123
  in uncontrolled hemorrhage, 180
  volume kinetics, 133
  volume replacement in infants, 69
colloid osmotic pressure (COP), 11, 138
  hydroxyethyl starch (HES), 139
  maintaining, to avoid tissue edema, 20
  reduced, crystalloids and, 139, 140
coload, in spinal anesthesia, 46
  crystalloid vs. colloid, 48
  support lacking for, 48
colonic resection, 30, 36
colorectal surgery, GDT using esophageal Doppler, 95
compensatory mechanisms
  dilutional anemia tolerance, 184–5
  hemodilution, 112–13, 117, 184–5
  hemorrhage, and anesthesia, 178
continuous cardiac output, 83–4
coronary artery disease (CAD), 116
coronary blood flow, 115, 116
corrected flow time (FTc), 88, 94, 96
creatinine, 14
critically ill patients, 157–8
  anemia in, 161
  HES and renal failure risk, 145

  severe sepsis and septic shock, 157–8
  see also sepsis; septic shock
crystalloid fluids (crystalloids), 1–10
  advantages, 4
  adverse reactions, 137, 138
    acid–base imbalance, 140
    edema and excess tissue hydration, 139–40
    hemostatic disturbances, 141, 142
    local, 137
  for children, 67, 69
  colloid fluids vs., 15–16
    gastrointestinal surgery, 23, 24
    GDT, 96–7, 98
    hemostasis affected by, 116
    hypovolemic shock, 172, 173
    response to ANH, 115
    severe sepsis/septic shock, 161
    spinal anesthesia, 46–7
    in uncontrolled hemorrhage, 180
  coload in spinal anesthesia, 48
  composition, comparisons, 2
  definition, 1
  distribution, 97, 123, 139
  elimination, 15
  fixed administration with GDT of colloids, 140
  fluid kinetics modeling, 47
  gastrointestinal surgery, 23
  glucose solutions, 5–8
  in hypovolemic shock, 172, 173
  indication, 97
  for infants, 69
  isotonic, in uncontrolled hemorrhage, 179–80
  mannitol, 8
  massive fluid resuscitation, adverse effects, 139–40
  normal saline *see* normal saline
  overhydration with, adverse effects, 29
  plasma volume expansion, 122–4, 133, 139, 171
  preload, in spinal anesthesia, 46, 47, 48, 54

obstetric, 45–6, 47
preoperative, geriatric
    surgery, 52–3
in severe sepsis/septic shock,
    161
volume kinetics, 132–3
volume needed, 139
    over estimated, 97
weight gain in elderly, 52,
    140
see also glucose solutions;
    Ringer's solution
cystoscopy, 148

D5W fluid, 5
daily fluid requirements, 18–19
day surgery, 56–64
    adverse events, 61
    benefits, 56
    discharge criteria, 61
    drugs impact on fluid
        balance, 61
    elderly patients, 56–7
    intermediate, clinical trials of
        fluid therapy, 58
    key messages, 62
    outcomes and safety, 56,
        61–2
    perioperative fluids, 58–61
    postoperative fluids, 61
    preoperative fasting, 57
    preoperative nutrition
        correction of deficits, 57–8
        energy loading, 58
dehydration, 52
    abdominal surgery, 29
    children, 67
    iatrogenic, gastrointestinal
        surgery, 29
desmopressin, 189
dextran (DEX), 12–13
    anaphylaxis risk, 13, 123,
        143–4
    clinical use, 13, 123–4
    hemostatic disturbances due
        to, 141, 142, 143
    hypertonic solution with, in
        hemorrhagic shock, 74
    low-molecular weight
        dextran-1, 144
    metabolism, 144
    pharmacokinetics, 13, 123
    plasma volume expansion,
        123–4
    rheological effect, 15
    safe use, 144

solutions commercially
    available, 13
Dextran 40, 138
Dextran 70, 123, 138
dextrose
    intraoperative, children,
        67, 68
    postoperative fluids for
        children, 70
diuresis
    osmotic *see* osmotic diuresis
    promoting/monitoring, 21
diuretics, TUR syndrome
    treatment, 154
DO$_2$
    critical, 185–6
    "luxury" (over-supply of
        oxygen), 185
dobutamine, 163
dopamine, 163
Doppler-guided monitoring
    see esophageal Doppler
        monitoring (EDM)
drugs
    impact on fluid balance, day
        surgery, 61
    pharmacokinetics, 131

early, aggressive goal-directed
        therapy (EGDT), 158
    clinical trials, 158, 159–60
    importance of speed/timing,
        159
    principles and benefits, 159
echocardiography,
        transesophageal, 86–8
    costs, advantages and
        contraindications, 87
    multiplane probe, 87
    pulmonary artery catheter
        use vs., 87
edema, 120
    adverse effects of infusion
        fluids, 139–40
    cerebral *see* cerebral edema
    crystalloids in plasma
        volume expansion, 123
    fluid replacement in sepsis,
        160
    mechanisms, 121, 122
    perioperative fluid excess, 92
    pitting, 4
    prevention, colloid osmotic
        pressure, 20
    sequelae, 123
elderly patients

cardiac output in spinal
        anesthesia, 46–7
colonic surgery, liberal vs.
        restricted fluids, 53
critically ill patients, 158
day surgery, 56–7
    restrictive vs. liberal
        fluids, 58
definition, for trials, 52
fluid retention, 52
orthopedic surgery,
    restrictive vs. liberal
        fluids, 53
perioperative cardiovascular
        events, 57
spinal anesthesia in, 46–7, 48
    hypotension, 45, 46
    weight gain and fluid
        overload, 52, 140
see also geriatric surgery
elective surgery
    fluid status assessment, 51
    fluid types to administer,
        51
see also specific surgery types
electrocautery, irrigating fluids,
        148
electrolytes
    glucose solutions with, 2,
        5, 6, 7
    isotonic hydrating solutions
        for children, 68
    requirements by children, 66
encephalopathy,
        hyperammonemic, 150
endothelial cell edema, 73
energy loading, preoperative
        nutrition, 58
Enhanced Recovery after
        Surgery (ERAS)
        programs, 96
ephedrine, 54
epidural anesthesia *see* spinal
        anesthesia
epinephrine (adrenaline), 163
    stage II of hypovolemic
        shock, 168
esophageal Doppler monitoring
        (EDM), 51, 86, 87–8
    cardiac output calculation,
        88
    contraindication, 40
    corrected flow time (FTc),
        88, 94, 96
    in GDT *see* goal-directed
        therapy (GDT)

esophageal Doppler monitoring
(EDM) (*cont.*)
intraoperative fluid
management, 51
intra-abdominal surgery,
37, 39
limitations, 88
principles/methods, 93
protocols, 88
volume status assessment,
86, 87–8
ethanol, 1, 127
irrigating fluid absorption
measurement, 152, 153
Evans blue, 128, 130
evaporative loss, 23
extracellular fluid (ECF)
expansion
mannitol, 8
Ringer's solutions, 4
hypo-osmotic irrigating
fluids effect, 150
volume, 127
body weight relationship,
129
children, 65
measurement, 129
normal adult, 127
tracers, for measuring, 127
extracellular fluid (ECF) space, 1
extravascular space, 120

factor XIII concentrate, 189
"fast-track surgery," 52, 53
fasting, preoperative routines,
57
fluid deficits in children, 67
revised guidelines, 57, 62
children, 66
fatigue reduction, day surgery,
61
fibrinogen, 189
FiO_2 (inspiratory oxygen
fraction), 188
Flotrac/Vigileo, 38, 85, 98, 108
fluid challenge
Frank–Starling, 93, 104
in severe sepsis/septic shock,
162
fluid compartments, 127, 132
fluid "efficiency," 129–31
measurement, 130
hemoglobin dilution
concept, 130
hemoglobin levels, 130
tracers, 130

fluid exchange
see microvascular fluid
exchange
fluid intake (oral)
postoperative, in children,
70
preoperatively, 57
fluid kinetics *see* volume
kinetics
fluid losses
children, 67, 68
see also hypovolemia
fluid overload
adverse effects, 29
avoidance strategy, 140
colloids, 139
crystalloids, 139–40
perioperative
complications, 92
in elderly, 53
postoperative, 51, 54
pulmonary surgery, 54
see also hypervolemia
fluid retention, 51
elderly, 52
fluid status assessment, 51
fluid volumes
calculation, using tracers,
127
kinetics *see* volume kinetics
measurement
anthropometry, 128–9
bioimpedance, 128
sodium method, 129
tracers, 127–9
sizes, normal, 127
"fluids and catheter treatment
trial," 161
Frank–Starling fluid challenge,
93, 104
Frank–Starling relationship/
curve, 85, 93, 97, 98
absorption of irrigating
fluids, 151
cardiac function affecting,
104, 105
description, 105
in hemorrhage, 177
preload dependence, 104,
105
respiratory variations in
arterial pulse pressure,
105
fresh frozen plasma (FFP), 189,
190
frusemide, 154

FTc (corrected flow time), 88,
94, 96
functional body fluid spaces,
132
functional hemodynamic
parameters, 103–6
algorithm for monitoring in
surgery, 109
fluid responsiveness in septic
shock, 162
monitoring, clinical outcome
and, 108
see also arterial pressure
waveform analysis;
pleth variability index
(PVI); pulse pressure
variation (PPV); stroke
volume variation (SVV)

gas exchange, hemodilution
and anesthesia effects,
114
gastrointestinal surgery
accelerated care protocols, 29
laparoscopic, 24–5
liberal vs. restrictive fluids in
elderly, 53
open abdominal, fluid
therapy, 23–4
"rules-of-thumb" for
perioperative fluids,
23–5
laparoscopic surgery, 25
open abdominal surgery,
24
gelatin (GEL), 15, 124
anaphylactoid/allergic
reactions, 144
hemostatic disturbances due
to, 142, 143
HES comparison, 143
metabolism, 144
plasma volume expansion,
124
preloading, in spinal
anesthesia, 47
products and types, 144
volume replacement in
infants, 69
general anesthesia, "rules of
thumb" for fluids, 21
geriatric surgery, 52–3
perioperative fluid
management, 53
postoperative fluid
management, 53

preoperative fluid
management, 52–3
see also elderly patients
Glasgow Coma Scale,
hypertonic fluid
administration, 75–8
glucose
isotonic hydrating solution
effect (pediatric), 68
renal threshold, 7
glucose-free solutions, for
children, 68
"glucose loading," 6
glucose solutions, 5–8
adverse reactions
cerebral damage, 6
local, 137
volume overload and
hypertension, 139
clinical use, 6
composition, 2
contraindications, 6
dosing and requirements, 7
electrolytes with, 2, 5, 6, 7
hyperosmolar, adverse
effects, 139
hypertonic, 6
hyponatremia due to, 7
insulin with, 6
intraoperative fluids for
children, 67–8
"nitrogen-sparing effect,"
6, 7
osmolality, 137
perioperative, in day surgery,
61
pharmacokinetics, 5–6
rebound hypoglycemia, 7–8
volume kinetics, 134
glycine solution, 150
elimination and absorption,
150
in TURP, 149
glycosuria, 139
"Gly-Gly" phenotype, 172
goal-directed therapy (GDT),
37, 51, 91–102
in abdominal surgery
see intra-abdominal
surgery
background to, 91
benefits, 92, 99, 108
colloids, with fixed
crystalloid
administration, 140
definition/description, 91

early aggressive *see* early,
aggressive goal-directed
therapy (EGDT)
early, supranormal oxygen
delivery, 91–2, 93, 99
mechanisms, 92
esophageal Doppler for, 93–6
guidelines, 95
improved outcome,
studies, 96
inotropes and vasodilators
with, 96
limitations, 96
recommendations, 96
hypovolemic shock, 172
limitations, 92, 99
modern, individualized
volume optimization,
92–9
arterial pressure waveform
analysis, 97–8, 108
crystalloids vs. colloids,
96–7, 98
technologies (other), 98–9
see also pulse pressure
variation (PPV); stroke
volume variation (SVV)
monitors for volume status,
93
guidelines, fluid management,
21–2
esophageal Doppler for
GDT, 95
intraoperative fluids for
children, 68
postoperative fluids for
children, 70
see also "rules-of-thumb"

Haemaccel™, 69
Hartmann's solution *see* lactated
Ringer's solution
head injury, albumin-related
mortality, 12
head-up tilt (HUT), 166, 167,
170
heart rate
AAA surgery, 168
hypovolemic shock, 166, 167
stage II, 168–9, 170
stage III, 170
hematocrit (Hct)
critical, 185
in dilutional anemia
tolerance, 185
hemodilution, 112–19, 172

acute normovolemic
see acute normovolemic
hemodilution (ANH)
anesthesia effects, 113, 114,
115, 188
compensatory mechanisms,
112–13, 117, 184–5
crystalloids, effect on
coagulation, 141
hemostasis affected by, 116,
141, 189
hypovolemic, 188
limits, 113–16
cardiac conditions,
115–16, 186
DO_{2crit}, 185–6
hemostasis and, 116, 141,
189
normovolemic, 184, 185
limits, 187
tolerance to, 115, 185
see also anemia, dilutional
hemodynamic instability, 19
hemodynamic monitoring, 108
invasive *see* invasive
hemodynamic
monitoring
non-invasive *see* non-
invasive guidance, fluid
therapy
hemodynamic parameters
fluid administration in intra-
abdominal surgery, 38
functional *see* functional
hemodynamic
parameters
hemoglobin
critical value, tissue
oxygenation, 113, 125,
185, 187, 189
critically ill patients, 161
postoperative, mortality,
186
dilution concept, 130
fluid "efficiency"
measurement by, 130
measurements, volume
kinetic analysis, 131,
134
normal, plasma volume
expansion and, 125
recommended levels, 20
restrictive vs. liberal
transfusion strategies, 20
hemolysis-induced renal
failure, 148

hemorrhage
  cerebral blood flow and oxygenation, 171
  massive, procoagulatory drugs, 190
  pale skin and sympathetic activity, 169–70
  perioperative setting, 178
  uncontrolled, 177–83
    adjuvant therapies, 182
    blood transfusions, 180
    choice of resuscitation fluid, 179–81
    coagulation management, 189
    deliberate hypotensive see under hypotension
    goal of resuscitation, 181
    guidance on resuscitation, 181–2
    normothermia vs. hypothermia, 182
    oscillation of blood pressure, 179
    pathophysiology, 177–8
    plasma administration, 181
    primary resuscitative fluid, 181
    recommended management, 181–2
    in surgery, anesthesia and, 178, 179, 181
    in trauma, 179, 181, 182
    Type-O red blood cells, 180
hemorrhagic shock, 157, 177, 178
  hypertonic fluid effects, 73, 74–5, 180
  summary of trials, 76
  isotonic crystalloid fluids, 179–80
  late signs, 177
  see also hemorrhage, uncontrolled
hemostasis, 178
  ANH and, 116, 141
  in shock and injury, 180–1
  see also coagulation
hemostatic disturbances, fluid-associated, 141–3
  colloid-associated, 141–3
  crystalloid-associated, 141, 142
  mechanisms, 141

see also coagulopathy
hepatic surgery, 39
  hypertonic fluids in, 78
Hetastarch, 13, 73, 142
high-flow, low-pressure state, 181
hip surgery, "rules of thumb" for perioperative fluids, 22
HSD (hypertonic saline dextran), effect on ARDS, 74
hydroxyethyl starch (HES), 13, 14, 124
  130/0.4 preparations, 144
    safety aspects, 145
  anaphylactoid reaction rate low, 143
  anti-inflammatory effects, 20, 26
  bleeding association, 142
  clinical use, 14, 124, 141
  colloid osmotic pressure, 139
  first generation, hemostatic effects, 142
  gelatin comparison, 143
  in hemorrhage, 188
  hemostatic disturbances due to, 116, 141–3
  hyperoncotic, 14
  in hypertonic saline, 14
  metabolism, 144
    incomplete, tissue deposition, 144
  in neonates, 69
  pharmacokinetics, 14, 124
  in plasma-adapted solutions, 142, 145
  plasma volume expansion, 124
  preloading, in spinal anesthesia, 47
  preparations, characteristics, 141
  pruritus due to, 144–5
  renal failure risk after, 145
  third generation, hemostatic disturbances, 142–3
  volume replacement in infants/children, 69
    coagulation, effect on, 69
    quantity and types, 69
hyperchloremic metabolic acidosis, 46, 140
  normal saline causing, 1, 46, 150, 180

hypercoagulable state, dextran counteracting, 143
hyperdynamic state, 160, 162, 163
hyperglycemia, 139
  perioperative, in children, 67–8
hyperosmolar solutions, volume overload and hypertension, 139
hypersensitivity, reaction to iv fluids, 143–4
hypertension, adverse effect of iv fluids, 138–9
hypertonic fluids, 73–81
  in aortic surgery, 78
  benefits, 73
  in brain injury, 73, 74
    prehospital administration, outcomes, 75–8
  in cardiopulmonary bypass surgery, 78
  clinical trials, 74–8
    hemorrhagic shock, 74–5, 76
    traumatic brain injury, 75–8
  in hemorrhagic shock, 73, 74–5, 76
  in hepatic surgery, 78
  intraoperative studies, 78–9
  intracranial pressure reduction, 74, 75
  mechanism of action, 73–4
  in spinal surgery, 78
  types, 73
  in uncontrolled hemorrhage, 180
  see also hypertonic saline
hypertonic saline, 3, 73
  adverse reactions
    local, 137–8
    volume overload and hypertension, 139
  in aortic reconstruction, 78
  in aortic surgery, 78
  in hyponatremia, 7
  for increased intracranial pressure, 75
  osmolality, 137–8
  prehospital administration, outcome in brain injury, 75–8
  TUR syndrome treatment, 153

volume kinetics, 132, 134
hypertonic saline dextran
    (HSD), effect on ARDS,
    74
hypervolemia
    absorption of irrigating
        fluids, 150–1
    adverse effect of iv fluids,
        138–9
    see also fluid overload
hypo-osmolality, 151
hypoalbuminemia, 12
hypocalcemia, 182
hypoglycemia
    glucose solutions, 6
    preoperative, in children, 67
    rebound, 7–8
hyponatremia, 150
    absorption of irrigating
        fluids, 151
        treatment, 153–4
    acute, management in
        children, 70
    brain damage, 153
    glucose solutions inducing, 7
    postoperative, in children, 70
hypotension
    anesthesia-induced, 21, 22
    deliberate, in resuscitation,
        178, 179, 181
        barriers/problems, 179
    drug-induced, 4
    hemorrhage in trauma
        patients and, 179
    maintenance, in hemorrhage,
        178–9
    in spinal anesthesia
        see spinal anesthesia
hypothermia, 140, 141
    benefits in resuscitation, 182
    dilutional anemia tolerance,
        188
hypovolemia, 120
    central, 168
    consequences, 92
    fluid status assessment and,
        51
    increased transcapillary
        escape rate, 122
    plasma volume expanders
        see plasma volume
        expansion
    prevention, perioperative
        fluids, 19
    reversal, Ringer's solutions, 4
    signs, 104

Starling curve, LV stroke
    volume, 98
tissue oxygenation and
    hemodilution effect,
    114
hypovolemic shock, 166–76
    AAA surgery, 168
    "cardiac arrest" in, 168
    cardiac output, 170, 171–2
    central blood volume
        see central blood
        volume (CBV)
    central venous pressures,
        170–2
        normovolemia definition,
        171
    characteristics, 166
    heart rate and arterial
        pressure, 166
    hypertonic fluid benefits, 73
    pre-shock, 167
    stage II, 168–70
        Bezold–Jarish reflex, 170
        bradycardia, 168–9
        pale skin and sympathetic
            activity, 169–70
        to stop bleeding, 169
    stage III, 168, 170
    volume treatment, 166,
        171–2
        aim, 172
        choice, 172–3, 174
        titration for
            normovolemia, 172
hypoxia, tissue, 185
hysterectomy, hypertonic
    saline, 78

immunosuppressive response,
    hypertonic fluids, 73–4
indications and challenges, of
    fluid therapy, 18–21
    basal fluid requirement
        provision, 18–19
    microvascular blood flow
        enhancement, 19–20
    oxygen transport adequacy,
        20
    promoting/monitoring of
        diuresis, 21
    tissue edema prevention, 20
indocyanine green (ICG), 128
infants
    fasting guidelines, 66
    guidelines for intraoperative
        fluid therapy, 68

volume replacement, 69
    albumin, 69
    crystalloids, 69
    gelatins, 69
    hydroxyethylstarch
        preparations, 69
    lactated Ringer's solution,
        69
    see also children; neonates;
        premature infants
inflammation
    early vs. late septic shock,
        158
    prevention in trauma, 20
inflammatory cytokines,
        hypertonic fluid effects,
        73
infusion fluids
    dilutional anemia tolerance,
        188
    as drugs, ix, 131
    warming, importance, 140,
        141
    see also colloid fluids
        (colloids); crystalloid
        fluids (crystalloids)
inotropic agents, 82, 159, 163
inspiratory oxygen fraction
        (FiO$_2$), 188
insulin, glucose solutions with, 6
interstitial fluid space, 3, 4, 11
interstitial fluid volume, 1, 127
    measurement, 128
    normal adult, 127
intra-abdominal surgery, 29–44
    clinical trials, "fixed" fluid
        volumes, outcome,
        30–7, 39
    improved outcome with
        liberal fluids, 36–7
    improved outcome with
        restricted fluids, 30–6
    outcome differences
        lacking, 36
    PVI monitoring, 108
    summary of trials, 31
    clinical trials, goal-directed
        fluid volume, outcome,
        37–9, 108
    benefits, 39
    colloid boluses, 40
    Doppler-guided fluid
        management, 37, 39
    hepatic surgery, 39
    optimization protocol, 38
    restricted fluids vs., 38–9

intra-abdominal surgery (*cont.*)
summary of trials, 33
duration, effect on fluid
balance, 37
inadequacy of predefined
strategy, 40
"rules of thumb" for fluids, 29
criticisms of, 29–30
summary of findings,
39–40
timing of fluid
administration, 40
see also gastrointestinal
surgery
intracellular fluid (ICF)
hypo-osmotic irrigating
fluids effect, 150
volume, 127
measurement, 128, 129
normal adult, 127
intracellular fluid (ICF) space,
1, 6
intracranial pressure
increase, causes, 122
reduction by hypertonic
fluids, 74, 75
reduction by mannitol, 8, 75
intraoperative period
fluids for children
see children
hypertonic fluids, 78–9
"rules of thumb" for
perioperative fluids, 21
intra-abdominal surgery,
29
laparoscopic
cholecystectomy, 24
open gastrointestinal
surgery, 24
orthopedic surgery, 22
vascular surgery, 26
intrathoracic blood volume
(IBV) *see* central blood
volume (CBV)
intravascular volume, 18, 51,
85
deficit, before surgery, 19
overload, colloid infusions,
139
replacement, in children, 67
invasive hemodynamic
monitoring, 82–90, 92,
103
arterial waveform pulse
contour cardiac output
see pulse contour
analysis

dynamic indices *see* arterial
pressure waveform
analysis
echocardiography, 86–8
esophageal Doppler
see esophageal Doppler
monitoring (EDM)
pulmonary artery
catheterization
see pulmonary artery
catheterization (PAC)
transpulmonary
thermodilution cardiac
output, 84
iodinated albumin, 127–8, 130
iohexol, 127
irrigating fluids, 148–56
absorption, 148
fluid comparisons, 151
incidence and
presentation, 149
measurement, 151–3
mechanisms, 148–9
pathophysiology, 150–1
prevention, 153
treatment, 153–4
types of fluids used, 150
see also transurethral
resection (TUR)
syndrome
complications, 148
composition, 148
extravasation, 149
massive, management,
154
hemolysis-induced renal
failure, 148
types, 150
iso-osmotic fluid, 1
isotonic solution, 1
intraoperative, for children,
68
normal saline, 1–3
perioperative, 58
postoperative fluids for
children, 70

Jehovah's Witnesses, 114, 186

knee surgery
perioperative restrictive vs.
liberal fluids, 53
"rules of thumb" for
perioperative fluids, 23

labor, 8
lactate

in resuscitation in
hemorrhage, 182
in Ringer's solution, 3
serum levels, intra-
abdominal surgery,
38–9
lactated Ringer's solution, 3
composition, 2
perioperative, in day surgery,
58, 62
in uncontrolled hemorrhage,
179–80
volume kinetics, 132
volume loading, 5
volume replacement in
infancy, 69
laparoscopic cholecystectomy
see cholecystectomy
laparoscopic gastrointestinal
surgery, 25
"rules of thumb" for fluids,
25
left ventricular end-diastolic
area, 87
assessment by
transesophageal
echocardiography, 87
left ventricular end-diastolic
pressure (LVEDP), 98
left ventricular end-diastolic
volume (LVEDV), 82,
87
esophageal Doppler
monitoring, 88
left ventricular preload, 82–3,
85
liberal fluid regimens
day surgery, 58
description, 52
in elderly, restrictive fluids vs.
colonic surgery, 53
orthopedic surgery, 53
laparoscopic
cholecystectomy
outcome, 37
LiDCO, 84–5, 98
lithium dilution, calibrated
pulse contour analysis
by, 84–5
liver transplantation, 39, 78
lower body negative pressure
(LBNP), 166, 170
lower limb surgery, "rules-of-
thumb" for fluids, 25
lymphatic system, 120,
121–2
stimulation, 125

malnutrition, preoperative
    management, 57–8
mannitol, 8, 75, 150
    elimination and absorption
        effects, 150
    hypertonic, 154
mass balance equation, 129
mean arterial pressure (MAP),
        167
    in EGDT, 159
    noradrenaline use, 163
    reduced central blood
        volume, 167
    reduced, stage II of
        hypovolemic shock,
        168, 173
    in uncontrolled hemorrhage,
        179
    see also arterial pressure
mechanical ventilation, 104,
        106
metabolic acidosis
    hyperchloremic
        see hyperchloremic
        metabolic acidosis
    hypochloremic, 1
    normal saline inducing, 1,
        11, 46, 150, 180
microvascular blood flow
    see blood flow
microvascular fluid exchange,
        120–6
    inside brain, 122
    lymphatic system, 121–2
    outside brain, 120–1, 122
    2-pore theory, 121, 124
    see also hypovolemia;
        plasma volume
        expansion
moderate-risk surgery, 103
    pulse oximeter waveforms,
        106
morbidity, perioperative, 92
mortality, high-risk surgery, 91
muscular relaxation, dilutional
        anemia tolerance, 188
myocardial function,
        dilutional anemia
        tolerance, 188

neonates
    albumin use for volume
        expansion, 69
    HES use, 69
    see also infants
neutrophil action, 73
NICOM, 99

nitric oxide, 112
non-invasive guidance, fluid
        therapy, 103–11
    functional hemodynamic
        parameters, 104–6
    see also pulse pressure
        variation (PPV)
    pleth variability index
        see pleth variability
        index (PVI)
    plethysmographic waveform
        (ΔPOP), 103, 106,
        107
    preload dependence
        determination, 104
    pulse oximeter waveforms,
        106–7
    static parameters, 104
    static vs. dynamic
        parameters, 104
    see also pulse oximeter
        waveforms
nonlinear least squares
        regression, 131
non-steroidal anti-
        inflammatory drugs
        (NSAIDs)
    day surgery, 61, 62
    impact on fluid balance, 61
noradrenaline
        (norepinephrine),
        163
    stage II of hypovolemic
        shock, 168
normal saline, 1–3
    adverse effects, 3, 180
    composition, 2
    hyperchloremic metabolic
        acidosis due to, 1, 46,
        150, 180
    for infants, 69
    irrigating solution, 150
        adverse effects, 151
    postoperative fluids for
        children, 70
normovolemia
    hemodilution
        see hemodilution
    maintenance, in anemia
        tolerance, 188
    plasma volume expanders
        for see plasma volume
        expansion
    "rules-of-thumb," 19, 26
    in vascular surgery, 26
nutrition, preoperative
    day surgery and, 57–8

energy loading, 58
obstetric spinal anesthesia
        see spinal anesthesia,
        obstetric
obstetric surgery, fluid
        management, 54
oedema see edema
oncotic pressure, plasma,
        124
    reduced, 70, 123
oozing, 13
optimal fluid strategy, 18
    gastrointestinal surgery,
        23–4
    see also under goal-directed
        therapy (GDT)
orthopedic surgery
    GDT using esophageal
        Doppler, 96
    restrictive vs. liberal fluids in
        elderly, 53
    "rules of thumb" for
        perioperative fluids,
        22–3
osmolality, 1
osmolality-associated adverse
        effects, 137–8
osmotic diuresis, 7, 8
    glycine solution absorption
        causing, 150
osmotic pressure, colloid
        see colloid osmotic
        pressure (COP)
overhydration
    adverse effects, 29
    see also fluid overload
oxygen consumption
    hemodilution and anesthesia
        effects, 114
    increased, ANH, 113
    myocardial, 115, 116, 188
    VO_2, 185, 186
    oxygen supply-
        dependency, 185
oxygen delivery, 103, 185
    critical DO_2, 185–6
    factors affecting, 186
    myocardial, 115, 116
    optimization, 103
    over-supply (luxury DO_2),
        185
    supranormal, early GDT,
        91–2, 99
    targets, 91
oxygen dissociation curve,
        113

oxygen, inspiratory fraction (FiO$_2$), 188
oxygen saturation
central venous (ScvO$_2$), 159, 162
measurement, pulse oximetry, 107
venous see venous oxygen saturation (SvO$_2$)
oxygenation, tissue
adequacy, fluids for, 20
criticisms of hypothesis involving, 29
hemodilution effects, 112, 113–14
increased by liberal fluid use, 36
increased, hemodilution effect, 113–14
efficacy, 114–15
intra-abdominal surgery, 36, 40

parasympathetic activation, hypovolemic shock, 168
pediatrics, 65–72
see also children; infants
pentastarch, 13, 144
perfusion index (PI), 107
perioperative fluids
day surgery, 58–61
geriatric surgery, 53
importance, 18
indications see indications and challenges
optimization, 18
principles, 19, 158
volume, 58
see also more specific topics
pharmacokinetics
albumin, 11–12
crystalloids, 97
dextran, 13, 123
drugs, 131
glucose solutions, 5–6
hydroxyethyl starch (HES), 14, 124
infusion fluid kinetics and, 131–4
mannitol, 8
Ringer's solution, 3–4
starch, 14
phenylephrine, 54
physiotherapy, 125
PiCCO, 85, 86, 98
pitting edema, 4
plasma

administration, 15, 184, 189
in trauma, 181
adverse reactions, 15
composition, 2
dilution, after infusion, 131
fresh frozen, 189, 190
in plasma volume expansion, 15
plasma colloid osmotic pressure see colloid osmotic pressure (COP)
Plasma-Lyte A, 2, 5
in uncontrolled hemorrhage, 179–80
plasma volume, 127
body weight relationship, 129
measurement, 127–8
normal adult, 127
plasma volume expansion
adverse effects, 124
colloid fluids, 11, 122–4, 138
albumin, 11–12, 123, 124
dextran, 13, 123–4
gelatin, 124
hydroxyethyl starch, 14, 124
reducing need for, 124–5
crystalloid fluids, 122–4, 133
efficiency of fluid, 129–31
ideal/"target," 134
normal arterial pressure and, 124
reduced renal clearance effect, 133
responders and non-responders, 134
Ringer's solution, 4
effectiveness, 133
pleth variability index (PVI), 103, 107–8
monitoring, clinical outcomes, 108
plethysmographic waveform see pulse oximeter waveforms
polycythemia, neonatal, 69
polyionique B66, 68
ΔPOP, 106, 107
2-pore theory, 121, 124
positive-pressure ventilation, 85, 97, 104
postoperative complications, "minor," 103
postoperative fluid management

in children/infants see children
day surgery, 61
geriatric surgery, 53
"rules of thumb," 21–2
laparoscopic surgery, 25
open gastrointestinal surgery, 24
orthopedic surgery, 22
vascular surgery, 26
postoperative nausea and vomiting (PONV), 169
day surgery, 62
laparoscopic gastrointestinal surgery, 24
prevention, 24–5
postoperative pain management, day surgery, 62
potassium, serum levels, absorption of irrigating fluids, 151
pre-eclampsia, 46, 48
preload dependence, 104, 105
assessment, 104
importance, 105
definition/description, 104
premature infants
albumin use for volume expansion, 69
volume replacement, 69
preoperative assessments, children, 66–7
preoperative fluids
geriatric surgery, 52–3
"rules of thumb," 21
laparoscopic surgery, 25–6
open gastrointestinal surgery, 24
orthopedic surgery, 22
vascular surgery, 26
pressure breathing, 166
protein exchange, microvascular, 120, 121
mechanisms, 121
convection, 121
passive, 121
2-pore theory, 121, 124
protein-sparing effect, 6, 7
pruritus, 144–5
hydroxyethyl starch (HES), 144–5
pulmonary artery catheterization (PAC), 82–4

continuous cardiac output, 83–4
early, GDT, 91
thermodilution cardiac output, 83
transesophageal echocardiography vs., 87
usage, trends, 82
pulmonary artery occlusion pressure (PAOP), 162
pulmonary artery wedge pressure (PAWP), 82–3
pulmonary capillary wedge pressure (PCWP), 104
pulmonary edema, 29, 54, 123
fluid volume relationship, 54
rapid infusion of Ringer's solution, 4, 5
pulmonary surgery, fluid management, 54
pulse contour analysis, 84
calibrated, 84
by lithium dilution (LiDCO), 84–5, 98
by thermodilution (PiCCO), 85, 86, 98
continuous, 84–5
contraindications, 84
fluid responsiveness in septic shock, 162
non-calibrated, 84, 85
pulse oximeter waveforms, 106–7
amplitude (ΔPOP), 106, 107
components, 106
fluid responsiveness prediction, 107
principles, 106
respiratory variations, 106–7
pulse oximetry, oxygen saturation measurement, 107
pulse pressure, 38
pulse pressure variation (PPV), 86, 97, 103
applications, conditions for, 106
fluid responsiveness in septic shock, 162
mechanical ventilation effect, 104
monitoring, clinical outcomes, 108
respiratory variations, pulse oximeter, 105, 106
tidal volume impact, 106

red blood cells (RBCs)
hemostasis and, 116
labeling, mass calculation, 128
reduction, hemodilution, 112
transfusions, 180, 184
velocity, 113
reflection coefficient, proteins, 120, 121
regression equations, 129, 131
rehydration, 19
renal damage, absorption of irrigating fluids, 151
renal failure
colloid-associated, 145
critically ill patients, 158
hemolysis-induced, 148
renal function, children, 65
renal insufficiency, Ringer's solutions cautions, 5
renal threshold, glucose, 7
respiratory systolic variation test, 86
restrictive fluid regimens
description, 52
intra-abdominal surgery effect on outcome, 30–6
GDT fluid volume effect on outcome vs., 38
perioperative, in elderly, 53, 58
resuscitation
cardiac, hypovolemic shock and, 168, 169
children, hydroxyethyl starch (HES), 69
deliberate hypotension in see hypotension
hypertonic fluids in see hypertonic fluids
massive, crystalloid adverse effects, 139–40
in severe sepsis see sepsis
in uncontrolled hemorrhage see hemorrhage
Resuscitation Outcomes Consortium, 75
right ventricular filling, 83
Ringer's solution, 3–5
acetated, 132
adverse effects, 4, 5, 29
in brain injury, 5
clinical use, 4
composition, 2
chloride, 141
lactate and acetate, 3

dosage/infusion volume, 4–5
for infants, 69
lactated see lactated Ringer's solution
pharmacokinetics, 3–4
Plasma-Lyte A see Plasma-Lyte A
plasma volume expander, effectiveness, 133
preloading, laparoscopic cholecystectomy, 24–5
in spinal anesthesia, 47
volume kinetics, 132–3
"rules-of-thumb," ix, 18–28
for adequate colloid osmotic pressure, 20
for adequate oxygen transport, 20
for basal fluid requirements, 19
general principles, 18–21
intra-abdominal surgery, 29
for normovolemia and hemodynamic stability, 19, 26
to prevent hypovolemia, 19
to prevent trauma-induced cascade systems, 20
procedure-specific, 22
gastrointestinal surgery see gastrointestinal surgery
orthopedic surgery, 22–3
vascular surgery, 25
to promote/monitor diuresis, 21
for rehydration in fluid deficiency, 19
standard (perioperative fluids), 21–2
see also guidelines, fluid management

SAFE study, 161, 180
saline
hypertonic see hypertonic saline
physiological (isotonic) see normal saline
sepsis, 157
HES avoidance, 14
severe, 157–65
anesthesia in, 158
crystalloids vs. colloids, 161
definition, 157

sepsis (*cont.*)
  early fluid resuscitation,
    158–60
  fluid responsiveness, 162
  later fluid resuscitation,
    160–1
  positive fluid balance and
    edema, 160
  summary/key messages,
    163
  vasopressors and inotropic
    agents, 163
septic shock, 157–65
  anesthesia in, 158
  children, 67
  definition, 157
  early vs. late, 158
  fluid management, 158, 160
    crystalloids vs. colloids,
      161
    early, 158–60
    later, 160–1
    summary/key messages,
      163
  fluid responsiveness, 162
  hydroxyethyl starch in
    children, 69
  vasopressors and inotropic
    agents, 163
shock
  cold *see* hemorrhagic shock
  warm *see* septic shock
smoking, 149
sodium
  isotonic hydrating solution
    effect (pediatric), 68, 70
  for measuring irrigating
    fluid absorption, 151,
    152, 153
  postoperative fluids for
    children, 70
sodium method, 129
sorbitol solutions, 150
spinal anesthesia, 45–50
  cardiac output affected by,
    46–7
  colloid fluid preloading,
    47, 48
  coload, vs. preload, 46, 48
  crystalloid fluid preloading,
    45–6, 47, 48, 54
  with gelatin or HES, 47
  crystalloids vs. colloids,
    46–7, 54
  coload, 48
  in elderly, 45, 46–7, 48
  hypertonic fluids in, 78

hypotension in, 45, 47, 54
  elderly, 45, 46
  etiological factors, 45
  fluid management
    summary, 48–9
  non-obstetric, hypotension
    in, 46
  obstetric, 45–6, 48
    hypotension, 45–6, 47, 54
  recommendations of fluids,
    49
  "rules of thumb" for
    perioperative fluids, 21
    knee surgery, 23
    orthopedic surgery, 22
  timing of fluid
    administration, 48
spinal surgery, intra-aortic
  hypertonic fluids, 78
starch, 13–14
  adverse effects, 14
  clinical use, 14
  pharmacokinetics, 14
  preparations/formulations,
    13–14
  see also hydroxyethyl starch
    (HES)
Starling curve *see* Frank–
  Starling relationship/
  curve
Starling fluid equation, 120, 121
sterile water, 148, 150
steroids, impact on fluid
  balance, 61
Stewart–Hamilton equation, 83
stroke, acute, 6
stroke volume (SV), 38, 87
  increase in preload, 104
  increased, hemodilution
    effect, 113
  maximization, GDT for
    see goal-directed
    therapy (GDT)
  optimization, Starling curve,
    93, 96
  pulse contour analysis, 84
  'recruitable', in GDT, 93, 94
  Starling curve *see* Frank–
    Starling relationship/
    curve
stroke volume variation (SVV),
  104
  measurement, 86, 97
  monitoring, clinical
    outcomes, 108
"Surviving Sepsis Campaign",
  159, 161, 162, 163

sympathetic activation
  hypovolemic shock, 167,
    168
  reduced, hypovolemic shock,
    168, 169–70
  in severe hemorrhage, 169,
    170
systemic inflammatory
  response syndrome
  (SIRS), 157
systemic vascular resistance
  (SVR), 162, 163
systolic pressure, 38, 85, 86
systolic pressure variation, 86
  fluid responsiveness in septic
    shock, 162

T cells, hypertonic fluid effects,
  73–4
tachycardia, in hypovolemic
  shock, 170
temperature-associated adverse
  effects, 137, 138
tetrastarch, 142
thermodilution, calibrated
  pulse contour analysis
  by, 85, 86
thermodilution cardiac output,
  83
  transpulmonary, 84
thermodilution curve, 83, 84
"third-day" transient circulatory
  overload, 140
third space, 23, 29, 67, 97, 134
  uncontrolled hemorrhage,
    resuscitation, 179
thyroid surgery, 58, 133, 134
tidal volume, 106
tilt table experiments, 166, 167,
  171
timing of fluid administration
  EGDT, 159
  intra-abdominal surgery, 40
  spinal anesthesia, 48
tissue deposition, adverse
  reaction, 144–5
tissue edema *see* edema
tissue hydration, excessive,
  139–40
tissue oxygenation
  see oxygenation, tissue
tonicity, 1
total body water, 127, 129
  children, 65
tracer methods
  fluid "efficiency"
    measurement, 130

fluid volume measurement, 127–9
limitations of use, 128
transcapillary escape rate (TER), 120, 121
increased, 122, 124
transcapillary fluid exchange, 20, 120–1
2-pore theory, 121, 124
transcapillary/transvenular hydrostatic pressure, 121
transcervical resection of the endometrium (TCRE), 148, 149
measurement of fluid absorption, 151
transcytosis, 121
transesophageal echocardiography see echocardiography
transfusion-related acute lung injury (TRALI), 15, 190
transfusion-related cardiac overload (TACO), 189, 190
transpulmonary thermodilution cardiac output, 84
transurethral resection of the prostate (TURP), 148, 149
bipolar resection technique, 153
glycine solution, absorbed fluid, 149
irrigation fluid absorption prevention, 153
transurethral resection (TUR) syndrome, 148
death from, 151
fluid absorption measurement, 151–3
irrigating fluids causing, 150, 151

pathophysiology, 150–1
prevention, 153
symptoms, 149
treatment, 153–4
transvascular fluid exchange, 120–1, 122
see also microvascular fluid exchange
trauma
crystalloid vs. colloid fluids, 15, 16
hemorrhage, 179, 182
blood pressure target, 179
see also hemorrhage
prevention of coagulation/cascade activation, 20
tricuspid valve regurgitation, 83

vagal activity, hypovolemic shock and, 169
vascular surgery, "rules of thumb" for fluids, 25, 26
vasoconstriction, in hemorrhage in trauma, 179, 182
vasodilatation, 3, 133
vasodilator peptides, 46, 47
vasopressin, 169
vasopressors
avoidance, plasma volume expansion and, 124
in septic shock, 163
in spinal anesthesia, 48–9
Venofundin, 14
venous oxygen saturation (SvO$_2$)
fluid responsiveness in septic shock, 162
hypovolemic shock, 171, 172, 174
inter-individual variation, 172
vesicle transport, 121

volume effect, infusion fluid, 129
volume kinetics, 127–36
anesthesia/surgery effect, 133
clinical use, 134
colloid fluids, 133
crystalloid fluids, 47, 132–3
distribution, compartments, 131, 132
elimination, 131, 133
"functional" fluid spaces, 132
glucose solutions, 134
hemoglobin measurements for, 131, 134
hypertonic saline, 134
modeling, crystalloids distribution, 47
"nonfunctional" fluid spaces, 134
volunteer studies, 132–3
volume status, assessment bedside, 82
invasive see invasive hemodynamic monitoring
volumetric fluid balance, irrigating fluid absorption, 151–2, 153
Voluven, 14
von Willebrand factor, 142, 143, 189
von Willebrand-like syndrome, 142, 143

warming, infusion fluids, 140, 141
water isotopes, 127
water requirements, children, 66
weight, fluid volumes relationship, 129
weight gain, 29, 30, 51
crystalloid fluids in elderly, 52, 140